Scheduling an Appointment with Your Doctor

Schedule an appointment with your doctor right away if you experience any of the following (Chapter 2):

- A new firm lump or mass in your breast
- Your nipple suddenly becomes inverted (goes in) or dimpled
- Discharge from your breast other than milk that comes out on its own
- You're being treated for an infection of the breast and it doesn't get any better or any worse after a week or two

Don't panic but don't delay!

Preparing for a Mammogram

If you're scheduled for a mammogram (Chapter 5)

- Find out before your appointment whether your insurance covers the procedure.
- Only go to a facility that's certified by the Food and Drug Administration.
- If you've had a mammogram in the past, bring the pictures and the doctor's report with you.
- Wear warm slacks, the machine is cold.
- Stay calm. Remember, out of 1,000 mammograms, 998-999 are not cancerous. Why worry if you don't have to?

Picking a Treatment, Almost any Treatment

If you're diagnosed with breast cancer, your treatment options depend on various factors and may include

- **Surgery:** Everyone with breast cancer has some form of surgery (Chapter 10). You may have a:
  - **Lumpectomy:** Removing the cancerous lump and some of the surrounding tissue.
  - **Mastectomy:** Removing the breast tissue.
  - **Reconstructive surgery.** Surgery to rebuild your breast. You decide if and when you want it.
- **Radiation therapy:** Radiation involves beaming *x-rays* or *gamma rays* at the cancer cells to damage or destroy them (Chapter 11).
- **Chemotherapy:** Chemotherapy is a combination of medications (Chapter 12) that reaches *all* the parts of your body, and kills the cancer cells that may remain after surgery and radiation. Its purpose is to prevent a recurrence of the cancer and to increase your chances of survival.
- **Hormone therapy:** Hormonal treatments such as tamoxifen (Chapter 13) are used both to prevent and treat breast cancer.

Being Sent for a Biopsy

Here are some helpful hints for your biopsy appointment (Chapter 5):

- Not all biopsies are the same; some can be done with a needle in the doctor's office while others require a small surgery. Ask your doctor's office which kind you'll be having.
- If you are having the surgical kind, have a friend bring you in and drive you home again.
- Don't panic. Remember, being sent for a biopsy does **not** mean that you have cancer. It's just a more accurate way of checking any suspicious cells to see whether they are *malignant* (cancerous) or *benign* (not cancerous). Three-quarters of biopsies done as a result of your doctor feeling a lump in your breast turn out to be not cancerous.

BESTSELLING
BOOK SERIES

Breast Cancer For Dummies®

Cheat Sheet

Introducing Your Treatment Team

Many professionals will be involved in your diagnosis and treatment. Your doctors include

- **Primary care doctor:** Refers you to breast cancer specialist.
- **Pathologist:** Looks at your tissue samples to determine whether they're cancerous.
- **Radiologist:** Determines the extent of your cancer using mammography, ultrasound, and more. May also do a biopsy.
- **Medical oncologist:** Helps you decide on which drug treatment is best for you. Will be in charge of your medical treatment for cancer.
- **Radiation oncologist:** Administers your radiation treatment.
- **Surgical oncologist:** Does biopsy, and operates on you for a lumpectomy or mastectomy.
- **Plastic or reconstructive surgeon:** Reconstructs your breast.
- **Anesthesiologist:** Gives you anesthesia (knocks you out — in a good way) during surgery.

Other members of your team include

- **Nurse:** Assists in your care before and after treatment.
- **Social worker:** Helps you emotionally, with problem solving, with insurance, and with other logistics.
- **Radiology technologist:** Positions you for X-rays and mammograms.
- **Physical therapist:** Helps your body heal by showing how to move, stretch, and exercise.

Keeping in Contact

Use the following chart to keep important names and numbers on hand.

Contact	Name/Address	Number
Partner's work/cell phone		
Partner's backup		
Children's school		
General doctor		
Medical oncologist		
Hospital		
ER		
American Cancer Society	www.cancer.org	1-800-ACS-2345
Y-Me National Breast Cancer Organization	www.y-me.org	1-800-221-2141

For Dummies: Bestselling Book Series for Beginners

Breast Cancer

FOR

DUMMIES®

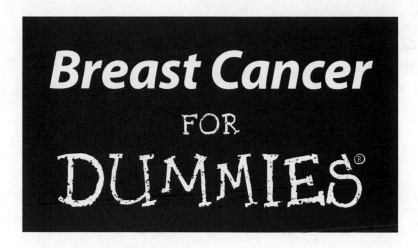

Breast Cancer FOR DUMMIES®

by Ronit Elk, PhD, and Monica Morrow, MD

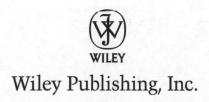

WILEY

Wiley Publishing, Inc.

Breast Cancer For Dummies®

Published by
Wiley Publishing, Inc.
111 River Street
Hoboken, NJ 07030
www.wiley.com

For general information on our other products and services or to obtain technical support, please contact our Customer Care Department within the U.S. at 800-762-2974, outside the U.S. at 317-572-3993, or fax 317-572-4002.

Wiley also publishes its books in a variety of electronic formats. Some content that appears in print may not be available in electronic books.

Library of Congress Control Number: 2003101673

ISBN: 0-7645-2482-8

Manufactured in the United States of America

10 9 8 7 6 5 4 3 2 1

1O/SR/QX/QT/IN

is a trademark of Wiley Publishing, Inc.

About the Authors

Ronit Elk, PhD, received her PhD in psychology from the University of Cape Town in South Africa. Soon after immigrating to the United States, she joined the faculty of the Medical School at the University of Texas in Houston. During her ten years in academia, Dr. Elk was awarded many research grants from the National Institutes of Health, published numerous scientific articles, and made countless presentations. Her life changed in the summer of 1997 when her father died following a protracted illness. Three months later she buried her mother, and shortly thereafter her husband was diagnosed with a terminal illness. "In less than two years, I lost those whom I cared about the most. All of them died of cancer, and the anguish I experienced was indescribable. However, in time, like so many others before me, I was able to transcend the pain, heal, and grow. I came to understand that the combination of my life-transforming experiences, together with my professional background placed me in a unique position. I could now contribute on a professional and personal level. I cannot think of a more wonderful organization to be a part of than The American Cancer Society." As scientific program director in the research department of the American Cancer Society (ACS), Dr. Elk has contributed to the substantial increase in funding for research into prevention and early detection of cancer, ensuring a good quality of life for survivors, and decreasing the disproportionate burden of cancer among the poor and underserved. Dr. Elk travels widely giving inspirational talks on cancer and survivorship.

She started her company, The Corporation of Courageous Chics, as part of her mission to inspire women to recognize their courage in the face of the many challenges they face. She designs, markets, and sells inspirational gifts for women, all based on the butterfly's metamorphosis. *Just like the small, soft caterpillar that can so easily be stepped on and squashed, we women sometimes find ourselves in vulnerable situations. Yet we don't give up, and accept the challenge before us. And then there are times when we just curl ourselves into our cocoon, being still and silent. Yet even at this time when we withdraw from the world, we dare to believe in a more hopeful future. The most difficult part is finding the strength and knowing how to break out of the cocoon, something we have to do for ourselves. But when we do, we emerge transformed into the magnificent butterfly that we are, free to fly, to soar, and to choose our path. Indeed, we "Women have no limits."* To see Ronit's inspirational gift line or to book her for a motivational talk, visit www.courageouschics.com.

Monica Morrow, MD, is professor of surgery at Northwestern University and director of the Lynn Sage Breast Center at Northwestern Memorial Hospital in Chicago, Illinois. She graduated magna cum laude from Pennsylvania State University and received her MD degree at Jefferson Medical College in Philadelphia. Her surgical training was at the Medical Center Hospital of Vermont, and she served a surgical oncology fellowship at Memorial Sloan Kettering Cancer Center in New York.

Dr. Morrow's career has been devoted to the diagnosis and treatment of breast cancer. She is the surgical editor of a major breast cancer textbook, the editor of a text on Management of The High-Risk Woman, and has authored more than 200 scientific publications on breast disease. She is coleader of Northwestern's Specialized Program of Research Excellence in Breast Cancer. Dr. Morrow is a former director of the Cancer Department of the American College of Surgeons and served as executive director of the American Joint Committee on Cancer. She regularly serves on national and international consensus panels to define state-of-the-art care for breast cancer. She has been honored as a Distinguished Alumni of Penn State and received the "Women Making a Difference Award" from the State of Illinois in 2003. Her husband is V. Craig Jordan OBE, PhD, DSc, the distinguished breast cancer scientist known as "the father of tamoxifen."

Dedication

We dedicate this book to countless courageous women whose lives have been altered by breast cancer. You endure more than anyone should have to and yet continue in the battle, supporting others through the journey and displaying a bravery that's acknowledged and respected by all. For leading the way — we thank you.

Authors' Acknowledgments

I wouldn't have reached this point in my life if not for my family. *Imim* is what I called my mother, a woman so gentle that even on those rare occasions when she was angry, my sister and I would laugh, wrap our arms around her, and nuzzle against her soft cheeks. It was her undeniable love for us that kept me grounded, connecting me to my core. I love you so much Imim and miss you more than I even dare admit. *My father* was unquestionably an impressive man who inspired awe and admiration in all who met him. His remarkable intellect and commanding presence no doubt contributed to his appointment as the Israeli Ambassador to so many countries. It was he who inspired me to become an outspoken defender of human rights and a determined and disciplined leader. *Harold "Haiwy,"* my husband and best friend, brought tranquility, tenderness, and a love of human beings to our lives. With you miracles weren't just possible, they happened. Even as you continue your journey into the next dimension, I know that our spirits remain connected. My kids *Allon* and *Talya* are the two people I love and admire the most in the world. They opted for paths least trodden, helping others rather than leading a familiar and comfortable life. As they begin their journeys into adulthood, I beam with pride for these two incredible human beings. My sister *Orly* dismissed my many doubts with her no-nonsense advice: "Oh, stop worrying, of course you're going to finish this book. And then you'll start something else!" My chosen sister, *Kerry,* and I speak the same language, and when her adorable son Liam was born, she gave me the honor of becoming "Granny Nonit." The Cohen clan in Nashville has accepted me as one of their own; braiding the hair of those adorable little girls is so much fun. *Dr. Ruth Lax* has been a friend of the family, since long before my grandparents arrived in Israel, barely escaping the Holocaust. When my parents died, she was there for me regardless of day or night.

Living continents away from my relatives, my friends are now my family and to each I owe a debt of gratitude. *Sue McCray* and I walk side-by-side through thick and thin. She never stopped believing in me and the mission of Courageous Chics. It's her extraordinary management and tireless strategizing that made the vision reality. *Rael* and *Barbara Elk* have generously shown their support for the company. *Karen Storthz* has been with me at each of my many hospitalizations (even after I threw up all over her). *Cyndi* and I spent wonderful times creating art (in between burping our babies). An accomplished writer, she has encouraged me every step of the way. My special bond with *Van Lofton* has been made even deeper now that her granddaughter, Paris, is my precious godchild. *Phillip Nguyen* showed me how the human spirit can triumph; *Niobi Ngozi* taught me how to laugh from a place deep inside. *Michael O'Donnell* supported me during so many of Harold's visits to the emergency room, and our daily talks nourished us both; *Alice Anne O'Donnell,* the gentle doctor everyone calls upon, regardless of problem or hour, was so generous during tough times. If not for *Joan McKirachan,* therapist extraordinaire, so much would not have been possible.

Since moving to Atlanta, I've made some special friends. *Edie Cohen,* a brilliant writer, challenges my mind and opens my spirit. *Rabbi Josh* welcomed me back into the fold. *Rebecca Green,* and her adorable *Sarah,* have become family. *Abby Drue* is a fellow "wise-woman," and *Paul Glickstein, Barry Roseman,* and *Patrick Crane* are guys any girl would be proud to count as friends. *Alda Bernald, Rhonda Collins, Eve Nagler,* and *Greta Greer* are colleagues who've become friends. Our roars of laughter often heard along ACS corridors, we continue plotting and planning a better world for all. I am blessed to have the best boss in the world, *Dr. John Stevens,* a dedicated, caring, and ethical human being.

My deepest gratitude goes to my agent *Elizabeth Frost-Knappman* for believing in me and for being so positive; to my editors *Natasha Graf* and *Alissa Schwipps* — no matter what the challenge, you worked toward finding a solution; to *Holly Grimes* for assisting with the endless logistics; and to *Burton Korman* for his invaluable assistance and calming influence (and the never-ending faxes). Our deepest gratitude goes to the *survivors,* who so generously shared their experiences, understanding, and wisdom.

Publisher's Acknowledgments

We're proud of this book; please send us your comments through our Dummies online registration form located at www.dummies.com/register/.

Some of the people who helped bring this book to market include the following:

Acquisitions, Editorial, and Media Development

Senior Project Editor: Alissa D. Schwipps

Acquisitions Editor: Natasha Graf

Copy Editors: E. Neil Johnson, Chrissy Guthrie

Acquisitions Coordinator: Holly Grimes

Technical Editor: Ruth O'Regan, MD

Editorial Managers: Christine Meloy Beck, Jennifer Ehrlich

Editorial Assistant: Elizabeth Rea

Cover Photos: © Will Ryan/CORBIS

Cartoons: Rich Tennant, www.the5thwave.com

Production

Project Coordinator: Nancee Reeves

Layout and Graphics: Carrie Foster, Stephanie D. Jumper, Tiffany Muth, Jacque Schneider, Mary Gillot Virgin

Special Art: Kathryn Born, Medical Illustrator

Proofreaders: Laura Albert, Susan Moritz, Kathy Simpson, Brian H. Walls, TECHBOOKS Production Services

Indexer: TECHBOOKS Production Services

Publishing and Editorial for Consumer Dummies

Diane Graves Steele, Vice President and Publisher, Consumer Dummies

Joyce Pepple, Acquisitions Director, Consumer Dummies

Kristin A. Cocks, Product Development Director, Consumer Dummies

Michael Spring, Vice President and Publisher, Travel

Brice Gosnell, Publishing Director, Travel

Suzanne Jannetta, Editorial Director, Travel

Publishing for Technology Dummies

Andy Cummings, Vice President and Publisher, Dummies Technology/General User

Composition Services

Gerry Fahey, Vice President of Production Services

Debbie Stailey, Director of Composition Services

Contents at a Glance

Table of Contents

Introduction

You felt it. You had a mammogram that detected it. Your lover found it. You've been diagnosed. If you or someone you love has been diagnosed with breast cancer, you're probably confused, afraid, shocked, or even angry. Or you may be all of the above. First, come to terms with your diagnosis. Give yourself the time that you need.

After you've come to grips, you also need to get a grip on the facts. Let this book become your trusted manual. Discover more about the cancer with which you've been diagnosed, explore your treatment options, find ways to make this new part of your life easier. Let shared experiences serve as your knowledgeable guide and anchor to help you make wise and confident choices.

Let us begin by offering you some good news. If your mammography results indicated an abnormal area in your breast, remember that 90 percent of breast lumps and calcium deposits turn out to be benign (noncancerous).

Think of breast cancer as a journey and this book as your roadmap. Have you already been diagnosed? In that case, remember this:

- Breast cancer is not a death sentence. Most women diagnosed with early stage breast cancer can look forward to enjoying a healthy, full life (see Chapter 8).

- Every woman diagnosed with breast cancer is different. Not only are you unique as a person, but so, too, is your particular form of cancer (see Chapter 7), your treatment options (see Chapter 9), and your prognosis (see Chapter 8).

- Every day more is discovered about how to prevent (see Chapter 3), detect earlier (see Chapters 4 and 5), and more effectively treat (see Chapter 9) breast cancer. You can play an active part in your own treatment.

- You are not alone. More than two million women in the United States today are breast cancer survivors. We don't know how many others there are in other countries, as many don't keep statistics, but wherever you are, there is someone else who's been there before. Many gladly provide you with support on your journey. Thousands of groups and programs across the country offer support, and chances are, one is close to your neighborhood.

About This Book

Think of this book as a trusted friend, a guide who knows and understands this path that you're on and can lead you through the information and choices truthfully and accurately in simple, easy-to-understand terms.

All the information in this book is based on the most recent research findings, the clinical expertise of oncologists, and the invaluable experiences of the women who have walked this road before.

Our purpose is to give you the facts, answer all your questions, and talk to you about some of the things that others may not feel comfortable addressing (like how to resume intimacy after your surgery). We hope that this book helps you feel like you have a sister who's a doctor, a sister who tells you what to expect every step of the way, who gives you the best advice she can, and guides you along the way. (Of course, there is absolutely no replacement for advice about *you* from your own doctor.) Our hope and belief is that because of this close family connection, you'll feel empowered to know and understand what's going on in your body, so that you can become a part of your own treatment team and make decisions along with your doctors and your family.

You don't have to read this book all at once if you don't want to. Just check out the Table of Contents or Index and then turn to the sections you specifically want to find out about and refer to other parts of the book as you need them. Mark the pages that you find most helpful and come back to them later, scribble in the margins, and highlight your favorite sections. This is *your* road map. Use it as you wish.

Foolish Assumptions

We make several assumptions about you:

- You, or someone close to you, has found a lump in her (or even his) breast or has been diagnosed with breast cancer.
- You want to find out all you can about what your diagnosis means for you.
- You want to know what to expect and when you'll be well again.
- You want to understand what you need to know about breast cancer, but you don't want to wade through mountains of complicated medical jargon.

✔ You want to know enough so that you know what questions to ask, what to expect, and be able to be a part of your treatment team.

✔ You aren't a specialist in the field, which means that you want the information explained truthfully and in a way that's easy to understand.

Regardless of why you're reading this, here are some assumptions you can make about us: We've made every effort to provide you with the most up-to-date information, in an accurate and truthful manner, presented in what we trust is a caring but nonpatronizing approach. We hope that you find it helpful.

Conventions Used in This Book

The following conventions are used throughout the text to make things consistent and easy to understand:

✔ All Web addresses appear in `monofont`.

✔ New terms appear in *italics* and are closely followed by an easy-to-understand definition.

✔ **Bold** is used to highlight the action parts of numbered steps.

✔ Sidebars, which look like text enclosed in a shaded gray box, consist of information that's interesting to know but not necessarily critical to your understanding of the chapter or section's topic.

Who better to understand your journey than someone who has walked this path before? So many survivors wrote in, gave their advice, and offered to help. Their words of wisdom, labeled by the "Survivors' Secrets" icon appear throughout the book, and we have no doubt that they'll be sources of comfort, support, and insight as you go through treatment. Their words serve as a reminder that you never have to walk this path alone!

How This Book Is Organized

You'll arrive at several landmarks during your journey through *Breast Cancer For Dummies*. From tests to diagnosis to treatment to support to coping with your new life, this book covers each leg (or breast, as is the case) of the trip.

Part I: Will My Hair Fall Out? Coming to Grips with Breast Cancer

If you or a loved one has been diagnosed, or if you're a woman, especially a woman older than 30, read Part I. You may think that you're pretty familiar with your breasts, but there's so much more going on inside them then you may know. These chapters help familiarize you with your bosom buddies.

You can't prevent breast cancer, but you can reduce your risk of developing the disease. Being aware of your particular risk factors is one way. Finding cancer early is another key. Doing so improves your chances of having successful treatment, and most important, finding cancer early greatly improves your survival rate. In this part, we walk you through breast self-examination, physical examination, mammography, and other lifesaving strategies. This section can literally save your life.

Part II: All Kinds of Oses — Diagnoses, Prognoses, and Treatment Options

This part describes tests and what their findings mean for you. We discuss what breast-cancer staging means, because determining the particular stage of your breast cancer is critical in determining your treatment options. The chapter on prognosis answers the question in the back of every woman's mind: "Will I die?" (Did you know that most women who are diagnosed early actually survive breast cancer?) Finally, you'll find out about the many treatment options available to you and how you can make the best choices for you and your family.

Part III: Buckling Up — Traveling Through Treatment

You mean I have a choice of what treatment I have? Yes, ma'am. Your options depend on many different factors, but you have the right to explore these options and participate in making the decisions. In this section, we describe the nuts and bolts of what you can expect during each form of treatment, including surgery, radiation, chemotherapy, and/or hormonal therapy. We cover everything you need to know about the most up-to-date treatments that are available, and we provide you with strategies for evaluating your options.

We also make recommendations for how best to deal with difficult parts of each treatment (as if you didn't know there'd be some of those). Losing a breast or both breasts isn't easy, and in this section, we discuss your choices in the matter and alternatives you can consider with regard to reconstructive surgery.

Part IV: Living Life After Diagnosis

When you've been diagnosed with breast cancer, no matter what treatment you undergo, looking after yourself is essential. Of course, that's easier said than done. In this part, we show how every woman, no matter how busy or how many demands she has upon her time, can find ways to meet her own needs.

Asking for help may be difficult, but building your own cheerleading squad may be just the ticket. We show you how in this part. Your family will likely be part of the squad, and so will friends, neighbors, and colleagues. Many people don't know how to respond, what to say, or what to do. In this part, we provide caretakers and friends with helpful hints that make the patient's life easier and even contribute to her or his recovery.

While you're getting support from family and friends, you're likely making enemies with your insurance company. We've dedicated a chapter to understanding your rights within the health insurance and legal systems.

Finally, finding out how to deal with the reality of the dreaded "r" word, *recurrence,* without becoming obsessively anxious, sometimes becomes a tightrope act. We share with you the myriad ways women with breast cancer have resumed full and active lives after treatment. Welcome to the inspiring world of breast cancer survivors!

Part V: The Part of Tens

This part gives you helpful information in handy groups of ten (or more). Here we offer such useful lists as ten hospitals offering clinical trials, and ten-plus services and agencies that are ready and willing to help you along the way.

Icons Used in This Book

Icons in this book are like the various keys on your key chain. Each one opens a different door.

This icon makes your life easier. The information that accompanies it can save you time.

This icon points out important information about which you need to be aware, so pay close attention whenever you see this icon: Your health — mental or physical — may be in jeopardy if you don't take heed.

This icon highlights ideas or information that you won't want to forget. By flipping through this book and looking for all the Remember icons, you can quickly read the most important information in each chapter.

You can skip this jargon-filled text if you prefer, but check them out whenever you want the juicy details.

This icon refers to words of advice, support, and wisdom especially for you from other breast cancer survivors.

Where to Go from Here

Keep this book nearby during your journey to recovery. Read what you need at the time, and leave the rest for later. Highlight parts that you find relevant to you; doing so makes them easier to find when you need to refer to them again.

Cut out, dog-ear, or otherwise mark the pages with information about which you have questions for the doctor, and then be sure to bring the book with you on medical visits. Share the book with your family and friends (better yet, let them get their own book to highlight), so that they better understand your journey and how best to be there for you. Refer them first to Chapter 20, which is intended specifically for them. When you no longer need it, keep this book somewhere safe, because it can serve as your memento of a road bravely traveled.

Part I:
Will My Hair Fall Out? Coming to Grips with Breast Cancer

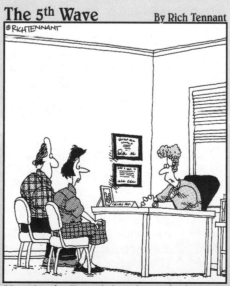

The 5th Wave   By Rich Tennant

"I realize the diagnosis is serious and raises many questions, but let's try to address them in order. We'll look at various treatment options, make a list of the best clinics to consider, and then determine what color ribbon you should be wearing."

In this part . . .

You've felt a lump and you're terrified. Is it or isn't it cancer? Chapter 2 is a lifesaver, showing you how to examine your breasts, identify lumps, and essentially get acquainted with their external contours and incredible internal milk factory. You'll recognize when something doesn't feel right, and if it's cancer, the key to a good outcome is catching it early. Chapter 3 discusses the risk factors for developing breast cancer and shows you how to know which of them put you at high risk but can't be changed and which risks can be lowered, so you can begin taking action. Shocked and afraid upon learning that you have breast cancer, Chapter 4 answers all those nagging questions about the various types of breast cancer, whether it's remained where it started or invaded other cells, and how these factors affect your treatment options and projected outcome. Dealing with your dilemma one step at a time makes your journey much less overwhelming and much more manageable.

Chapter 1

Tackling Breast Cancer One Step at a Time

*B*reast cancer. Just hearing those words is enough to send a shiver down any woman's spine. Everyone has known at least one friend or family member with the disease, and tragically, so many people have had a loved one who fought bravely, but in the end, lost her battle with the disease. You probably felt deeply for those women and their families, and most likely helped them in one way or another.

But this time, it's different. If you picked up this book, you're likely the one who felt a lump in the shower the other day or had a mammogram that your doctor said looked suspicious and now wants you to have more tests. Or maybe the worst thing you can imagine has happened: Your doctor just told you that you have breast cancer, and you're still in shock. Questions are whirling through your head:

✔ How bad is it?

✔ Am I going to die?

✔ What treatment do I have to go through?

✔ Who's going to look after my kids? My job?

✔ Does my insurance cover this stuff?

✔ How am I going to manage?

And when you're in shock (which is a completely normal reaction under these circumstances), processing information becomes difficult. You can hear the doctor's words, but they seem to fly right over your head. You just can't seem to grasp what he or she is saying. You heard "breast cancer" and something about "surgery" and "prognosis," and that's where everything stopped.

If you or someone you love has been diagnosed with breast cancer, you've come to the right place. We'll guide you through the process of getting better every step of the way, from diagnosis all the way to the rest of your life.

Staring Right Back at the Shocking News

The impact of the news that you have breast cancer may feel overwhelming at the moment. The key to dealing with this overwhelming news is tackling it one step at a time; taking it piece-by-piece, in little chunks. You may think that you need to act immediately, but that seldom is the case, and your doctor will let you know when it is. Chapter 4 gives you the basics about breast cancer; that's a good place to start getting a grip on what's happening. And check out Chapter 18, which tells you what to expect in terms of emotions and how you can deal with them.

Searching for Treatment

You have time to read about your treatment options and who will serve as members of your treatment team. Chapter 9 talks about treatment options and your team (just call yourself coach). In fact, Part III features chapters that describe the different treatment options, how effective they are, and what their side effects are like. You discover more about which route you may wind up taking: chemotherapy, radiation, or hormone therapy. And what about surgery? Chapter 10 talks about the different surgical options and describes who the candidates are for each of those options.

Take the time to think and feel. Give yourself a week or two to find out about your cancer and what it entails (what kind of cancer it is, what stage it's in, whether it's spread to your lymph nodes or other organs, and so on), consider all your options, and then begin working on your treatment plans.

Predicting Your Prognosis

You need to realize that part of the reason you're suffering from uncontrollable fear and anxiety is that you don't know what you can expect to happen. Understanding your particular diagnosis can help you feel more empowered. Chapter 6 helps you read your pathology report, and Chapter 8 helps you get into the nitty-gritty by answering that nagging question: "What are my chances?"

The three important factors that you need to recognize when talking about your predicted outcome or *prognosis* are that

- ✔ No one, not even your own doctor, can tell you for sure what your *exact* prognosis is.

- ✔ The percentages are just projections, not absolutes. They're based on how large numbers of women in similar circumstances have done in the past. And besides, many other factors can influence your individual prognosis.

- ✔ Prognosis is measured in 5-year, 10-year or 20-year blocks. That doesn't mean that you'll live only 5 (or 10 or 20) years; it's just a way of measuring outcomes. The *survival rate* tells you what percentage of women with breast cancer live *at least* 5 or 10 years after being diagnosed. But remember that many of these women live much, much longer.

The full details about the five stages of breast cancer can be found in Chapter 7. Knowing about the particular stage of your breast cancer points to what your treatment options are and what your prognosis is likely to be.

Talking with Family and Friends

So you're a wreck. What about your partner? And the kids? They know that something's wrong.

Straight talk is the best policy. Be upfront with your partner and other members of your family, talking about your fears. Chapter 19 can help you do just that. Your partner, family, and friends are all so intent on helping you that you wonder just how you're going to be able to help them do that. Sit them down with Chapter 20, which we've written just for them. And what about the kids?

Sharing your journey: Surveying the statistics

More than two million cancer survivors live in the United States. Yes, that means women who have gone through the journey you're about to embark upon and who have not only survived but also thrived. Most of these courageous women have gone on to lead meaningful, productive lives. Some still are struggling to reach the five-year mark, and, of course, some are like you; they've just been diagnosed with the disease. No matter where on their journey they are, a community of survivors stands ready to share its wisdom, supporting you in your times of sadness and celebrating each of your many triumphs.

On the other hand, statistics are startling: Other than cancers of the skin, breast cancer is the most common form of cancer among women. In fact, one of every three cancers diagnosed in women in the United States is breast cancer. The American Cancer Society predicts that in 2003, about 211,300 women (and 1,300 men) will be newly diagnosed with *invasive breast cancer* (or cancer that has the potential to spread outside of the breast). Another 39,000 women will be diagnosed with *noninvasive cancer* (or cancerous cells that lack the ability to spread outside the breast).

If you're like most people, you're wondering, "Will I live?" As many as 39,000 women (and 400 men) died from breast cancer in 2002. It is the second leading cause of cancer deaths among women. But here's some good news: *Most women do not die from breast cancer,* and your journey won't be the same as anyone else's. Your individual prognosis (outcome) depends on many factors, and in Part II of this book, we discuss the probable course of your disease and your recovery. The chances are good that you'll make a full recovery and go on to live a full and fulfilled life, especially if your cancer is detected early.

If you don't tell the kids what's going on, they'll let their imaginations provide them with the answers, and you can bet they'll think of something much worse than anything you could have thought of. But how are you supposed to tell them without scaring them? Fortunately, child psychologists have studied this for many years, and in Chapter 21, we provide you with many helpful insights and suggestions.

Seeking Out Others

After you know where you're headed, you can seek help. Countless support groups and programs are in place across the country to provide you with the help you need, and most of them are staffed by cancer survivors. Don't hesitate about getting in touch with them. We list many of these helpful resources in Chapter 23, and be sure to check out Chapter 20, where we tell you where and how you can build support. Take a look at many of the Survivors' Secrets (they're marked with a special icon) throughout this book for words of inspiration from breast cancer survivors who've been in your shoes and know the ropes.

In addition to person-to-person contact, consider complementary therapies. So many breast cancer survivors have found that yoga, meditation, and breathing exercises have sustained their spirits and strength. That's why in Chapter 14 we describe some of these methods, so you can choose the one that's right for you. After you find the ones that fit your needs, use them and see how wonderful they make you feel.

Taking Care of Business

The final step before beginning your treatment is getting everything in your life in order, so you can focus only on getting better. As tough as that may sound, the reality is that money, insurance, and your job must be addressed even though you may not feel like facing those issues right now. That's why in Chapter 17 we review your insurance benefits, help you plan your financial future, and tell you which laws afford you what kind of protection and where and how to apply for financial support.

Moving Forward with the Rest of Your Life

So you've completed your treatment, and now, you're wondering what happens next. A long, wonderful journey lies ahead, but the two stumbling blocks that you need to watch for are the fear of recurrence and rekindling intimacy with your partner.

Being afraid of a recurrence is natural, but handling that fear wisely is another story. It is possible to predict your likelihood of recurrence, but realizing that *not* all recurrences are the same is just as important. Your prognosis of recovery after a recurrence varies according to the type and extent of the recurrence. All these aspects of your encounter with breast cancer are discussed in Chapter 16, including how to fight a recurrence if you ever do have to face it.

Somewhere between juggling your new outlook post-treatment and stifling your fear of recurrence, you realize that you have a partner and a remaining sense of sexuality! Although you may know it's time to reconnect, intimacy following breast cancer surgery and treatment can be intimidating for many. Don't let that stop the joy that being close with your partner can bring. In Chapter 19, we candidly discuss the stumbling blocks and embarrassing moments, but more important, we explain how to move beyond those roadblocks to experience once again the ecstasy that joining together can bring.

Chapter 2

Getting Hands On with Your Breasts

Remember as a girl all that giggling with your best friends about the lacy bra your mother finally got you? It, of course, pinched and itched, but you were just so proud. Remember the first time someone you cared for deeply caressed your breasts, and you thought you'd just melt away? Regardless of what your particular recollections are, everyone has memories associated with their breasts.

Despite the significance of their breasts in their lives, most women don't examine them the way they need to on a monthly basis.

Being Best Friends with Your Breasts

Breasts come in all shapes and sizes. In fact, most women don't have identical breasts. Each is slightly different in size. The part of the breast with which most people are familiar is the outside. The *areola* is the darker area of the breast surrounding the *nipple,* as shown in Figure 2-1. The shape and size of the areola varies between women, with blonde women usually having lighter ones and darker women having darker ones. Breasts vary a lot, despite the way Hollywood likes to present them. Fewer people are familiar with the internal part of the breast, which houses many things, including fat and breast tissues.

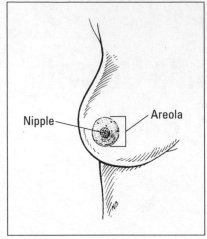

Figure 2-1: External view of a woman's breast.

Looking at lobules and ducts

A marvelous and miraculous process takes place within the breast — milk is made. Instead of having to go to the store, women produce and distribute baby food that can keep a baby alive and help it grow up to be strong and healthy.

Breasts make this miracle happen. I describe this system as the tree of life. Spread throughout the breast are milk-producing *lobules,* which are glands. They're spread throughout the breast like leaves are spread all over a tree. These lobules are connected to the delicate milk-carrying *ducts* that resemble the delicate branches of a tree. Just as the dainty branches come together on a tree to form the larger branches, so, too, do the ducts join together to form the major ducts. The major ducts then lead to the nipple, the tree trunk. Fat carefully cushions these milk-producing miracles. (Who says that all fat is bad?)

Connective tissue holds this precious package together. *Connective tissue* is a gelatin-like substance that's present throughout the body. The only muscle present in the breast is in the nipple and around the lobules, all of which is designed to get milk easily to baby. The lack of muscle within the breast is why with time your breasts tend to sag, and no amount of exercise can prevent that from happening.

Blood and lymphatic vessels

In addition to a milk-producing gland system, breasts also contain a large supply of nerves, blood vessels, and *lymphatic vessels.* Blood vessels carry blood throughout the body and nerves help you feel things. The *lymphatic system* is like the garbage disposal system of the body. Its job is to remove dead cells, bacteria, and other harmful agents from the body. (Our bodies knew about recycling long before it became fashionable!) These agents are ultimately dumped from the lymphatic system into the blood stream where they're removed from the body by the kidneys. Unfortunately, both the lymphatic system and the blood can carry cancer cells from where they started to other parts of the body.

But the lymph vessels also do something else. Whenever they find something threatening, such as undesired bacteria or a virus or a cancer cell, they deposit it in the *lymph nodes*. These small, bean-shaped extensions of the lymph vessels are collections of immune system cells. The nodes, good little soldiers designed to protect your body, make antibodies that fight the attacking enemy. If breast cancer cells start moving away from where they started, they often travel through the lymphatic vessels. As soon as they reach the lymph nodes, there's a higher risk that they've also entered the blood stream, and from there, they may continue on their destructive journey to other parts of your body. For example, when breast cancer cells have entered the axillary lymph nodes, the likelihood that breast cancer cells also have entered the blood stream is greater (compared with tumors that have not entered the axillary lymph nodes). Chapter 3 provides you with a full description of this process. Lymph nodes become extra important when you're suspected of having breast cancer because they enable your doctors to know the risk of whether the cancer has spread. Chapter 7 talks about this topic in depth.

The lymph nodes that drain the breast are shown in Figure 2-2. The *supraclavicular nodes* are above the collarbone; *axillary lymph nodes* are in the axilla (or armpit); and the *internal mammary nodes* are beside the sternum (breast bone).

SURVIVORS' SECRETS

Susan G.

"I was just too busy what with my job and the kids and everything. Who has the time, right? Boy, was I wrong! I was in the shower, rushing as usual, but then I felt this lump and I was like — 'Hey, this wasn't here before, was it?' At first I just wanted to forget about it, you know, put it out of my mind. But I just couldn't, so I made an appointment right away to see my doctor. And you know what? Every day I thank the Lord for helping me make the right decision. It was the decision that saved my life. If I could give you just one bit of advice it would definitely be, 'Please see your doctor as soon as possible; it will save your life.'"

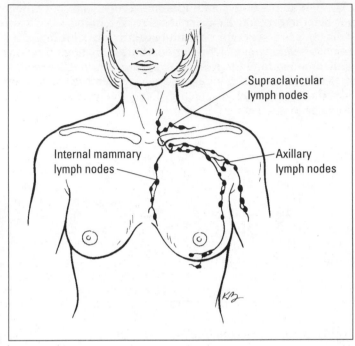

Supraclavicular
lymph nodes

Internal mammary
lymph nodes

Axillary
lymph nodes

Figure 2-2:
Lymph
nodes and
lymphatic
vessels:
What a
system.

Taking Matters into Your Own Hands: Breast Self-Exams Can Save Your Life

Breast self-examination is considered a good-news, bad-news scenario. The bad news (I prefer hearing it first): More women are being diagnosed with breast cancer today than were 20 years ago. In fact it's the second most common form of cancer among women (after skin cancer).

Now for the good news: More women than ever are now surviving breast cancer. Although this good-versus-bad situation may sound like a contradiction, it isn't really. More women *are* surviving for two main reasons:

✔ Mammograms can detect cancer earlier than before.

✔ Treatments for breast cancer are constantly improving.

Simply put, the earlier that breast cancer is found, the better the chances for successful treatment. And successful treatment means a better chance for survival.

One of the first steps toward finding cancer early is doing monthly breast self-examinations (see Table 2-1 for some self-examination do's and don'ts). Examining your breasts once a month helps you become familiar with the lay of the land and, as such, whether anything is different from one exam to the next. If something *is* different, you notice it immediately. Breast self-examination is easy to do, it's free, and best of all, it can save your life. Sounds like a good enough reason, doesn't it? If you don't do it for yourself, then think about doing it for your family.

Table 2-1	Do's and Don'ts of BSEs
Do	*Don't*
Examine your breasts at the same time each month.	Do not examine your breasts just before your periods (unless you want to give yourself a heart attack) because your breasts may be full of lumps and bumps at that stage.
Use the flat part of your fingers to examine your breasts.	Do not use your whole hand to examine your breasts.

When examining your breasts, getting comfortable is important. Maybe you can lock the door . . . whatever feels best to you. As you look at and feel your breasts, remember that you're looking for

- Changes in the way your breasts usually feel
- Lumps
- Signs of redness or puckering of the skin
- One breast that's *unusually* larger than the other
- Nipple discharge

Here are some steps you can take to properly examine your breasts while lying down:

1. **Lie down with a pillow under your right shoulder.**

   This helps flatten your right breast.

2. **Place your right arm behind your head.**

   If you have large breasts, use your right hand to support your breast while you examine it with your left hand.

3. **Use the finger pads of the three middle fingers on your left hand to feel for lumps in the right breast.**

A firm ridge located under your breast is completely normal.

- Press firmly.
- Vary the pressure from light to deep each time you touch it.

4. **Move your finger pads around the breast in the same way every time.**

    You can use either an up and down, around in a circle, or from the outside toward the center motion, but make sure that you do it the same way every time. Figure 2-3 shows a woman feeling in a circular pattern.

5. **Go over the entire breast and chest area, from the middle of the armpit to middle breastbone and to the collarbone.**

    The woman in the shower in Figure 2-3 shows a shaded area; that's where you need to check.

6. **Switch hands and repeat steps 1 through 5 to examine your left breast.**

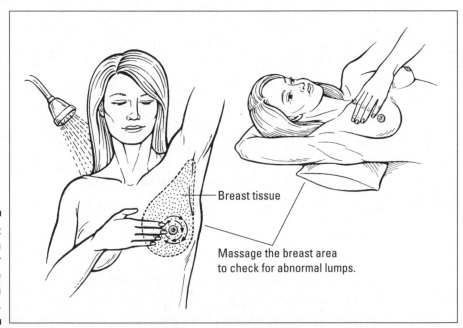

Figure 2-3:
Examining in the shower and while lying on the bed.

Breast tissue

Massage the breast area to check for abnormal lumps.

If you prefer performing the exam standing up in the shower

1. **Run a shower.**

Your soapy hands move over your breasts more easily. Don't forget that having a partner do a little quality check with you in the shower is fun every now and then.

2. **While in the shower, lift your left arm and put your left hand behind your head.**

3. **Check your left breast with your right hand (moving the pads of your fingers in either an up and down, around in a circle, or from the outside toward the center motion as described in the previous list of steps).**

4. **Check your right breast with your left hand.**

5. **After the shower, stand in front of the mirror with your hands by your sides.**

   See whether you notice any changes, such as dimpling or one breast being *unusually* larger than the other.

6. **Do the same with your hands raised above your head.**

Bumping into a Lump

While you were checking your breasts perhaps you found something different; you definitely felt a lump. Now you're just plain terrified. Well, you're not really sure it's a lump, it's sort of squishy and it moves, but wait a minute, it's also kind of firm. It seems to come and go. You felt it last month, and then you couldn't feel it any more, but now it's back. If you hold your arm just like that . . . no, no, yes . . . just like that, yes, there it is.

Try not to panic. Remember these important facts:

- Ninety percent of breast lumps are *benign* (or noncancerous).
- Lumps that come and go are nothing to worry about.
- When you're younger than 40 and you feel a lump, it's *very* unlikely to be cancer. Breast cancer is rare among young women (see more about breast cancer and age in Chapter 3).

Begging for benign

When you find a lump in your breast, it usually turns out to be one of the many benign (noncancerous) causes of lumps and cysts, including the ones listed in Table 2-2.

Table 2-2		Benign Growths		
Growth	*What It Is*	*What It Feels like*	*Who Is Prone*	*How the Growth Is Diagnosed*
Cyst	Fluid-filled duct	Round and smooth. Can move around and can change size during menstrual cycle, with potential pain or tenderness.	Anyone can get cysts. It's most common in women in their 40's and 50's.	Your doctor can identify a cyst by sticking a needle in, drawing out fluid, and making a diagnosis based on that (see Chapter 5).
Fibro-adenoma	Collection of stromal cells (cells that support the other cells in your breast)	Movable and rounded lumps, firm or hard.	Teenagers and young women.	Surgically removed or diagnosed with a needle biopsy (see Chapter 5) and monitored.
Fat necrosis	Dead fat cells	Hard, flat lump, irregular in shape. Clinically it feels like cancer (but isn't).	Women older than 50 or those with a breast injury.	You'll probably have a biopsy (see Chapter 5).
Infections	Bacteria	Swelling, redness, pain, fever.	Pregnant and breast-feeding women.	Antibiotics. Sometimes an abscess must be surgically drained. An infection around the areola can require surgical duct removal and antibiotics.
Intraductal papilloma	Tiny polyps in the ducts	Watery or bloody nipple discharge.	Anyone is prone.	They are not cancerous but must be biopsied (see Chapter 5) because discharge is present.

Growth	What It Is	What It Feels like	Who Is Prone	How the Growth Is Diagnosed
Mammary duct ectasia	Ducts are and clogged with dead cells from the duct lining	You may have a thick nipple discharge (like cheesy material), swelling, and inflamed area.	Most common in women over 50.	Biopsy (see Chapter 5).

Muttering about malignancy

So how can you tell whether it's cancer? A malignant lump is more likely to be firm and irregularly shaped. The most common signs of breast cancer are

✔ A new firm lump or a mass in your breast

✔ Swelling of your breast

✔ Dimpling of your breast

✔ Nipple redness or scaliness

✔ Retraction (when the nipple turns inward)

✔ Discharge of anything other than milk that squirts out on its own

✔ A lump that seems to be growing

Make an appointment to see your doctor whenever you find any of these signs. Remember that although statistically it's very unlikely to be cancer, being safe is your best course of action. Try to get an appointment with the doctor within the week. Your doctor probably will send you to get a mammogram and to see a breast surgeon. Depending on what the surgeon thinks, and what the mammogram shows, you may need a *biopsy* (where a sample of the lump is removed and analyzed by a pathologist) or an *aspirate* (where a needle is inserted into the lump to prove whether fluid is present) if your doctor thinks the lump is a *cyst* (fluid-filled lump). These procedures are described in detail in Chapter 5.

Knocking out cyst myths

If you're one of the many women who gets small cysts, you may be diagnosed with *fibrocystic disease*. Many women are told they have fibrocystic disease because their breasts are lumpy or tender at certain times of the month. This is *not* a disease, it's part of the normal response of your breast tissue to changes in your body's hormones. Pain and lumpiness have nothing to do with your risk of cancer.

Chapter 3

Understanding and Reducing Your Risk

*E*veryone's heard the terrifying statistics about breast cancer. In fact, probably only a few of you don't personally know someone who has suffered and maybe even died from it. Second only to skin cancer, breast cancer is the most common form of cancer and the second most common cause of cancer deaths (second only to lung cancer) in American females. What causes this dreadful disease? Unfortunately, scientists still don't know. All they can explain are some of the risk factors. Huh? Aren't risks and causes one and the same? Not really.

The *cause* of an illness is proof that a certain factor directly results in an illness. Smoking is a great example. The fact that smoking causes cancer of the lungs has been proven unequivocally. On the other hand, a *risk* is a factor(s) that increases your odds of developing a disease.

In this chapter we discuss the known risk factors in tandem with the unknown where breast cancer is concerned, how to determine whether you're at high risk for it, and what you can do to improve your odds against getting breast cancer.

Assessing the Odds

If you're a betting person, you may be asking what the odds of your getting breast cancer are. The answer, unfortunately, isn't so simple. You can't just look up what your particular risk factors are, list them on a page, add them together, and come up with a clear picture. Some factors carry more weight than others. Some factors may either aggravate or mitigate others. And, combinations of several factors are much more risky than combinations of others. However, having said all that, your doctor still may use a mathematical model of your risk factors to *estimate* your risk of breast cancer.

And that isn't all. You may exhibit many of the risk factors but never develop breast cancer (which although great, probably won't stop you from worrying). On the other hand, you may have no risk factors at all, aside from being a woman, and still get breast cancer. In fact, 50 percent of women who get breast cancer have no risk factors. It doesn't seem fair, does it?

The two general types of risk are

- ✔ **Absolute risk:** *Absolute risk* is the actual numeric risk that points to a particular segment of the population getting breast cancer during a specified time period. For example, a 40-year-old woman whose mother had breast cancer, who has had no children, and no breast biopsies has a 1.1 percent risk of developing breast cancer in the next 5 years, and an 18.8 percent risk of developing it by age 90.

- ✔ **Relative risk:** Relative risk compares the incidence of breast cancer in women with a particular risk factor. For example, a woman with a sister who has breast cancer has twice the risk of developing breast cancer as the woman with no risk factors. Put another way, the woman whose sister has breast cancer has 100 percent higher risk of developing breast cancer than the woman without any risk factors. So, the higher the score where relative risks are concerned, the greater is the risk of members of that group getting breast cancer as compared with a group whose members don't have those particular risk factors. To find out how this is pertinent to one individual, relative risk needs to be converted to an absolute risk. In short, your absolute risk is the one you need to know.

Facing Risks You Can't Change

Unfortunately, with breast cancer, you just can't do anything about *most* of the most important risk factors: being a woman and getting older! However, knowing what they are nevertheless is important. If you know you're at high risk, you can ask your doctor about getting mammograms at an earlier age, for example.

Sex

Breast cancer is such an overwhelmingly female disease that sometimes sex isn't even mentioned as a risk factor. It's just taken for granted. Breast cancer occurs in males (see the "Breast cancer in men" sidebar in this chapter for more information); however, in the United States, approximately 44,000 women get breast cancer annually compared to only 1,500 men.

Getting older

Other than being a woman, the most common risk factor for breast cancer is getting older. Fifty percent of a woman's lifetime risk for developing breast cancer occurs after age 65, and 80 percent of breast cancers occur in women older than 50.

When you're 20, your chances of developing breast cancer are rare: 1 in 2,044 (so rare that mammograms aren't even recommended unless you're at high risk). But when you're 70, your chances are 1 in 24.

Don't be scared if you're younger than 40 and feel a lump. It's very unlikely to be cancer; in fact, most lumps in young women are not cancerous. Nevertheless, ask your doctor. In the rare case that you are diagnosed with cancer, your prognosis depends on the type of cancer, how far (or not) it has spread, how you respond to treatment, and several other factors.

Although you can't do much about getting older (other than getting wiser), women nevertheless *can* stay in good health and have regular mammograms and medical checkups. (See Chapter 5 where we describe this in full.) Although good health and regular checkups don't reduce your risk of developing breast cancer, they can help you keep closer tabs. When you find it early, you *significantly* improve your chances for an excellent outcome.

Medical history

Certain factors in your previous medical history have a direct bearing on your risk for getting breast cancer. They are

- ✔ **A history of breast cancer:** If you've had breast cancer once, your risk of developing breast cancer in the other breast (which isn't the same as recurrence, see Chapter 19) is increased three to four times; however, the absolute risk is very low: Only 8 percent of women who have had one breast cancer in 10 years ever get a second breast cancer. That's why vigilance and continued monitoring are so important.

> ✔ **Breast biopsy results with atypical cells:** Sometimes a breast biopsy doesn't find cancer but detects what are commonly referred to as *pre-cancerous conditions*. That means the cells are not like normal cells, they're *atypical*. In those cases, making sure that you have annual mammograms and breast exams by your doctor and that you routinely do your own monthly breast self-examinations is important. Table 3-1 explains the types of risks indicated by your specific biopsy results.

Breast cancer in men

Although breast cancer is 100 times more common in women, at least 1,500 men will be diagnosed with breast cancer in the United States in 2003. Four hundred men die of breast cancer each year, accounting for 0.22 percent of cancer deaths among men in the United States.

Many similarities exist between breast cancer among men and women, but several differences stand out. The most obvious relates to size of the breast. Because men have very little breast tissue, a mass is much easier for them and their doctors to feel, even when it's very small. Although women know about breast cancer, many men don't realize that they too can get this disease, so they often neglect a breast lump or think it's from something else. Likewise, because they have much less breast tissue, men have to have a mastectomy in most cases.

Most lumps in men are not cancerous, and can be caused by enlarged breast tissue, which can happen if a man is taking medications to treat a heart condition or high blood pressure, or if he smokes marijuana. (Yep, you heard right.)

Doctors used to think that men with breast cancer had a worse prognosis than women, but they've since found out that when the stage of the cancer of the man is compared with the stage of the cancer of the woman, the prognosis is the same. Similarly, the more that men are diagnosed early on, the more of them who will have a better outcome. As with women, what causes breast cancer in men isn't known.

However, doctors do know what risk factors increase the likelihood that men will get breast cancer. The good news is that most breast cancers in men have estrogen and progesterone receptors on their surface, and men do just as well taking *tamoxifen* (a hormone treatment) as women do.

The known risk factors for male breast cancer include

✔ Being older. Most men with breast cancer are diagnosed at age 65 or older.

✔ Having a family history of breast cancer. Twenty percent of men with breast cancer have close relatives (male or female) with breast cancer.

✔ For men with a family history of breast cancer, having a mutated BRCA2 gene (see "Inheriting the genes: Your ancestry" in this chapter) increases the risk further. Men with breast cancer need to strongly consider genetic testing for BRCA2.

✔ *Klinefelter's syndrome,* a congenital (you're born with it) condition that increases breast cancer risk. Women have two X chromosomes, and men have one X and one Y chromosome. Men with this syndrome have an extra X chromosome, which results in them having lower levels of the male hormone testosterone and higher levels of the female hormone estrogen, resulting in smaller testicles and infertility. This syndrome affects 1 in 1,000 men. About 3 percent of men with Klinefelter's syndrome will get breast cancer.

✔ Having severe liver disease like *cirrhosis*. Men with cirrhosis also have lower levels of testosterone and higher levels of estrogen, which increases the risk of developing swellings in the breast and breast cancer.

✔ Being exposed to radiation, particularly as treatment for cancer in the chest (such as Hodgkin's or non-Hodgkin's lymphoma), which increases breast cancer risk.

✔ Being treated for prostate cancer with estrogen-related drugs. This treatment slightly increases a man's risk of developing breast cancer.

✔ Being obese. Obesity is likely to be a risk factor for male breast cancer.

Because doctors don't know how to prevent breast cancer in men, the most important thing that can be done is detecting it early and beginning treatment immediately. Some men are embarrassed to go to the doctor, so, if you know a man with a lump in his breast, take him to the doctor yourself. It probably isn't cancer, but if it is, you can save his life.

Table 3-1	How Biopsy Results Affect Risk	
Biopsy Finding	*How It Affects Your Risk*	*More on the Matter*
Proliferative breast disease without *atypia* or *usual hyperplasia* (overgrowth of cells lining the ducts, but cells look normal)	Increases 1.5 to 2 times	The risk is relatively low. During a period of 15 years, only 4% of women with proliferative breast disease develop breast cancer, compared with 2% of women who don't have this disease. Doctors don't consider this factor alone a true risk factor.
Atypical hyperplasia (overgrowth of abnormal cells lining the ducts, but cells look normal)	Increases by 4 to 5 times	The risk is relatively low: 8% risk of developing cancer during a period of 15 years.
Fibrocystic changes without proliferative breast disease (for example, cyst or fibroadenoma)	Doesn't affect your risk at all	80% of lumps you feel fall into this category.

Family history

A family history of breast cancer has long been known as a risk factor. Women with family histories of breast cancer are at higher risk (1.5 to 3 times higher) of developing breast cancer when female family members who have had the disease are *first-degree relatives* (such as mothers, sisters, or daughters). The risk grows even higher when your family shows one or more of the following:

✔ More than one first-degree relative has had breast cancer

✔ A first-degree relative who developed breast cancer at an early age

✔ A relative who had breast cancer in both breasts

✔ A relative with ovarian cancer

✔ A male relative with breast cancer

If you have no first-degree relatives with cancer, having a more distant relative with cancer has little, if any, impact on your risk.

Before you start remembering all your distant cousins and aunts five times removed who you think had some form of cancer, you need to know that your level of risk depends on a variation of these factors:

✔ The *exact relationship* of your relative with cancer

✔ The age at which that relative was *diagnosed*

✔ The *number* of relatives with the disease

For example, if your mother was older when she was diagnosed and no other family history of breast cancer exists, your risk is not as high as having many close relatives who developed breast cancer early in life, which, of course, increases your risk.

One myth about breast cancer indicates that your risk is only increased when the affected relatives are on your mother's side of the family. That simply isn't true; your father's family is just as important in contributing to your risk.

Your ethnicity

Certain aspects of your ancestry continue throughout your life. All of us carry on customs and rituals, practices, and habits that have been passed down from one generation to the next. Risk predisposition based on your heritage hasn't been well studied in most ethnic groups (other than the Ashkenazi Jews, which we describe in the "Ashkenazi Jews and inherited genes" sidebar). What *is* known, however, is that differences in incidence rates of breast cancer are evident among different ethnic groups. For example

Ashkenazi Jews and inherited genes

Your doctor may ask you whether you're Jewish. Don't think he's being nosy, it's because 1 in 40 women of Ashkenazi (European) Jewish descent carry the BRCA1 and BRCA2 (breast cancer) gene, which is significantly higher than in the general population where only 1 in 500 to 800 people carry the gene. This means that Ashkenazi Jews (male and female) have a significantly higher risk of having inherited the gene, which puts Ashkenazi women at considerably higher risk of developing early-onset breast cancer.

The chances of finding a mutation in an Ashkenazi woman who has a personal history or family history or both, of breast or ovarian cancer or both, is *much higher than* in an non-Ashkenazi. Researchers looking at the genetic history of Ashkenazi Jewish women with breast cancer who were younger than 40, found that 20 percent or even more had this genetic mutation.

The risk is higher in Ashkenazi Jewish women even without family ties so if you're an Ashkenazi Jewish woman who has this personal history, talk to your doctor, get informed, and consider genetic counseling (which we describe in more detail later on in this chapter). If you are an Ashkenazi Jewish woman younger than 40, consider genetic counseling.

✔ In the United States the risk of developing breast cancer is highest among White women, followed by African American, then Asian American, then Hispanic, and lastly by Native American women.

✔ When combining women across all ages, White women are more likely to develop breast cancer than African American women. However, African American women who are younger than 40 have slightly higher rates of breast cancer than White women of the same age group. The distressing fact is that African American women are more likely to die from breast cancer than White women. The reason may be in part because breast cancers tend to be diagnosed at later stages in African American women, when the cancer is bigger and associated with a worse prognosis. Coming in later for treatment in this group of women may in part be due to lack of health insurance, a sense of fatalism and/or distrust of the medical establishment.

Inheriting the genes: Your ancestry

Genetic risk is when your genetic makeup (our bodies are made up of millions of different genes) includes an abnormal gene that predisposes you to developing an illness such as breast cancer. Genes are made up of thousands of different parts called *base pairs*. If even one part of a gene is altered (mutated), that gene can malfunction and thus predispose you to diseases. Some individuals are born with a mutated (abnormal) gene, which means they're at a higher risk of developing a disease than individuals with normal genes. The issue of genetic risk of breast cancer has received plenty of press, because scientists recently identified two genes that provide new insight into the genetics of breast cancer, not to mention an entirely new avenue of hope. (For a more detailed description of how genetic mutations increase the risk of developing cancer, see Chapter 8.) Now that we know where the mutations are that cause such a high risk of breast cancer, we can try to find treatment strategies to reduce risk.

The names of each of the two genes that are checked for mutations that increase the likelihood of developing breast cancer start with the letters BRCA, which stand for *br*east *ca*ncer (and you thought they were just trying to confuse you). Each one also is numbered:

- BRCA1
- BRCA2

All women and men have BRCA1 and BRCA2 genes, but the risk of cancer is only increased when the gene is abnormal and mutated. This type of mutated gene is present in all cells of the body, not just in the cancer. That allows a blood test to be done to determine who has the abnormal gene. If you have a BRCA1 or BRCA2 mutation, you have a 50 percent chance of passing that abnormal gene on to your children, whether they're male or female. The good news is that BRCA1 or BRCA2 mutations are responsible for only 5 percent to 10 percent of breast cancers (see "Testing for BRCA 1 or BRCA2 mutation" later in the chapter for more information about who should consider being tested). Most women, even those with a family history, do *not* have this mutation.

Although they're uncommon, mutations of the BRCA1 and BRCA2 are important because women who have these mutations are at *significantly* higher risk of developing breast cancer sometime during their lives. Their risk is 37 percent to 85 percent compared with a 12.5 percent risk in the general female population. Regrettably, the increased risk isn't all. They're also more likely to get breast cancer *early* in their lives.

 Women with BRCA1 and BRCA2 mutations also are at significantly higher risk of developing cancer in the other breast and developing other forms of cancer (such as ovarian cancer). Table 3-2 provides more information about these higher levels of risk. As scary as this news is, only 1 in 500 to 800 people have a mutation (alteration) of the BRCA1 gene, and fewer still have a mutation of the BRCA2 gene.

Table 3-2	Increases in Risk for Other Cancers Caused by BRCA1 and BRCA2 Mutations	
Mutated Gene	*Type of Cancer*	*Increase in Risk*
BRCA1	Primary breast cancer	37%–85%
	Second breast cancer	40%–60%
	Ovarian cancer	20%–40%

Mutated Gene	Type of Cancer	Increase in Risk
BRCA2	Primary breast cancer	37%–85%
	Ovarian cancer	10%–20%
	Male breast cancer	6%

Regarding the Risks You Control

There's not much you can do about being a woman (well, you can but who wants to?) or getting older (many have tried but few have succeeded). However, there are factors that can increase your risk for breast cancer that you *can* do something about. These include taking hormone-replacement medication, being obese after menopause, and drinking alcohol. Changing these factors can slightly reduce your risk for developing breast cancer.

Harmonizing those hormones

Absolutely no doubt exists whatsoever that reproductive hormones (substances in your body that control how you reproduce, become a woman, and so on) are key factors that affect a woman's risk of getting breast cancer. The two important reproductive hormones in women are *estrogen* and *progesterone*. The latest research indicates that progesterone is worse.

Menstruating, menopausing, and having babies in between

What's the common denominator between starting your periods (oh, those terrible cramps), having babies (oh, those contractions), and menopause (oh, those hot flashes)? Each event affects when and for how long the cells in women's breasts are exposed to female hormones estrogen and progesterone. The longer you're exposed to hormones, the greater your risk of developing breast cancer. The events and corresponding effects are

- **Menstruation:** The younger the age at which you begin menstruating, the higher your risk. For each successive year after age 11 that a female starts her menstrual cycle, the risk of getting breast cancer decreases by 20 percent. The younger you are when you start menstruating, the longer your body is exposed to female hormones.

- **Menopause:** The older you are when you stop menstruating, the higher your risk. Women who start menopause before age 45 experience *half* the risk of developing breast cancer as women who begin menopause after 55. The older you are when you stop menstruating the longer your body is exposed to female hormones.

✔ **Giving birth:** Not ever having children increases risk. The risk of getting breast cancer is 1.4 times higher for women who have never had children than for those who do. Women who have never been pregnant ovulate every month and have a greater exposure to female hormones.

✔ **Age at childbirth:** The younger you are when you have your first child, the lower the risk. The risk for women who have a child after age 30 is two to five times higher than for women who have their first child before age 18.

✔ **Breast-feeding:** Some studies suggest that nursing your baby longer decreases your risk of getting breast cancer. Unfortunately, you have to breast feed for very long periods (years) to significantly reduce your risk and even then it may only decrease your risk before menopause.

Let's put all this into perspective. Even though all this may raise your concern, remember that the risk of an average American woman developing breast cancer is only 2.5 percent for the entire 20-year period (between the ages of 35 and 55). Even if your risk doubles because of exposure to hormones, it's still just 5 percent!

What are you supposed to do about all these factors? Although you certainly can't change when you start your periods, you can

✔ Technically have an effect on when you arrive at menopause by considering an *oopherectomy,* surgical removal of the ovaries. (See "Calculating Risks" later in this chapter.) This is *only* a consideration for women with BRCA1/2 mutations.

✔ Choose whether you want to have a baby.

✔ Choose how old you'll be when you have a baby.

Even if you're at very high risk, you can't make these life-altering decisions strictly on the basis of trying to lower your risk for breast cancer. Also, you may be unable to become pregnant and therefore unable to affect your risk. So you can see that these methods are only somewhat within your control.

Here's hormones in your eye

Your risk of getting breast cancer also is affected whenever you take hormone replacement therapy (HRT) after menopause. HRT combines female hormones estrogen and progesterone and is given to women after menopause to reduce menopausal symptoms. The effects of these therapies include

✔ **Hormone Replacement Therapy (HRT):** Whenever you ask any woman older than 50 about HRT, you'd better be prepared to listen! Everyone has had an experience good or bad, one way or the other.

Two female hormones are used in HRT: estrogen and progesterone. Estrogen helps prevent menopausal symptoms, such as bone loss and heart disease. Progesterone helps prevent uterine cancer. Studies of HRT have found the following:

- The risk for breast cancer increases when you've been using HRT for more than five years. The biggest risk is seen when both estrogen and progesterone are given together. Pills containing estrogen alone (only used in women who have had a hysterectomy) appear to increase the risk of breast cancer to a lesser degree.

- The risk of getting breast cancer reduces after HRT is stopped.

- HRT increases your risk for breast cancer and does *not* have a beneficial effect on heart disease, which researchers previously thought was true. Researchers concluded that the negative effects of HRT outweigh the benefits, and so recommended stopping ongoing studies. HRT does help with hot flashes though and protects against osteoporosis and is probably safe to take for short periods (perhaps up to two years).

HRT today is recommended only for short-term relief of menopausal symptoms. Many other drugs can protect women against osteoporosis that don't increase breast cancer risk. Unfortunately, they don't help with night sweats or hot flashes, but there are other non-hormonal treatments available for these symptoms. Talk to your doctor about these alternative drugs. When making the decision whether to use HRT, discuss *your* risk factors with your doctor.

Keeping that weight down

Whenever you're at a dinner or another type of party and the topic of cancer comes up, the conversation inevitably drifts around to food and exercise. Some revelers are likely to argue that food and exercise have nothing to do with cancer and that the disease is on the rise because of all the pollution in the air. Others tell about an article they just read that says that if you eat right and exercise, you can prevent breast cancer. Well, the verdict is in:

- ✔ Women who are obese after menopause *are* at slightly increased risk of developing breast cancer.

- ✔ Excess weight significantly increases your risk of dying from cancer.

Being overweight increases your risk of dying from cancer, and accounts for 20 percent of cancer deaths in women. That means that close to a quarter of deaths from cancer in women can be attributed to excess weight. Startling, isn't it?

This just-published information is consistent in its findings: People who are overweight have a higher risk of death from *a whole range of cancers*. The findings are irrefutable:

- ✔ If you're a woman who's overweight, you have a much higher risk of developing cancers of the breast, uterus, cervix, and ovaries, and of dying from them.

- ✔ If you're a woman and you're obese, you have a significantly higher risk of death from cancer than normal weight women with cancer.

Losing weight could prevent one of every six cancer deaths in the United States! Yes, that's for the whole of the country, and yes, that includes all kinds of cancers, not only breast cancer, but it applies to you.

- ✔ You can decrease your weight by
  - Eating your veggies first
  - Eating more proteins first, which helps you feel full longer
  - Avoiding the local fatty fried fast-food drive-throughs
  - Working some physical activity into your routine (after consulting a doctor, of course)
- ✔ Increasing your intake of vegetables, fruits, and dietary fiber

  You can work more fruits and veggies into your diet by
  - Slicing fruit into your cereal
  - Blending fruit into a beverage

Lifting those legs

Exercising can decrease your risk of getting breast cancer. Although a relatively new area of research, several studies have found that premenopausal women who exercise have a lower risk of breast cancer than women who don't.

Exercising is a very effective way of losing weight and keeping fit.

Want some help? Then

- ✔ Take the stairs instead of the elevator.
- ✔ Be a far parker (in other words take a walk) at the grocery store, the mall, the restaurant, or at work.
- ✔ Take a walk around the block every time you're craving fatty foods.
- ✔ Get an exercise tape and do a little at a time until you feel comfortable.

✔ Join a gym and find the exercises or classes that you enjoy. Going with a friend helps makes it easier the first few times!

Bypassing the booze

Bypassing the booze can help decrease your risk of breast cancer. Some studies have found that drinking beer, wine, or hard liquor increases your risk for breast cancer. No, I'm not kidding, and this isn't just about women who are heavy drinkers. You can avoid alcohol by

✔ Steering clear of places that serve alcohol

✔ Slamming a spritzer instead

If you do drink, research suggests taking folic acid daily can help reduce the effects of alcohol and your chance of developing breast cancer.

Avoiding radiation

Exposure to radiation (for example radiation given to treat a cancer, not just a chest X-ray here and there) before age 40 clearly increases breast cancer risk. Exposure to even moderate doses of radiation increases cancer risk, but the risk for breast cancer increases only when radiation is directed specifically at the chest area.

The good news is that if you're exposed to radiation when you're older than 40, you have a minimal increased risk for breast cancer, because women's breasts are much more susceptible to damage from radiation when they're still developing. You don't have to worry about the levels of radiation in mammography (see Chapter 5), because they're so low that they won't increase your risk of breast cancer.

Other risks still unknown

A number of other factors have been suggested to increase breast cancer risk, but so far scientific proof for this is lacking. For example, the effect that environmental pollutants may have on breast cancer. Talk about controversial. One of the more famous examples is on Cape Cod and Long Island, where women have a high incidence of breast cancer. Environmental pollutants, such as DDT and other similar chemicals, are the suspected cause, but researchers found no evidence to support a link between those pollutants and breast cancer. More studies are planned.

Debunking urban myths

There's always something that will be suspected as a cause of breast cancer. In today's Internet-savvy world, information takes mere minutes to travel around the globe, and although that's extremely helpful in many circumstances, it can sometimes result in misinformation. Two such examples:

✔ **Underarm deodorants:** Internet messages recently raised considerable panic among women by saying that chemicals in underarm deodorants were absorbed through the skin, blocking the lymph system, causing toxins to accumulate in the breast, and resulting in breast cancer. This scenario is simply not consistent with the science of how cells become cancerous. Check out Chapter 4 for a more-detailed description of how cancer develops.

✔ **Underwire bras:** Another Internet message and at least one book suggested that underwire bras cause breast cancer by obstructing flow of lymphatic fluids. Please know that simply no evidence, either clinical or scientific, supports this claim.

Calculating Your Risk: Choosing a Model That's Right for You

Your doc can use two methods to calculate your actual breast cancer risk score. She asks you many questions about your medical and family histories, and then inputs this data into the especially designed computer program. All kinds of complicated formulas then calculate your score.

Understanding the models

The two models for calculating breast cancer risk are the Claus Model and the Gail Model (named after those who developed them). Which is right for you?

✔ **The Claus Model** considers only your age and your family history of breast cancer. It's the right model for you when your major risk factor is relatives with breast cancer and you don't have a genetic mutation.

✔ **The Gail Model** takes into account multiple factors that influence risk, such as your age, menstrual and childbearing history, the number and results of previous breast biopsies you've had, and your family history of breast cancer. The model gives you a five-year risk and a lifetime risk of developing breast cancer compared to a woman of your age and race who doesn't have risk factors. The Gail Model can be accessed at:

- The National Cancer Institute (NCI): You can order the free risk assessment tool, known as Risk Disk either by phone at 800-422-6237 or at NCI's Risk Assessment Web site (bcra.nci.nih.gov/brc/).

- Harvard University (www.yourcancerrisk.harvard.edu/)

Remember that neither of these models predicts risk in women with BRCA1 and BRCA2 mutations. For women who may have these mutations, the best way to learn about your level of risk is by genetic testing.

Testing for BRCA1 or BRCA2 mutation

The American Society of Clinical Oncology recommends that you consider being tested for mutated breast cancer genes (even when you *haven't* had breast cancer), if you have

- ✔ More than two first-degree relatives with breast cancer, and one or more with ovarian cancer, diagnosed at any age.

- ✔ More than three first-degree relatives with breast cancer diagnosed before they were 50.

- ✔ Two sisters diagnosed with breast or ovarian cancer before the age of 50.

- ✔ A first-degree relative who's had two breast cancers, two ovarian cancers, or breast *and* ovarian cancer.

Table 3-3 fills you in on some of the risk factors that point to a greater potential of having the mutated breast cancer gene.

If you think you may fit into this group, ask your physician to send you to a genetic counselor who can tell you your risk of carrying a breast cancer gene and the pros and cons of getting tested.

If you haven't been diagnosed with breast cancer, but a member of your family has, that family member needs to be tested first (even if it happens to be a male family member), whenever possible, because that is the individual who's immediately affected. If your relative with cancer doesn't have the gene, there's no point in you being tested.

Genetic testing for BRCA1 and BRCA2 gene mutations is now commercially available. However, before you think about taking this test, talk to your doctor about your risk factors. If the doctor shows you why you're not at high risk, consider not taking the test. If you are at high risk for a gene mutation, testing can provide you with important information on your level of risk of breast and ovarian cancer, and with information pertinent to your children.

Table 3-3	Factors That Can Determine Risk of Mutated Breast Cancer Gene	
If You...	*And You...*	*Then...*
Had breast cancer in *both* breasts between 40 and 50 years of age	Have a first- or second-degree relative who had breast or ovarian cancer *before* she was 50 years old	The chance of your having the mutated gene is 42%.
Are Jewish	Got breast cancer before you were 30 years old	The chance of your having the mutated gene is 33%.
Are not Jewish	Got breast cancer before you were 30	The chance of your having the mutated gene is 12%.

If you decide to have the test, undergoing genetic counseling is *strongly recommended* to help you weigh some of the risks and benefits of taking the test. Several reasons for making this recommendation include

✔ The test is expensive (at least $2,400 and more when other family members are tested), and not all insurance companies pay for it.

✔ The test is complicated, because each gene has more than 100 possible mutations.

✔ Not having the mutated gene *doesn't* mean that you don't have a breast cancer gene. Many more mutations have yet to be identified.

✔ If you test positive for the mutated gene, researchers still can't tell you for sure *whether or when* you may get breast cancer.

✔ If you have the mutated gene, you're likely to want to tell your family members. If you have it, they'll need to consider testing since they may have the mutation as well.

As you can see, the test raises as many questions as it provides answers. That's why genetic counseling is essential. To help you find the genetic counseling and testing center nearest you, contact NCI's genetic testing Web site at www.cancer.gov/cancerinfo.

Chapter 4

Rebellion of the Mutated Genes: Reviewing Breast Cancer

*W*hen you've just been diagnosed with breast cancer, you're shocked and afraid. You just want to go back to life before your diagnosis. You may not even feel like reading this (or any other) book. Feeling that way is okay; it's natural. Your life has just been turned upside down. Everything is different. You may think that you have to act immediately, but *you don't*. It's taken your lump years to grow to the point that it can be detected. Give yourself some time to think. Give yourself some time to understand your cancer, so you can find out what it means for *you* and *your family*. Getting an overview of breast cancer is a good place to begin.

The Lowdown on Cancer: What It Is, What It Does

I don't know about you, but I like to know about my body and what's going on inside me, especially when I've just been told there's something wrong with it. But who wants to know every single medical detail? (That's why we go to doctors, isn't it?) Still, having some basic understanding is great so that you can become a fully participating member of your treatment team. Thus, in this section, we give you a quick and easy overview of what causes cancer.

Ginger L.

"When I walked out of the doctor's office, I felt like I couldn't breathe, like there was no air. I couldn't sleep for three nights after that. I just couldn't sleep, so after I put the kids to bed, I stayed up all night, you know, just watching TV and stuff. But then I'd start crying, and my mind felt all confused and everything. I kept thinking 'I'm going to die. My God, I'm going to die. Who's going to take care of my kids?' I tell you, I was scared. I've never been so scared in my life. But then, when I finally called the Survivors Group, Sandra came over right away. That's when everything changed for me. I realized I wasn't alone. She sat with me, and she just held me. She brought over some books and told me to take my time reading them. She told me how important it was that I become a part of my treatment. She even highlighted some parts for me. When I saw my doctor the next week I knew what to ask."

Making copying errors: The tale of small and big mutations

All the cells in your body replicate themselves. When they do it right, they create mirror images of themselves. (They're so in love with themselves that they want to create another cell just like the first. There's no accounting for vanity!) After the mirror image is created, the cell divides into two and, voilá! . . . you now have a new cell just like the old one (see Figure 4-1).

Well, the same is true with the cells in your body, cells that comprise every single part of your body. These cells all follow the same pattern again and again, over and over: First they sit around doing nothing (*quiet phase*), and then they start to work. Their job is to create a mirror image of themselves (*synthesis*). Then, after they've rested some more (hey, copying every single detail of the cell is difficult, you try it!), the cell divides into two (*cell division/ mitosis*), so now you have a new cell just like the old one.

Copying and dividing cells is how you grow. Babies and young children obviously make many new cells, but as you get older, this process slows down considerably. Cells divide and multiply only to replace older cells that are worn-out, or injured, or dying. You know when you have a bruise? The darker area is where dead cells are being cleaned out so you can heal. A bruise is one instance where your body makes more cells to replace the ones that died.

Every time a cell creates the mirror image of itself, it must copy all the zillions of parts that comprise its overall makeup, and sometimes the cell makes a mistake. These errors are called *mutations*. Some mutations are minor; some are pretty major. What happens next depends on how serious the mutation is

✔ Some mutations *aren't* big deals. When a mutation causes you to be born shorter than everyone else in your super-tall family, you may get teased a lot, but that's about the extent of it. Because the cell doesn't pose a danger to your health, it is allowed to continue to duplicate itself.

✔ Some mutations *are* big deals. When the cell realizes that it has created another cell that's badly mutated, it kills itself. Yes, it commits suicide by dissolving (killing) the mutated cell, and then beginning to create new ones from the normal cells. You don't even know it's happening (and it can happen a lot throughout your lifetime).

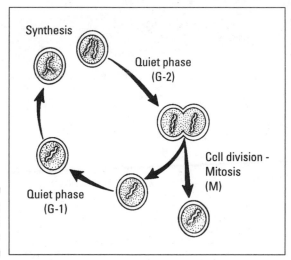

Figure 4-1:
The cell
cycle.

Every cell has *checkpoints* whose job is making sure they stop every mutated cell. If checkpoints find a cell with a small mutation, the cell must first go back and get fixed before it can return to the checkpoint. If the cell mutation is a major one, it must commit suicide. Not even one mutated cell, or even a mutated part of the cell, is allowed through the checkpoint.

Sometimes, however, something terrible happens. One of the checkpoints becomes mutated and leaves open the gate for all the other mutated cells to pass through. As these mutated cells begin flowing, once they've passed the checkpoint, they grow and multiply like crazy. And as they multiply, they change or alter themselves, "Why should I look puny like my mom and dad? I'm gonna make myself as big and bold as the guy next door." Before long, many of the mutated cells take off in all directions, leaving the gate open for other cells that want to mutate and join them and changing themselves as they go along. Figure 4-2 illustrates the progression from normal cells (in this case, they're in the milk duct), to cancerous cells that remain in place (in situ) and on to cancerous cells that begin moving out (invasive).

What you now have is a bunch of bad cells replicating themselves. This situation is the one thing that all cancers have in common; they all are abnormal cells growing out of control.

Just knowing that all these cells are dividing up inside you under the supposedly watchful eye of the cell checkpoints is kind of scary. Even scarier, these are checkpoints that you trust with your life.

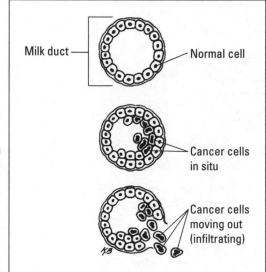

Figure 4-2:
Progression
of normal
cells to
invasive
cancerous
cells.

Gathering mutated cells mean tumors of all kinds

When many abnormal cells get together and settle, they form a *tumor* (an abnormal mass of tissue). The two kinds of tumors are *benign tumors,* which are noncancerous, and *malignant tumors,* which are cancerous.

Although tumors are more likely to be malignant when they're firm and have irregular shapes, and benign tumors are more likely to feel round or soft, you can't tell by feel alone whether a lump is cancerous. So *don't* panic when you feel a lump, but *do* see your doctor, get the tests your doctor recommends, and go from there.

Benign tumors

Cells that form benign tumors can divide and grow out of control just like cells in cancerous tumors, but — and this is the important difference — they don't spread to other parts of the body. So, although you'll still feel a lump, it's a lump that stays in the same place.

For example, normal cells that are produced in the *lobules* (the part of the breast that produces milk) are supposed to remain in the lobules, doing their job, which essentially is making sure that they're ready at a moment's notice to begin producing milk when the woman becomes pregnant. If some of the lobule cells become a little mutated and grow too big to fit into their own skins, they form a lump. That lump is not cancerous, but only a doctor and special tests can say for sure. That's why seeing your doctor whenever you feel a lump is so important.

Malignant tumors

Malignant tumors are cancerous tumors made up of abnormal, mutated breast cells. These cells are capable of going to parts of the body where they don't normally live and of growing rampantly out of control.

Using the same example of normal cells in the lobules, suppose that these cells mutate, start to grow, and grow fast. These mutated cells either spill out of the lobules into surrounding breast tissue and then swim via the *lymph vessels* (more on those in Chapter 2) into the *nodes* under your arm, or they spill into your blood stream and out to other parts of your body, all the while growing and multiplying like crazy.

Causing the mutation: Genetics or environment?

When you ask doctors what causes lung cancer, they can give you a pretty definite answer: Smoking triggers cancer by altering a gene in the cells, and when that happens, the altered gene causes cells to divide out of control and spread where they're not wanted. Knowing about this trigger mechanism makes explaining what causes lung cancer easy for doctors. Instead of having to do extensive research to find the specific gene that's been altered in lung cancer, doctors can focus on teaching people about the effects of smoking on cancer. Doctors know for sure that if their patients choose not to be exposed to tobacco smoke, their risk of developing lung cancer is dramatically reduced. Unfortunately, researchers don't yet have such simple answers when it comes to breast cancer. I wish we did, but the reality is that we don't.

A *gene* is the part of the DNA that contains all the hereditary information about you, like the color of your eyes, the color of your hair, your height, and whether you're susceptible to certain diseases.

Here's what is known about what causes breast cancer: Your genes definitely play a part. Researchers have even been able to identify two familial genes, *BRCA1* and *BRCA2* (explained in Chapter 3), that when altered or mutated significantly increase the risk of breast cancer in only a small number of women. If either your BRCA1 or BRCA2 gene is altered or mutated, you have a genetic tendency to develop breast cancer.

However, other than inheriting mutations of the two genes responsible for breast cancer, researchers still are not clear about what the root causes of the genetic alterations are. Is it something in the environment to which you've been exposed, such as pesticides or toxic fumes? Is it being exposed to a virus or something else that doctors don't know about? Or is it the food that you eat or your general health? Breast cancer researchers know that some interaction must be occurring between genes and the environment that causes them to mutate.

Additionally, researchers still don't know what to do to prevent the mutations of the genes. As we are writing this book, researchers are toiling day and night to help identify risk factors and ways to prevent women with these mutated genes from developing breast cancer (described in detail in Chapter 3).

Staying in Place or Running Rampant: Classifying Breast Cancer

You know how nothing in this world is simple, right? Well, neither is describing breast cancer. Actually, it's like describing yourself. You can just portray your physical appearance, or you can express aspects of your personality, or, if you dig deeper, you can convey your innermost feelings, and you can expand on it (or not). How you describe yourself just depends on who is asking and why. The same is true with breast cancer. Several aspects of your cancer have a huge impact on your *prognosis* (predicted outcome). Some of these factors include whether the cancer stayed in one place, spread to more distant parts of the body, how fast it spread, and so on. In this section we describe a few of the more important factors. In Chapter 8, we discuss your prognosis, and in Chapter 9, we review your treatment options.

One of the first ways breast cancer is described is by the exact part of the breast in which it started. (For a great description of all the parts of the breast, see Chapter 2.) It's like people saying, "I'm from New York, but I've lived in Texas for the last four years," or "Me? I was born in Louisiana and

Carcinoma means cancer

You know that doctors use many big Latin words (wish they wouldn't but that's the reality) to explain what they think you don't want to hear. Well, they refer to the most common kinds of cancer as "carcinoma." You'll hear that term often. So every time you hear the word "carcinoma," just substitute the word "cancer."

Here's one more tip about names that mean cancer: Even when a cancer spreads, it is still named after the part of the body where it started. In other words, when it starts in the breast and spreads to the lungs, it still is called breast cancer.

I'll die in Louisiana." You get the picture. Breast cancer usually begins either in the *ducts* (the passages that connect the lobules with the nipple — 85 per cent) or *lobules* (the glands that produce milk). That's why you'll hear terms like *ductal carcinoma,* which simply means breast cancer that started in the ducts of the breast. Similarly, *lobular carcinoma* means cancer that started in the lobes of the breast. (Easy when you know how, huh?)

Exploring types of localized breast cancers

If you've ever overheard breast cancer survivors talking, you'll hear them throwing out words like, "Was it *in situ* or *infiltrating*?" No, they're not speaking in a foreign language (although technically Latin is like a foreign language to many, if not most, people). Instead, they're talking about something that's very important in breast cancer . . . whether it has stayed put or spread. That factor is ever so important in determining your prognosis. Localized cancers of the breast are called *in situ,* which means the cancer is confined to the part of the breast where it started.

Lobular carcinoma in situ (LCIS)

When a cancer starts in the lobes of the breast and the cancer cells remain where they started, it's called *lobular carcinoma in situ,* commonly referred to as LCIS. Taking it one word at a time. *Lobular* means starting in the lobe, *carcinoma* means cancer, and *in situ* means it's remained right there in the lobe.

But guess what? LCIS isn't a cancer. Huh? Well, when LCIS was first identified, it was considered an early form of cancer, which is why it includes the word "carcinoma." Today most oncologists (cancer doctors) don't consider LCIS a true breast cancer, but instead they think of it as an abnormal growth of cells in the lobules. Doctors currently are talking about changing the name completely, but you know how things change slowly. So, for now, the word carcinoma remains in the name.

That said, these abnormal cells nevertheless indicate that you're at risk of developing invasive breast cancer sometime in the future. Even if LCIS is diagnosed in one breast, you're at risk of developing cancer in *both* breasts. Although this risk is only 1 percent per year, it still is a risk, and that's why your doctor will continue to monitor you very carefully, just like women with other risk factors, like having a mother with breast cancer, are monitored. You won't know you have it even if you or your doctor examine your breast, or for that matter, even if you have a mammogram. LCIS usually is picked up only when you have a *biopsy* (when the doctor removes some breast cells to examine them, see Chapter 5) for something else. If LCIS is what you've been diagnosed with, take a deep breathe. (I'm sure you were worried, but worry no more.) You have just been given very good news. Make sure you get monitored on a regular basis, but for now, you have reason to celebrate.

Ductal carcinoma in situ (DCIS)

The other *in situ* (localized) cancer of the breast begins (and remains) in the ducts, and so it's called *ductal* (in the ducts), *carcinoma* (cancer) *in situ* (stays in place). However, unlike LCIS, the risk of a *recurrence* (or return) of cancer, including *invasive cancer* (in other words, beyond the duct cells) is high without treatment. In fact, researchers believe that if it isn't treated, DCIS will progress to an invasive cancer in most women. How fast it progresses and how long it takes to become an invasive cancer depends on many factors, like the type of the DCIS (yup, they come in a variety of types), your age, your health, and many other factors. That's why such a wide variety of treatments exist, all the way from a simple excision (cutting out the area), to a mastectomy (removal of the entire breast). Chapter 9 provides details about treatment. (See why comparing your treatment to someone else's isn't a straightforward approach.)

DCIS used to be very rare in the past, but *incidence rates* (the rate of new cases) have skyrocketed during the last 20 years. However, this dramatic increase doesn't reflect the fact that more women are developing DCIS, but rather it shows that it can be attributed mainly to the widespread use of mammography (see Chapter 5). Mammography enables doctors to detect DCIS, which is something they were unable to do before it came into widespread use.

Cancer in the ducts of the breast is rarely detected by self-exam or by the doctor's physical exam, but a mammogram can detect it. Even though this form of cancer is localized, it can become an invasive form of cancer if it isn't treated. Isn't that a good enough reason for you to schedule your regular screening mammogram?

Unfortunately, until recently, doctors had neither a good grasp of the natural history of DCIS nor a uniform way of classifying it. More important, doctors aren't yet able to predict which women with DCIS will develop a more serious invasive form of cancer at a later time. All these unknowns have resulted in considerable debate in the medical community regarding which treatment is best for women with DCIS. This debate makes determining what course of action to take very difficult for women with DCIS. (I mean, if the doctor doesn't know, who does?) Fortunately for everyone, Dr. Monica Morrow, a coauthor of this book, has pioneered a great deal of research on DCIS and has been instrumental in developing treatment guidelines that doctors worldwide are using when any of their patients are diagnosed with DCIS (see Chapter 8).

Invasive breast cancers

When cancer cells move out of the duct or the lobules into adjoining cells, they're called *infiltrating* or *invasive cancers* (no Latin here!) These cells eventually form a lump that is more likely to be felt during a physical examination, unless, of course, it's so small that it can only be picked up on mammogram (see Chapter 5). The two types of infiltrating cancers are again named after the part of the breast in which they start.

Infiltrating ductal carcinoma

The most commonly found kind of breast cancer (70 percent) is *infiltrating ductal carcinoma*. It is cancer that originates in the ducts and invades the surrounding breast tissue.

Here's how it develops: As the cancer cells that begin in the ducts start invading the fatty tissue around the duct, they stimulate the growth of fibrous, scarlike tissue that surrounds the cancer. The good news is that the fibrous tissue makes the mass easier to find by physical exam and on a mammogram. The other good news is that the actual cancer may be smaller than the size of the lump suggests.

Depending on the location of ductal cancer, it may cause the nipple to retract (pull in) or other symptoms like nipple discharge or skin puckering or dimpling. These symptoms may be caused by other benign (noncancerous conditions), but they are signals that require immediate investigation, so see your doctor.

The prognosis for infiltrating ductal carcinoma depends on a variety of factors, such as which organs it has spread to, how fast the cancer is growing, and how you respond to treatment.

Infiltrating lobular carcinoma

Less often (in 15 percent of breast cancers) infiltrating cancer originates in the lobes and is known as *infiltrating lobular carcinoma*. The lobular cancer cells stream out to the surrounding breast tissue. Unlike ductal cancer, infiltrating lobular carcinoma doesn't produce fibrous growth, which makes it more difficult to detect on a mammogram. That's why when it's first detected the lump is likely to be larger than ductal cancer. It also feels softer, more like a thickening than a lump. The prognosis for this form of cancer depends on a variety of factors, including which organs it has spread to, how fast the cancer is growing, and how you respond to treatment.

Rare forms of breast cancer

As if ductal and lobular carcinomas weren't enough, a few other rare forms of breast cancer exist, and we describe them in the following sections.

Medullary carcinoma

Medullary carcinoma is a rare form (5 percent) of infiltrating ductal cancer that has a relatively distinct boundary between the tumor cells and normal cells. Its other distinguishing characteristics are large-sized cancer cells and the presence of immune system cells at the edges of the tumor. Only 5 percent of women with breast cancer have medullary carcinoma, and the prognosis is slightly better than for other invasive forms of cancer. Although it's so named because it is the same color as the brain (medulla), medullary carcinoma has absolutely nothing to do with the brain.

More rarities

Another very rare form of breast cancer that begins in the mucus-producing cells is called *mucinous (mucus) carcinoma*. The prognosis for this form of cancer is better than for other more common invasive cancers.

In about 5 percent to 8 percent of breast cancer cases, a woman will have a cancer in both breasts, with both being the primary (original location) cancer. In other words, one isn't caused by the other. Fortunately, this disease is usually simple to detect, because when doctors find cancer in one breast, they do a mammogram of both. Sometimes a woman will have cancer in her other breast after she's been treated for cancer in the first breast. It's usually another primary (main) cancer. What it usually indicates is that you're more susceptible to developing cancer, but it doesn't mean your prognosis is worse. Your prognosis depends on the cancer itself.

Paget's disease

Named for Sir James Paget, the scientist/surgeon who first described it, Paget's disease is another rare (3 percent) form of cancer that starts in the breast ducts and then moves to the nipple and *areola*, the dark circle around the nipple. Common symptoms include a crusting and scaling or redness of the nipple and areola and sometimes areas of bleeding or oozing and burning or itching. Please don't panic if you have these symptoms. Often they are not caused by cancer, but rather by some other easily treated cause like eczema (talk about relief!). However, you must have a biopsy to find out whether it's cancer. This disease of the nipple is rare, found in only 1 percent of women diagnosed with breast cancer.

Tubular carcinoma

This disease gets its name because it's made up of cancer cells that look like little tubes. It is an infiltrating cancer, but it has a much better prognosis than infiltrating ductal or lobular cancers. It is found only in fewer than 10 percent of women diagnosed with breast cancer. This type of breast cancer *always* has estrogen and progesterone receptors.

Inflammatory breast cancer

Inflammatory breast cancer is a serious kind of advanced breast cancer, but fortunately it is very rare, affecting only about 1 percent of women diagnosed with breast cancer. It gets its name because it looks and feels as though the breast is infected, with the skin that looks red and feels warm. Because the skin of a breast with this disease often looks like the skin of an orange, it is called "peau d'orange," which, in French, means skin of an orange. You or your doctor won't likely even feel a distinct lump, but your breast is usually firm and swollen.

Here's the trick: Whenever you're put on an antibiotic (because the doctor thinks you have an infection of the breast) and there's no change in your condition within a week (it stays exactly the same), go back to your doctor immediately, and ask for a biopsy. Although it's very rare, it may be inflammatory breast cancer. A biopsy that indicates that you have inflammatory breast cancer shows cancer cells in the *lymphatic channels* (the lymphatic system, which is like the body's garbage disposal system) in the skin of the breast.

Phyllodes tumors

These tumors can manifest as a lump in the breast (they can be any size, a tiny speck on a mammogram or as big as a basketball), but believe it or not, it's very rarely malignant (cancerous.) Goes to show that not all lumps indicate cancer. Phyllodes tumors also are rare, because they don't start in the duct or the lobes of the breast. Instead they develop in the *connective tissue* (the tissue that supports and surrounds the ducts and lobules) of the breast. Fewer than 10 women a year in the United States die of this disease.

Finding Out How Far It Has Spread: Staging Breast Cancer

Knowing how far your cancer has spread and to what parts of your body is crucial, because your treatment options and your prognosis depend on it. Unfortunately, doctors don't have a way to determine your prognosis with absolute certainty, but one method for assessing it comes close. It's referred to as the stage system, and it tells you the size of the tumor, whether it has spread, and how far and to what part of the body if it has spread. The stage of your cancer can make a huge difference in your life, and who doesn't want to live? In Chapter 7, we describe how stages are determined and what they mean for you. In Chapter 8, we describe prognosis, and in Chapter 9, we explore your treatment options.

Part II:

All Kinds of Oses — Diagnoses, Prognoses, and Treatment Options

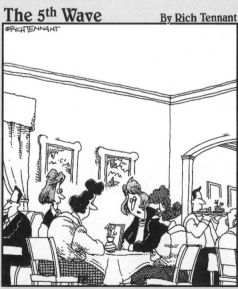

The 5th Wave   By Rich Tennant

@RICHTENNANT

"I saw my pathologist today and he was very
thorough in his recommendations. He said we
should start with the lobster bisque, have the
venison, and finish with the profiteroles."

In this part . . .

Feeling a lump isn't enough information for a diagnosis, so you may need several tests and/or small surgical procedures to determine your status. Knowing what to expect from each procedure (Chapter 5) enables you to be an active participant. The mysteries of the pathology report, which describes everything that can be seen under the microscope about your tissue sample, are unlocked and translated in Chapter 6, so you'll know what is (or isn't) wrong with you. If diagnosed with cancer, you probably want to know, "Am I going to die?" "It depends" may not be what you want to hear, but the truth is many factors determine your outcome and treatment options. Finding out in which stage of cancer you've been diagnosed (Chapter 7) helps you know the extent of and what to expect from the cancer, what your predicted outcome is (Chapter 8), and what treatment options are available (Chapter 9). Equipped with this knowledge, you're in great shape for becoming an integral member of your treatment team.

Chapter 5

Warming Up to Mammography, Sticking It Out During Biopsy

In This Chapter

▶ Picturing a mammogram

▶ Screening with mammograms

▶ Identifying abnormalities with mammograms

▶ Diagnosing with biopsies

Maybe your doctor has found a suspicious lump and is sending you to have a mammogram to get a more accurate picture. Or maybe after the mammogram, the *radiologist* (a doctor who reads and interprets X-rays, see Chapter 9) wants to do a *biopsy* to get more accurate information on the lump. A mammogram *suggests* but can't definitively *prove* that an abnormal finding is cancer. So, to determine whether it's actually cancerous, tissue needs to be taken from the lump (biopsy) and then viewed under a microscope. Being worried is natural, but please try to wait until you get the results before you start imagining the worst. Why begin worrying if it may not even be cancer? The mammogram and the biopsy are what help determine whether it is or it isn't

In this chapter, we describe the different types of mammograms (did you know there are more than one?) and give you the latest recommendations. We also talk about the different types of biopsies and what you can expect from them.

What's Black and White and Round all Over? Picturing a Mammogram

A *mammogram* is a type of X-ray, except that instead of taking pictures of your bones, it takes pictures of the soft tissue (breast tissue and fat, see Chapter 2), which is what your breasts are made of. The two types of mammograms are

- **Screening mammograms:** A screening mammogram is your regular annual screening. It's a picture of a breast of a woman with no problems to make sure that all is well.

- **Diagnostic mammograms:** A diagnostic mammogram is a more detailed set of pictures examining a suspicious lump that you or your doctor may have detected during a breast examination or an abnormality discovered during a screening mammogram.

Although mammograms are perhaps the most important advancement in breast cancer detection during the past 30 years, the realities of its use are that

- Most breast cancers cannot be prevented, but the earlier they're found, the better your likelihood for a successful treatment. Screening mammograms can find breast cancers earlier than most other methods of detection.

- Finding breast cancer early is the single most important way that you can prevent death from this disease. And mammography, at this point, is the best tool for that chore. Early detection also decreases the chance of your having to have a mastectomy, which we discuss in Chapter 10.

- Screening mammograms aren't perfect (find out more about that in the sidebar "Addressing the controversy: A false alarm" later in the chapter). Sometimes, they miss a cancer.

Amanda C.

"I will be sure to get a mammogram (an inside your body kind of picture) when I am older. Mom says it doesn't hurt. Because Mom had a mammogram, we caught her cancer early and the doctors could get it out before it spread to different parts of her body."

Mary G.

"I have to admit that I failed to seek medical attention for about two years. I knew I had a lump, and I ignored it. That was stupid. Late in October, I finally saw the doctor, had a mammogram and ultrasound and got the bad news. Within three days, I was in surgery."

For right now, however, a screening mammogram is the best way of finding breast cancer early. It can detect cancer in your breast *before* any physical symptoms develop. A recent study found a 30 percent reduction in the number of deaths attributed to breast cancer in women who were older than 50 and had regular breast exams and mammograms! A just released study found an even higher decrease in deaths, a decrease of almost 50 percent.

So how often should you have a screening mammogram? My recommendations are

- ✔ **Women ages 40 and older:** Have a mammogram (and a clinical breast exam) every year.
- ✔ **Women younger than 40 who are not at high risk:** No need to have a mammogram until you're 40.
- ✔ **Women younger than 40 and who *are* at high risk:** Talk to your doctor about when you need to begin screening. The time will vary and depends on your level of risk and the cause of your risk.

Thanks for the mammories

Mammo means breast in Latin, of course, and *gram* means picture. And what of it? Well, here's a bit of good news for a change. Only one or two screening mammograms out of every 1,000 actually lead to a diagnosis of cancer. The other 998 or 999 are normal. Think of all the ladies sitting in the mammography clinic waiting room with you, all wearing the same flimsy, dowdy hospital gowns (I wish someone would design gowns that are more attractive), and all silently thumbing through magazines as they wait to have their mammograms and just get out of there. If your clinic screens about 100 women a day, that means only three to six of the women who go through that facility during an entire month will ever be found to have breast cancer. All the rest won't.

You can also check out the new hot-off-the-press breast cancer screening guidelines released in June 2003 by the American Cancer Society. The ACS convened a panel of experts to find out whether the screening guidelines with which women have become so familiar needed to be revised. The new ACS recommendations, described in full on its Web site (www.cancer.org), take into consideration all the recent research findings and recommendations. The new guidelines now include recommendations for

- ✓ **Women at high risk:** Speak to your doctor about the possibility of screening.
- ✓ **Women younger than 40:** Have a clinical breast exam (see Chapter 2 for a full description) every few years.

Whenever you're going in for a screening mammogram, make sure that you find out whether your insurance company covers the procedure. You're covered when you have Medicaid. If you don't have any insurance at all, find out whether your state provides mammography coverage. See Chapter 17 for detailed information about how to access this information.

Having a mammogram can be a little cold

If you've never before had a mammogram, you need to prepare yourself for one thoroughly cold encounter. Besides having to get undressed and don a skimpy gown (open to the front, please), you bare your breasts and put them one-at-a-time onto a plastic plate for pressing.

By the way, when scheduling your mammogram, try to set it up at times other than your time of the month. After all, breasts can be particularly sensitive just before your period.

The woman in Figure 5-1 is undergoing a mammogram. The following list of steps walks you through a typical mammogram:

1. **You're taken to an office, given a gown, and asked to take your top and bra off.**

   Make sure that your gown opens to the front. You may also be asked to remove any jewelry around your neck that may interfere with the picture.

2. **You'll probably have to wait in the waiting room.**

   That's where you'll find other women sitting around in the same ugly gowns, reading magazines, and pretending to be totally engrossed in them, but all the while wishing their turn was already over.

3. **An assistant asks you to accompany her on a visit with the *mammography technologist* (the person who takes the mammography pictures).**

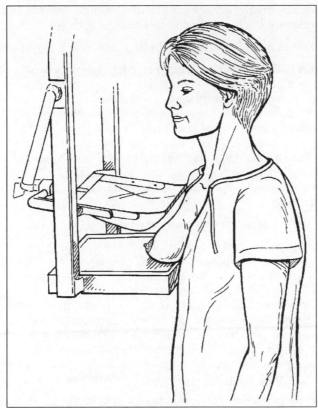

Figure 5-1:
Getting a
mammo-
gram can be
a squishy
situation.

Sometimes, the mammography tech comes for you herself; at other times, an assistant walks you to the technologist's office. Sometimes, you're the only one escorted to the room, but other times, groups of a few women at a time are taken there. (I hate that because it always seems to happen to me!) Depending on the size of the clinic, the room where the mammogram is done, the technologist may be either very close or far enough away to require a walk through some of the hospital corridors. (Yup, that's me again, clutching my gown as I walk with as much dignity as I can muster.)

4. **The technologist asks you about the possibility of your being pregnant.**

   She asks you whether you're pregnant, but you'll also see cautionary signs posted in the waiting room and the room where the mammogram takes place, clearly warning that if you are or even think you may be pregnant, you *must* tell the technologist, because X-rays can harm the fetus and are not prescribed when you're pregnant.

5. **The technologist, usually a woman (which can be comforting because your breasts must be properly positioned) adjusts you, your breast, and the machine in preparation for taking the mammogram.**

This step may involve what feels like quite a bit of tugging and pulling on your breasts or gently pushing your shoulder forward.

6. **One breast at a time is squeezed between plastic X-ray plates.**

The flatter that the breast can be pressed, the more accurate the picture. Placing your breast between two plates is a weird feeling, because when they say pressed, they really mean as squished as it can be (sometimes vertically, sometimes horizontally depending on the view required), and that's certainly not the way your lover or you would ever consider pressing your breast. Although many who've endured this procedure say that having a mammogram is "uncomfortable," that's really a euphemism. When your breasts are sensitive, having a mammogram sometimes can be downright painful. Fortunately, each picture only takes a few moments.

7. **Several different pictures usually are taken.**

The mammography technician inserts a different X-ray plate into the machine for each new photograph and then tells you to hold your breath, steps out of the room while the picture is being taken, in a matter of seconds tells you can breathe again, before releasing the breast. Remaining still is important so that the technician gets a clear picture. Breathing in and out can blur the picture, just like when you take a photograph. Then the technician may reposition your breast for another picture from a different angle. If your doctor asks for a specific view, a mark may be made on your breast, and you may have to be placed in a contorted position (again, for just a few moments).

8. **After the pictures are taken, you take a seat in the waiting room.**

The radiologist then makes sure that the pictures are clear. Come on now, how many times have you taken a picture and cut off a head or it came out blurry? It can happen here, too (very seldom but you want to be absolutely sure, don't you?). If the technologist can see all that she needs, you can go back to the changing room, get dressed, and go home. If another view is needed, the tech repositions you and takes another picture.

9. **You play the waiting game.**

You have to wait for the results, which usually are sent to your doctor when you have a screening mammogram. Your doctor's office then tells you how you'll get your results. The doctor's office either sends you a letter with the results or calls you if more needs to be done. If you haven't heard back from your doctor in about ten days, call and ask for your results. You don't want to fall through the cracks!

If you're having a diagnostic mammogram, the radiologist may talk directly to you about your results or to the referring doctor who then lets you know the results. Whether the radiologist or referring doctor explains your results depends on the hospital, the doctors, and the circumstances. No clear guidelines or rules exist.

> ## Mammogram fantasy
>
> During the mammogram, I usually visualize walk-ing on a beautiful beach, listening to the waves, and feeling the wind and sun on my face. I find that doing so gets me through those few short but uncomfortable moments with greater ease.

Reading the X-ray

How many movies have you seen where a doctor, usually young, male, and cute, firmly pushes a black-and-white X-ray film onto a lighted screen, peering at it with furrowed brow and hands plunged deep into the pockets of his white lab coat. Although not quite as melodramatic in real-life (that's the movies for you!), that scene is a common one, because it depicts how many radiologists go about interpreting X-rays (or *film,* as they like to call it). So, what does the radiologist see and look for on a mammography film?

X-rays are black-and-white images. Denser tissues and bones show up white, and less dense tissues show up in varying shades of gray. The less dense the tissue, the grayer (or darker) it appears on the X-ray.

Your breast's two main components, glandular tissue and fat, have different densities. These components and others are discussed at length in Chapter 2. Glandular tissue is dense, because it is made up of cells that stick together and, therefore, shows up white on an X-ray. Fat, on the other hand, is not as dense and shows up gray.

Similarly, malignant and benign lumps usually are dense. Like glandular tissue, they show up white on film. Young breasts consist mostly of glandular tissue, so being able to see lumps in younger breasts can be difficult, because the differences between white glandular tissue and white lumps are difficult to discern. As women age, they lose glandular tissue, so older breasts gener-ally consist of more fat, which is why mammograms are more effective for older women. White lumps are easier to see when contrasted with gray. After menopause, this contrast becomes even more distinctive because most of the glandular tissue is gone (unless you take estrogen, which maintains glan-dular tissue).

Results of screening mammograms are reported as either normal or abnor-mal; however, the results of each diagnostic mammogram are reported on standardized forms. Each diagnostic mammogram is encoded with a number from 1 (nothing abnormal) to 5 (very possibly cancerous) that is known as your BI-RAD score, which stands for Breast Imaging Reporting and Data System. (Actually, there's a 0 too, but that means they can't see it clearly and thus need to get other pictures.) See Table 5-1 for a description of each score.

These standardized reports were developed by the American College of Radiography for two reasons:

- To have a uniform way of interpreting the results of a diagnostic mammogram
- To allow data to be used to better follow up and monitor women's outcomes if they were diagnosed with breast cancer

These data are used in determining how accurate and helpful diagnostic mammography is (and they're the best we've got right now!).

Table 5-1	BI-RAD Scoring System	
BIRAD Score or Classification	*What does it mean?*	*Any further steps needed?*
0	An abnormality may be present, but it can't be seen clearly.	Additional images are needed.
1 (Negative)	Nothing abnormal.	No.
2 (Benign = not cancerous)	Benign-looking findings (such as benign calcifications, or lumps, described in Chapter 2) can be seen. These abnormalities lack the specificcharacteristics of cancer.	No. This score ensures that other doctors won't misinterpret the mammogram as showing something suspicious when it's benign.
3 (Probably benign)	What can be seen is likely to be benign and not expected to change over time. The risk of a malignancy is less than 2%.	Have another mammogram in 6 months to see whether any change has occurred that raises concern that the abnormality is malignant.
4 (Suspicious abnormality)	What can be seen doesn't definitively look like cancer, but the radiologist is concerned because a good probability exists that it may be.	Biopsy is recommended (see "Bringing on the Biopsy" later in this chapter).
5 (Highly suggestive of being malignant — cancerous)	What can be seen looks like cancer. High probability of cancer.	Biopsy is strongly recommended.

Hitting a bump in the road

For you to be able to physically feel a lump, it usually measures about one centimeter across. Look at a ruler: A centimeter is teeny tiny. A mammogram can pick up a lump that's half that size! That's pretty impressive in anyone's book.

Some lumps appear round and smooth and some don't. Lumps are classified in three general categories:

✔ **Cysts or fibroadenomas.** These benign lumps appear and feel smooth and round (Figure 5-2). A mammogram can spot them, but it can't tell the difference between a *cyst* (which is a fluid-filled sac) and a *fibroadenoma* (which is a solid lump made of noncancerous cells). You'll probably need an ultrasound (described in the next section), because it can diagnose cysts. You can find out more about noncancerous lumps in Chapter 2.

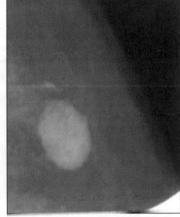

Figure 5-2:
A lump that looks benign (not cancerous) on a mammogram.

✔ **Cancers:** A lump with edges that appear irregular, jagged or that pulls inward, distorting the surrounding breast tissue, and has radiating strands may be cancerous (see Figure 5-3).

✔ **Calcifications.** These calcium deposits in the breast appear as tiny white spots on a mammogram. Calcifications can be

- **Macrocalcifications:** These calcifications are benign. They are larger deposits that arise because of normal aging of arteries or old injuries. (Remember the time you walked into the open closet door?)

- **Microcalcifications:** These calcifications are smaller than $\frac{1}{50}$th of an inch; hence the term *micro*. They appear in the mammogram as fine particles.

Some microcalcifications are associated with cancer or are precancerous. When scattered throughout the breast, they're unlikely to be cancer, and 80 percent of microcalcifications are *not* cancer. However, when a few tiny ones are clustered closely together (as in Figure 5-4 where they're branching, following the paths of the ducts, and clustering together), they may be a precancerous condition known as *ductal carcinoma in situ* (see Chapter 3 for a full description of this type of cancer).

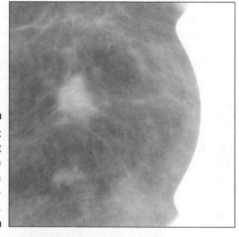

Figure 5-3:
A lump that looks like cancer on a mammogram.

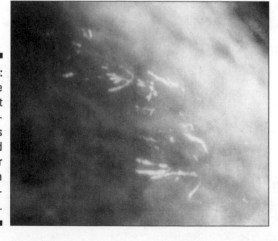

Figure 5-4:
Appearance of malignant microcalcifications (enlarged for a clearer view) on a mammogram.

You could also have an abnormal density, which refers to tissue that has a different consistency in one spot than in the remainder of the breast. Dense tissue can indicate overlapping breast tissue, noncancerous changes, or cancerous cells.

Using mammograms and other tools to diagnose cancer

A mammogram *suggests* but can't definitively *prove* that an abnormal finding is cancer. So, to answer the question of how you can you tell for sure whether any of the lumps, bumps, calcifications, or dense areas on a mammogram actually are cancerous, tissue needs to be taken from the lump and must be viewed under a microscope. For that to happen, you must have a biopsy, which I talk about in the section "Bringing on the Biopsy" later in this chapter, but before you have a biopsy a few other steps may be taken to try to rule out cancer.

Finding abnormalities with mammography

Screening mammograms show two views of the tissue in each breast: *craniocaudal* (top to bottom) and *mediolateral oblique* (from the side). Whenever something suspicious is seen on a screening study, doctors call it an *abnormality* and send you off to have a *diagnostic mammogram* or perhaps even an ultrasound.

Diagnostic mammograms may include several of these additional views of your breast:

- ✔ **A magnification view:** This process magnifies the area under suspicion, making it much easier for the radiologist to see and assess it more clearly. This view is especially useful for microcalcifications (see the previous section).
- ✔ **A spot compression view:** Pushing on part of your breast enables the radiologist to have a much clearer view of the edges of the lump, which helps the doctors to distinguish between just overlapping breast tissues and densities that are more suspicious.

Detecting cysts and differing densities with diagnostic ultrasound

An ultrasound is a painless imaging procedure that sends high-frequency sound waves through whatever's placed in front of it. The waves bounce back whenever something (like a breast lump) gets in the way. You may have had an ultrasound when you were pregnant. Isn't it miraculous when you see your little one sucking its thumb or moving its little fists? Anyway, these bouncing sound waves are converted by a computer into little digital dots on a video display terminal and then recorded as an image on X-ray film. (Isn't technology something?)

Ultrasound examination can't pick up microcalcifications the way that a mammogram can. On the other hand, however, it can distinguish between a solid lump and a fluid-filled cyst, and it doesn't use radiation the way the mammogram does.

SURVIVORS' SECRETS

Cyndi K.

"My greatest inspiration is my beautiful 97-year-old grandmother, Rosa, who had a mastectomy more than 50 years ago. . . . 'Yes, I still miss my right breast,' she says. 'And yes, there are moments when I feel sad about not being complete . . . but I'm alive; I'm lucky to have the cancer behind me. And really, honestly, there is more to life than my right breast." The earlier you're diagnosed, the greater the possibility of complete recovery. So what are women waiting for?"

From *There's More to Life Than My Right Breast*

Ultrasound testing is very useful for finding this distinction in every woman. However, it's an especially useful tool when there's a questionable lump and you have dense breasts, because it's capable of detecting differences in density between the lump and breast tissue. Mammograms can't do that. In addition, an ultrasound may provide better definition of the size and other borders of the lump.

The procedure lasts between a few minutes to half an hour. The technician or the doctor puts gel on your breast and moves the arm of the machine (sometimes called a wand) over the lump, while looking at a screen to accurately locate the abnormality so that a good image can be viewed and recorded.

Finding out where you're headed

After one or more of these diagnostic tests, your doctor recommends one of three courses of action:

- **No further testing is necessary:** The original suspicious finding is clearly not of concern because it shows no evidence of being cancer. Therefore, you don't need any more tests at this time. (Yes!) Come back in one year for your regular mammogram. Go home and play with the kids.

- **Wait and then repeat the mammogram:** Sometimes, when your lump or calcification has only a very low chance (1 percent to 2 percent) of being cancerous, based on its appearance and a finding that it hasn't grown or changed since the previous mammogram, the radiologist may ask you to wait six months and then return for a repeat mammogram. You may ask: "If I wait so long, won't the cancer spread out of control by then?" Cancers grow very slowly, and studies indicate that *wait-and-repeat mammograms* are a safe and effective way of avoiding unnecessary biopsies.

- **Biopsy:** This recommendation means that cells or tissue will be extracted from the suspected area of your breast. The tissue then is examined under a microscope. Viewing tissue cells under the microscope is the only way of determining for sure whether they are malignant when it isn't clear from just looking at the X-rays.

The doctor's rule of thumb is: Anything that has more than a 1 percent to 2 percent risk of being cancer, based on its appearance on the mammogram or ultrasound, gets biopsied.

Getting accurate results

Mammograms can be difficult to read because many different definitions of normal exist. Normal breasts look different on an X-ray the same way they look different in real life. Every woman's breast is different; some have more fat and others more breast tissue and the way these differences are distributed can be different too. Furthermore, a mammogram isn't like an X-ray of a fracture, where you can see a separation of the bone. In mammograms you see many different things, such as the fat and the glandular tissue, calcifications, and more. That's why having considerable specialty experience is necessary to accurately assess a mammogram.

The Food and Drug Administration certifies all mammography facilities that meet its standards. These standards include provisions for specialized training for staff members and a system for making sure that follow-up investigations are conducted whenever any abnormal finding is reached. You can help ensure a more accurate mammogram by

✔ **Going to an FDA-certified facility.** If the certification isn't prominently displayed (as it should be), ask to see the facility's certificate.

✔ **Attending a facility that either specializes in mammography or does many mammograms each month.**

✔ **Having a *baseline* (first) mammogram and then one mammogram every year thereafter.** Subsequent mammograms can be compared with the baseline mammogram. This technique helps tremendously, especially when you find a clinic that you like and can have your mammogram done there each year. That way

- You don't have to worry about any changes that may be caused by slight differences in the way clinics take the pictures or the type of machinery that's used.

- You can just imagine how relieved you'll feel when a microcalcification that showed up on your last mammogram is also discovered by the radiologist in the exact same spot, and more important, the exact same size, when comparing the new film with the one from the previous year.

✔ **Bringing the X-ray pictures and reports of your previous mammograms and/or biopsies that you've had before to the clinic.** The comparison is invaluable!

✔ **Bringing old films with you whenever you move or change facilities.** I once had to argue with a clinic that claimed the film was its property and wouldn't release it initially. It's amazing how effective a little strong-arming can be!

✔ **Not wearing deodorant or talcum powder on the day you have your mammogram.** Chemicals in them sometimes show up as calcifications, and heaven knows, you probably have enough problems to worry about without adding any more!

Mammography centers give specific instructions to patients on what to avoid on the day of the exam.

Addressing the controversy: A false alarm

Although screening mammography is a great tool for finding cancer early and saving lives, few things in life are perfect, and neither is mammography. It, too, has drawbacks. In spite of researcher's attempts to find solutions, two main problems remain:

✔ Breasts of women younger than 40 consist mostly of dense breast tissue, which makes seeing abnormalities on mammograms difficult.

✔ *False positives* occur. Sometimes, a mammogram shows a lump that radiologists think may be cancerous, but when the surgeon or radiologist biopsies the tissues, no cancer is found.

In early 2002, a controversial article that was published in a medical journal (and widely reported on television and in the news media) concluded that mammography screening was not beneficial. This report caused an enormous stir, confusion, and near panic in some cases.

However, after a detailed analysis of studies done around the world, scientists concluded that evidence demonstrates that mammography lowers the death rate in women with breast cancer. The studies acknowledge some risks associated with mammography and that false positives sometimes result in women undergoing unnecessary biopsies and possibly even unnecessary surgeries, but those risks decrease as women get older.

Since the controversial study was reported, several other studies have discovered that mammography screening reduces the number of deaths from breast cancer. For example, a huge study of mammography screening services in Sweden, which included a third of *all* the women in that country, found that among women older than 40, the number of deaths caused by breast cancer was reduced by 44 percent through the use of mammography. You don't have to be a rocket scientist to figure out that this study reconfirms that mammography saves lives.

However, controversy attracts large audiences and breeds good ratings, and that's probably why the press and television made such a big fuss over the controversial study. Moreover, little doubt exists that the media did a great disservice to women by reporting the controversy without putting it into the proper perspective.

As a result, many women now are confused about whether mammography is beneficial. They don't know what to believe anymore. If they don't believe that an annual mammogram can help save their lives, they may not go in for screening. At this moment, your mother, sister, your neighbor, or your best friend may be walking around with a tiny precancerous calcification, and if she has a mammogram during which it is detected, it can be dealt with early on and successfully. However, if she's lost confidence and doesn't have a mammogram, the calcification can continue growing undetected and result in more serious consequences.

Bringing on the Biopsy

Whenever you're sent off to the hospital or clinic to have a biopsy for a lump in your breast, it doesn't mean that your doctor knows for sure that the lump is cancer. It depends on the level of suspicion. For example, if your BI-RAD score is 4, it indicates a *suspicious abnormality* (which may or *may not* be cancer), but the only way to know for sure is by doing a biopsy. A biopsy is the only safe and effective way of knowing for sure which suspicious lumps can be left safely alone and which ones must be removed.

During a biopsy, a sample of tissue is removed from the breast in one of four ways. Two kinds of biopsies (see Figure 5-5) make use of a needle (breasts A and B), and two require surgery (breasts C and D). We discuss the different kinds of biopsies in the sections that follow. Your doctor chooses the appropriate kind of biopsy, depending on the size of your lump, how it feels, and where it is inside your breast. Be sure to ask your doctor which kind you're scheduled for.

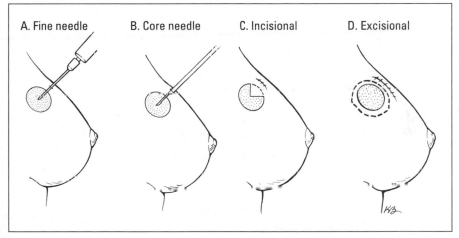

A. Fine needle   B. Core needle   C. Incisional   D. Excisional

Figure 5-5:
Types of biopsies. Biopsies C and D require surgery.

Being told that you need to have a biopsy can make you anxious, but as you're waiting for the results know that it's very unlikely that you have cancer. Remember that 70 percent to 80 percent of biopsies that were done because doctors found an abnormality on your mammogram (when you couldn't feel a lump or anything) are *not* cancer. That's a huge proportion of benign results, don't you agree? Even when the biopsy reveals that you have cancer, the earlier you catch it, the better your chances of a good outcome.

SURVIVORS' SECRETS

Cyndi K.

"I've just been to the gynecologist for my annual checkup. After eight weeks of a hectic tour promoting my latest book, I'm in maintenance mode: The car's in for service, the carpets are being cleaned, my hairdresser is booked, and today I went for the physical. As I was leaving, the gynecologist suggested that I have a mammogram.

'I think I feel a cyst in your right breast,' he said. I came straight home and called to make an appointment for a mammogram. Now, I have to wait 10 days. I'll try not to think about it too much."

From *There's More to Life Than My Right Breast*

Feeling fine: Fine needle aspiration

If you have a lump that's discovered upon a physical examination of your breast, the doctor may order a *fine needle aspiration* (FNA) — *aspiration* means withdrawing, in this case, cells — which is the least invasive of all biopsies. This procedure usually takes place in a surgeon's office and takes only a few minutes.

A *fine needle* is similar to the kind that is used to draw blood, but it's thinner and removes (or aspirates) only a few cells from the lump. When having an FNA

1. **You undress from the waist up.**

2. **You lie down on a table and cover up with a sheet, except for the breast needing the biopsy.**

   This is just like having blood drawn except that you're lying down.

3. **The nurse or surgeon cleans your breast with alcohol swabs to remove risk of infection.**

4. **The surgeon numbs your breast with a local anesthetic, which is administered via a needle.**

5. **The surgeon inserts a fine needle into the lump to retrieve a few cells.**

6. **You get dressed and go back to your life.**

7. **The cells are sent to a pathologist, who examines them under a microscope to determine whether they're cancerous.**

8. **The pathologist sends the results to your surgeon (see more on this in Chapter 6).** Most places don't give immediate results, although a few do.

Unfortunately, this procedure sometimes misses cancers, because the needle isn't actually stuck into the lump but rather into nearby breast tissue or because too few cells are obtained to make a diagnosis. Similarly, when your results are positive for cancer, an FNA cannot distinguish between *in situ* or invasive cancer (see Chapter 3 for a description of the types of breast cancer), which means that you may need to have an additional biopsy, such as a core needle, incisional, or excisional biopsy (all described in the following sections). On the other hand, in experienced hands, an FNA is more than 95 percent accurate.

Getting to the point: Core needle biopsy

A *core needle biopsy* (CNB) is similar to the FNA, except that the needle is slightly larger and extracts small pieces of tissue called *cores*. As with the FNA, this procedure can be done in the surgeon's office under local anesthetic. Although CNB is a little more invasive than FNA, it nevertheless can provide more detailed information. CNB is the most common form of biopsy because it provides accurate information but causes less discomfort than surgery and doesn't leave a scar.

In the case of a lump or calcifications that can't be felt but have been detected by a mammogram, the doctor won't know where to insert the needle. However, the doctor can use one of two methods to guide the needle to its destination:

- **Ultrasound:** Ultrasound (See "Detecting cysts and differing densities with diagnostic ultrasound" section earlier in this chapter) can be used to guide the needle to the right place because the surgeon can see exactly where to insert the needle. This process can be done in the surgeon's office or in the X-ray department at a hospital or a breast-imaging center. It usually takes 15 minutes to half an hour, and here's what usually happens:

   1. **You lie on your back.**

   2. **The doctor applies a gel lubricant to your breast.**

   3. **The ultrasound wand is placed on your breast to locate the exact spot of the lump.**

   4. **Local anesthetic given.**

   5. **The needle shows up on the ultrasound screen as it's inserted to extract a core of cells.**

- **Stereotactic biopsy:** When ultrasound can't visualize the abnormality, like with calcifications, the doctor (usually a radiologist, occasionally a surgeon) may use a stereotactic biopsy machine. This type of X-ray machine is designed specifically for doing biopsies and shows the inside of the breast so that the doctor knows exactly where to place the needle into the abnormal area being biopsied.

The stereotactic machine and its pictures are identical to a regular mammography machine and its pictures. However, this machine contains a computer that uses a mathematical formula to locate the lesion in the breast. The procedure almost always is done in the X-ray department. When you have a stereotactic breast biopsy, you generally follow these steps:

1. **Lie on your belly on the X-ray machine.**

2. **Your breast falls through an opening in the table onto an X-ray plate.**

3. **Just like a regular screening mammogram, your breast gets squashed (not great, but think of the benefits!)** The machine is like a regular mammogram machine; it doesn't move or make any noise.

4. **At this point in the procedure, your patience comes into play, because you must lie absolutely still for as long as 45 minutes while the doctor finds the exact problem spot.**

   Use those relaxation techniques I talk about in the "Mammogram fantasy" sidebar in this chapter. Imagine that you're sitting on a magnificent beach, shaded by palm trees, and watching the crystal-clear turquoise water in front of you. . . . Or, if you prefer, you can picture yourself on top of a majestic red-earthed mountain in Sedona with only the sound of the gentle breeze and perhaps a bird soaring overhead. Chapter 16 offers a menu of several relaxation techniques.

5. **When the abnormal area is located, local anesthesia is given and a biopsy needle is inserted into your breast and directed toward that spot to extract cores of tissue.**

   The local anesthesia (which can burn but only for a few seconds) will take care of any pain during the procedure. After having it, you may suffer from a little bruising, but it should clear up quickly.

Sucking it up for surgical biopsy

A *surgical biopsy* refers to the removal of the lump by *excision,* or through surgery. A surgical biopsy is performed when a core needle biopsy won't work, or it's been done but hasn't provided a definite answer about whether cancer is present. Most *excisional biopsies* can be done in the office, surgical center, or through the outpatient department of a hospital under local anesthesia, although you may want to choose an intravenous (IV) sedative to get you through it.

Whether you can eat or drink before the procedure depends on the type of anesthesia you're being given. Ask your doctor. If you have sedation or general anesthesia, you need someone to drive you home.

During an excisional biopsy

1. **You put on a gown and lie on the operating room table.**

2. **Your breast is cleaned with antiseptic paint to reduce infection. A sterile drape is put in front of your face, so that you don't see the operation.**

3. **The doctor feels the lump and administers local anesthesia to the area of the lump to make it numb and then makes the incision.**

4. **The lump is removed and the incision is sewn up and bandaged.**

   A biopsy can be a lumpectomy *if* the edges of the tissue taken out are free of cancer cells. Usually, when an excisional biopsy is done, the surgeon tries to take a rim of normal tissue. That way, if the diagnosis is cancer, the lumpectomy is already done!

In the case where a lump is discovered but can't be felt, and a core needle biopsy isn't possible, you may have to have wire *localization* before the surgery. The wire localization biopsy, shown in Figure 5-6, is similar to a core needle biopsy in that the radiologist uses either ultrasound or stereotactic mammography to insert a fine wire attached to a tiny hook into your breast at the site of the calcifications or lump. The wire shows the surgeon where specifically to cut. Instead of sampling cores of tissue, the rest of the surgery is just like an excisional biopsy.

I (Ronit) had this procedure done and no one explained what he or she was doing. I couldn't figure out why I had to walk to the operating room with all these needles and wires sticking in my breast. I thought it was so funny. Of course, the anesthetic helped my humor!

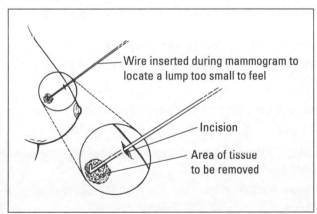

Figure 5-6:
Wire
localization
biopsy.

Wire inserted during mammogram to locate a lump too small to feel

Incision

Area of tissue to be removed

You'll be able to go home soon after the biopsy. If you have any pain, most patients find that acetaminophen is enough to take care of it. Don't take aspirin or nonsteroidal anti-inflammatory medication like ibuprofen or naproxen sodium, because they can increase your chances of bleeding or bruising.

Although probably small, you'll have a scar. Discussing this factor with your doctor before the surgery is helpful, so that you understand exactly what to expect.

Receiving the results from the pathologist takes a few days. The pathologist sends them to your surgeon) who then discusses them with you. Biopsy results are discussed in detail in Chapter 5.

Asking questions to prepare yourself for a biopsy

If you're going in for a biopsy, you're probably going to have plenty of questions. Ask the doctor who will be performing the biopsy to describe the procedure to you. The nurse will also probably give you a written handout of guidelines.

Never be afraid to ask questions. Even when you get a handout that explains the procedure, sometimes having someone verbalize (or even draw a picture of) the information is simply easier. People process information differently, and getting a doctor or surgeon to speak in layman's terms can sometimes be tough.

The answers to the following questions vary depending on what kind of biopsy you have. Follow your doctor's instructions carefully.

Asking the surgeon about the biopsy procedure

Before you have your biopsy, you may want to ask your doctor the following questions so that you know what to expect.

- ✔ What type of biopsy do you recommend? Why?

- ✔ Where will you do the biopsy?

- ✔ What exactly will you do? How long will it take? Will I be awake or knocked out during the biopsy?

- ✔ Can you draw me a picture that shows me the approximate size of the incision and the size of the tissue you'll remove?

✔ Will the resulting hole affect the shape of my breasts? Will it show afterward?

✔ Where will the scar be? What will it look like?

✔ When can I go back to work? Take care of my kids? Am I allowed to lift things?

Asking the nurse about postsurgical care

Often the nurse is the best person to answer the more practical postsurgery questions for you since nurses are the ones who deal with this aspect of care.

✔ Can I drive home afterward or will I need someone to drive me?

✔ When can I take off the bandage?

✔ How do I care for the incision?

✔ When can I take a shower?

✔ Will the stitches dissolve or do I need to come back to have them removed?

Asking your doctor about outcome

The most important question is, of course, about the results. Your surgeon will probably bring up these issues, but in case that doesn't happen, or in case you were too anxious to remember (taking notes is a good idea), don't be afraid to ask:

✔ When will I know the results?

✔ Will you call me or should I call you?

✔ Will you or someone else explain the biopsy results to me?

Chapter 6

Decoding Your Pathology Report

. . . .

. . . .

Medical reports can be intimidating. They seem to be filled with obscure terminology (there's that Latin again), complex text, and a whole series of indecipherable numbers. When the report is talking about your body, attempting to understand these reports is especially frustrating (and maybe even frightening), and it feels like you're always the last one to know.

Your *pathology report* tells you two things: First, whether you have cancer, and second, the extent of the cancer. How is this finding made? It's done by the pathologist (think microscope), who looks at the cells that are taken out of your breast. If you have a biopsy (Chapter 5), the pathologist can determine whether the extracted cells are cancer. If you have surgery (look ahead to Chapter 10), the pathologist can determine the size of the cancer, whether it has spread to your lymph nodes, and whether it was all removed. So the pathology report holds the keys to your diagnosis, prognosis, and treatment, and is the one piece of paper (actually it's probably two or three pages) that you probably will want to see (or at least go over so your doctor can explain the findings to you).

After you know all that, you can begin discussing your next steps with your doctor and family. By understanding what your findings mean, you'll be in a better position to discuss your treatment options with your medical team. In this chapter, we walk you through the nuts and bolts of the report so you can not only read it but also understand what the findings mean for *you*.

Drink up

"When I (Ronit) was pregnant, I remember looking at the report of my ultrasound, which was prescribed because of complications that I was experiencing. The bottom line of the report read, 'Decreased liquor.' 'What?' I thought. 'They want me to drink less alcohol? How can that be when I don't even drink, not even a glass of wine.' I was shaking with indignation (and fear) when I went to see my doctor, who explained that *liquor* was the fluid that surrounded the baby in the uterus, and that what the report referred to were concerns about this fluid. Oops! I felt so stupid that I forgot to be worried about the implications of the real findings. Everything turned out okay, by the way, and my son is now a strapping young man who towers over his mother."

Looking Under the Microscope

Have you ever been underwater diving or snorkeling? There's another world beneath the calm surface of the water that you can't see when you're lying on the beach or even swimming. The same is true for your body. Under the surface of your skin is an exciting world that you can't see with the naked eye, but the pathologist, with his powerful microscope, can. When looking at tissue samples that are taken from your body, the pathologist is searching for certain factors that ultimately help to determine what your diagnosis and prognosis will be. (The implications of what each of the pathologist's findings mean for your prognosis are explained in detail in Chapter 7.)

The pathologist looks for

- Evidence of cancer in the cells of the breast.
- If cancerous cells are found, the pathologist looks further to find out

  - The type of cancer

  - The size of the cancer

  - How aggressive the cancer is

  - Other aspects about the cells that have direct implication for your treatment options

  - Whether any cancer cells can be found on the edges (or *margins*) of the tissue removed (When there are cancer cells on the margins, that means not all of the cancer was removed during surgery.)

  - Whether any of the cells in each (one by one) of the lymph nodes shows any evidence of cancer

Reviewing the Report

The pathology report is comprised of several parts. Although the order of the information may vary slightly, the report usually looks like the example shown in Figure 6-1. Refer to the sample report as you read this chapter.

The pathology report is sent directly to your doctor, because that is who discusses these findings with you. Ask for and keep a copy of the pathology report. Take notes as the doctor goes through it with you. When you've had time to digest the information, you can go back and ask more questions.

Identifying information

The *identifying information* section of the report refers to details that ensure your specimen doesn't get mixed up with anyone else's and other information that helps keep a careful track of the specimen as it moves from your surgeon's office to the pathologist's office and back again. The basics are given here, including your name, birthday, sex, social security number, the medical record number, the specimen number, when the tissue was taken (the "obtained on" date), when the lab received the sample, and when the report was written by the pathologist (the "reported on" date). The example report also indicates that a special report, Faxitron, (an X-ray of the lumpectomy) was done. The photographs entry refers to photographs of the specimen or drawings made of it by the pathologist

Clinical information

Your surgeon (the person who does the operation, either the surgical biopsy, discussed in Chapter 5, or a lumpectomy or mastectomy, discussed in Chapter 10) fills out the *clinical information* section of the pathology report form, listing all the pertinent medical information, so the pathologist can carry out the most accurate series of tests. Measurements of the tumor are given in centimeters (length, width, and if a third dimension can be measured, height).

The example report shows that Rhonda had a diagnosis of cancer on the core biopsy, which is where cells are taken from the breast with a needle (see Chapter 5), and is undergoing surgery now to determine the extent of the cancer. (Dr. Monica Morrow, the surgeon and one of this book's coauthors, performed a core biopsy, and the pathologist examined the tissue from the core biopsy to see whether it was cancer.)

1. *Identifying information*

Patient: Rhonda Brooks	**Specimen #:** S01-24680
Medical Record #: 98765432/1	
Social Security #: 123-45-6789	**Birth date:** 01/01/1952 (Age: 50)
Sex: F	
Obtained on: October 25/01	
Reported on: October 28/01	
Attending Physician: Monica Morrow, M.D.	
Special Studies: Faxitron	
Photographs: Diagram Attached	

2. *Clinical information*

The patient is a 50 year old female with a core biopsy diagnosis of breast cancer, left, undergoing wire localization lumpectomy, sentinel lymph node biopsy, and axillary lymph node dissection of left breast.

3. *Gross description*

A. Received in saline labeled "sentinel node, left axilla" are two lymph nodes with attached Fibrofatty tissue measuring 1.8 x 1.6 x 0.3 cm in aggregate. Both the lymph nodes are bisected and appear grossly negative for tumor. The specimen is representatively submitted as follows:

   1. One lymph node, bisected

   2. The other lymph node, bisected

B. Received fresh in a faxitron and labeled "left breast lumpectomy" is a 5.0 x 3.5 x 1.0 cm fragment of Fibrofatty tissue. The specimen is oriented as follows: Short suture = superior, long suture = lateral. The specimen is inked as follows: Anterior surface is inked yellow, posterior surface is inked green. The specimen is serially sectioned from superior to inferior and reveals a single hard discrete lesion with ill-defined margins measuring 0.8 x 0.7 x 0.6 cm. The lesion is located 0.2 cm away from the deep margin. The remainder of the specimen reveals fibrocystic changes. A biopsy site is identified next to the lesion. The specimen is entirely submitted as per attached diagram in a total of 13 cassettes.

4. *Final diagnosis*

A. Left axilla sentinel lymph node, excision:

   Two lymph nodes, negative for carcinoma.

B. Left breast, lumpectomy

   Infiltrating ductal carcinoma, Grade 1 of 3, measuring 1.0 x 0.7 x 0.6 cm.

   Ductal Carcinoma in-situ, cribriform, minor component.

   Invasive carcinoma within 1 mm of inked deep margin and 2 mm from the inked anterior margin

   Separate focus of atypical ductal hyperplasia.

Figure 6-1:
An example pathology report.

5. *Summary*
   Breast Cancer Staging Summary
   (Microscopic Findings Combined with S01-25423)

Infiltrating Tumor Type:	Ductal
Grade:	1 (1A, 1N, 1MC)
Size:	1cm on core 8, 1.0 x0.7x 0.6cm
In-Situ/Intraductal Tumor Type:	Ductal, cribriform
Grade:	1
Size:	Minor component
Margins:	Close (see above)
Vascular or lymphatic invasion:	Not demonstrated
Total lymph nodes:	2
Number positive:	0
Extranodal invasion:	N/A
Dermal lymphatic invasion:	Not demonstrated
Nipple involvement:	Not demonstrated
Tumor Marker Studies	
ER/PR/p53/CERB-2:	ER/PR-positive, p53/CERB-2-negative
DNA/ploidy:	Upon request
Tumor bank:	Yes
Mammographic lesion:	Mass
Procedures Done:	Lumpectomy with sentinel node biopsy

Doctors may use shorthand to refer to the location of the tumor on the pathology report. Table 6-1 gives you the 411 on what these acronyms mean.

Table 6-1	The 411 on Location Shorthand
Shorthand	*What it means*
RUOQ	Right breast; Upper, outer quadrant
RLOQ	Right breast; Lower, outer quadrant
RUIQ	Right breast; Upper, inner quadrant
RLIQ	Right breast; Lower, inner quadrant
LUOQ	Left breast; Upper, outer quadrant

(continued)

Table 6-1 *(continued)*	
Shorthand	**What it means**
LLOQ	Left breast; Lower, outer quadrant
LUIQ	Left breast; Upper, inner quadrant
LLIQ	Left breast; Lower, inner quadrant

Gross description

A *gross description* isn't "gross" because it's yucky; it's just an *overall* description — you know, like the overall paycheck that you'd rather have.

 Yes, the gross part of the report is grossly difficult to decipher, but don't worry, this information is for your doctor and not the stuff that determines your prognosis or treatment. Also, the summary section (described later in this chapter) is much easier to understand (thank goodness) and includes the same information in shorter, more digestible bits so you can skip straight to that.

In the gross description, the pathologist describes what the tissue looks and feels like before examining it under the microscope. The description isn't that meaningful to you, because it's just a description of the tissue *before* it's examined under the microscope. The gross description section also gives the exact source from which the tissue sample or samples were taken. In Figure 6-1, the report notes that Rhonda had two tissue samples taken — one from her left breast ("left breast lumpectomy") and one from the lymph nodes under her left arm ("sentinel node, left axilla are two lymph nodes"). Her left! And not the doctor's left.

A few words in the sample report that require a little more explanation are

   ✔ **Sutures** are stitches put in by the surgeon and used to mark the different sides of the specimen. The surgeon places a stitch at some of these places (usually two) on the specimen:

     • *Superior:* Top

     • *Inferior:* Bottom

     • *Anterior:* Front

     • *Posterior:* Back

     • *Medial margins:* Middle edges

     • *Lateral:* Side edge

The placement of the sutures tells the pathologist exactly how the sample fits into your body (in other words, *specimen orientation*). The pathologist then marks the specimen with special ink that can be seen under the microscope. (In this report they're inked in black, yellow, blue, and green.)

✔ *Unfixed* means the opposite of *fixed,* which means put into a preservative solution. The preservative, which is usually formalin, makes the tissue easier to cut into small slices.

✔ *Fibrofatty* refers to the fibrous fatty cells of which most women's breasts are composed. (It doesn't mean you're overweight.) Chapter 2 talks more about your breasts and what they're made of.

✔ *Serially sectioned* means that the sample was cut *(sectioned)* in a certain direction in this case, top to bottom.

✔ Slices of tissue are placed in small containers called *cassettes.* This procedure helps the pathologist keep precise tabs on exactly which tissues are put where. In the Figure 6-1 example, the specimens are placed in 13 cassettes.

✔ *Grossly unremarkable* means the tissues look normal to the naked eye, and *grossly negative* for tumor means that to the naked eye, the tissue looks like there is no tumor.

✔ The lymph nodes are cut in half or *bivalved* and may be cut into more pieces called *sections,* depending on the size of the abnormality, so that they can fit into the processing cassettes. See Chapter 7 for full lymph node details.

Final diagnosis

The *final diagnosis* section is, of course, the bottom line. Depending on what it says, you know whether you can celebrate or begin discussing surgical treatment options with your doctor.

This section is where the pathologist lists all the findings that will have a bearing on the final diagnosis, including

✔ The type of cancer you have (described in Chapter 3)

✔ The grade of the cancer, which indicates how fast it is growing (see Chapter 7)

✔ The extent (if any) of lymph node involvement (Chapter 7 shows how this affects the stage of your cancer, and Chapter 8 explains the effect of this on your prognosis)

In Rhonda's case, she has been diagnosed with *infiltrating ductal carcinoma*, a cancer of the duct that can spread. The cancer has been completely *excised*, or removed, which is certainly grounds for celebration. The pathologist also found other cells with *atypical ductal hyperplasia*, abnormal cells that are *not* cancer. The news about Rhonda's lymph nodes is excellent. Her cancer has not spread (*metastasized*) to any of the nodes nor were any abnormalities found in them.

Summary

Everything in a nutshell: You may want to read this part of the report first because it's quick and easy to understand. All the information listed here are measures of the extent and type of the cancer. Extent and cancer type are explained in detail in Chapters 6 and 7, but Table 6-2 provides you with some summaries (of the summary, if you will).

Table 6-2	Pathology Report Summary Information	
The category	*What the sample path report shows*	*What it means*
In-Situ/Intraductal Tumor Type	Ductal	Cancer that has begun in the ducts of the breast and has invaded other cells.
Grade	1	Grade is an attempt to measure how fast-growing or aggressive the cancer is. *Grade 1* cancers consist of relatively normal-looking cells that aren't growing rapidly and are arranged in small tubules. *Grade 2* cancers have features between Grades 1 and 3. *Grade 3* cancers are the highest grade, cells don't look like normal cells, and they tend to grow and spread more aggressively. The news here is great!
Size	1.0 x 0.7 x 0.6 cm	The size of the tumor based on viewing it on the microscope slides (not always the same as the gross size). This one is tiny.
Margins	Close	Whether any cancer remains on the edges of the tissue removed. It was close to the margins.

The category	What the sample path report shows	What it means
Vascular or Lymphatic invasion	Not demonstrated	Whether the cancer has invaded the lymph vessels or the blood vessels in the breast. Not demonstrated means no. This is good news.
Total lymph nodes	2	This refers to the number of lymph nodes that were removed and sent to the pathologist.
Number positive	0	This refers to the number of lymph nodes that were found to have cancer in them. None!
Extranodal invasion	N/A	This refers to cancer that's growing through the boundary of the node, but because, in this case, no nodal involvement was discovered, this wasn't examined.
Dermal lymphatic invasion	Not demonstrated	Was there invasion (spread) to the dermis (skin) outside of the lymph node? No!
Nipple involvement	Not demonstrated	Was there any cancer in the nipple area? No!
Tumor marker studies		This is the heading for a series of tests to measure certain aspects of the cancer cell itself.
ER/PR (estrogen/ progesterone)	Positive	The cancer cells have a receptor for estrogen and progesterone, which means 1. A better prognosis, and 2. This kind of cancer can be treated with tamoxifen or other antihormonal drugs.
p53	Negative	This is a protein in the cell whose job is to suppress tumors. Sometimes it gets mutated and then allows tumors to grow. In this case it is not mutated.

(continued)

Table 6-2 *(continued)*

The category	What the sample path report shows	What it means
CERB-2	2-negative	HER-2/*neu* (which also is called CERB-2) is a protein in the cancer cell that gives the cells instructions to make too many copies of itself. These cancers tend to grow and spread more aggressively than other breast cancers. But, the good news is that they can be treated with a drug called Herceptin, which prevents the HER2/*neu* protein from stimulating breast cancer cell growth. Good news here, it's negative.
DNA Ploidy	In this hospital, this test is not routine but is done only if requested. Your report may have it, so we include the definition here.	*Ploidy* indicates how much DNA is in the cancer cells. If there's a normal amount, the cells are called *diploid*. If the amount is abnormal, the cells are called *aneuploid*. Some studies have found that aneuploid breast cancers tend to be faster growing and more likely to come back, while others have not found this (that's why it isn't a routine test in all hospitals).
Tumor bank	Yes	This refers to whether the patient agreed to donate her tissue to the tumor bank (in which cancerous cells are collected) for future research. She did.
Mammographic lesions	Mass	This refers to whether a lesion was visible on mammography. In this case a mass was visible.
Procedures Done	Lumpectomy with sentinel node biopsy	

Chapter 7

Who Knew That All Cancer Is Also a Stage?

In This Chapter

▶ Discovering how to foresee your journey

▶ Putting the pieces together

▶ Tuning in on the tumor, nodes, and metastasis

▶ Predicting your path

"*H*ow bad is it?" "Am I going to die?" "What treatment am I going to need?" These questions are some of the first ones you'll be asking after your doctor confirms that you have breast cancer. Unfortunately, the answer you're likely to hear is, "It depends," and that can be frustrating. However, it's the truth. Your situation depends on whether the cancer has spread *(metastasized)* or remains in one place *(in situ),* and if it *has* spread, it depends on exactly where and how extensively it has spread. It also depends on other aspects, such as how fast the cancer's growing, your age, your general health.

Even with so many unknowns to deal with, there must be some way of putting all this information together so that everyone, doctors and patients alike, can calculate how extensive your cancer is (or isn't) and, based on that information, explain to you what your treatment options are and what your *prognosis,* or projected outcome, is likely to be.

You're right. There is a way. It's called *staging,* and it's a system that tells you how extensive your cancer is according to established measurements and guidelines. This chapter helps you understand how doctors determine the stage that your particular cancer is in, what the different stages are, and what all this information means to you.

Breast cancer has five stages, numbered 0 through IV, with 0 being the least advanced and IV being the most advanced stages. You'll hear your entire treatment team frequently referring to the stage of your cancer, so being at least a little familiar with it may be helpful to you. Knowing the stage of your cancer also helps you answer the most important question that I'm sure is in the back of your mind, "Will I die?" (Determining your prognosis is described in Chapter 8.)

Understanding the Staging System

Systematically being able to detect all the cancer cells in your body simply would be a wonderful accomplishment, and, ideally, knowing everything possible about your particular cancer cells would enable your treatment team to develop a treatment that was tailored specifically for you. Unfortunately, at this point, a means of assessing your cancer with 100 percent accuracy doesn't exist because methods of determining whether any microscopic cancer cells have spread and exactly where they are simply haven't been devised. The best system that's available right now is the staging system, and we tell you upfront that it isn't perfect.

Experts continually are working in teams to improve the staging system (including our very own Dr. Monica Morrow, a coauthor of this book). In fact, a revised system was launched in January of 2003; although it is an improvement over prior systems, even the new system isn't 100 percent accurate. For right now, staging is the best system we have, and it's the system everyone uses, including hospitals, insurance companies, your medical team, and breast cancer survivors.

Putting the pieces together

The staging system works like a jigsaw puzzle with lots of little pieces. Only when you put them all together can you see the whole picture.

Step 1: Tests, tests, and more tests

You undergo a series of tests, and the results are all put together to form one picture of how extensive your cancer is. Actually, the test results form two related pictures.

✔ The first one, *clinical staging*, is like a rough sketch that's drawn from the preliminary information doctors can gather before you have any kind of surgery to assess how extensive your cancer is. Clinical staging helps doctors determine what kind of surgery and treatment you may need, but it's based only on clinical findings, which are discussed in the next subsection.

✔ The second picture, *pathologic staging,* adds many more of the pieces to the initial sketch by taking the findings seen under the microscope (see Chapter 6) into account. Pathologic staging is based on the results of clinical staging combined with the more accurate information that the pathology report can provide, such as the exact size of the cancer, and whether it has spread to the *lymph nodes* (the glands under your arm). Like with a painting, by sketching the rough outline in soft pencil, you can sort of see where the picture will take you. However, until you have all (or at least most) of the painting done, there are many different ways it can turn out. It's the same with finding out about the stage of your cancer — first you outline the sketch and then add the pieces of information to make the whole picture.

Clinical staging

Clinical staging includes taking your medical history, examining your breasts, and undergoing one or more of a range of tests that begin determining whether the cancer has spread to more distant parts of your body *(metastasized),* whether it has moved out of where it started but has not metastasized *(invasive),* or whether it's still in one place *(in situ).* This kind of staging forms the basis for your surgeon's evaluation. The different tests that you'll undergo usually are prescribed in a particular order because each is dependent on findings from the one before. The following tests are among the more common ones prescribed during clinical staging.

✔ **Mammograms:** You're likely to have *mammograms* (an X-ray) taken of both breasts to find out whether you have cancer in the other breast and to better understand the extent of the lump that's been found. This kind of mammogram is a procedure that helps provide a clearer picture of whether the lump is cancerous. That's why it's called a *diagnostic mammogram.* It's different from a *screening mammogram* (the kind everyone generally thinks about when they talk about mammograms), which screens women to find out whether there's anything suspicious. We describe the differences in full in Chapter 5.

✔ **Blood tests:** Blood tests that measure normal enzymes in your bones and liver may be conducted. Abnormal blood test results may be an indication that the cancer has spread, and so more extensive tests, such as bone scans or CAT scans or MRIs, may then be conducted.

✔ **Chest X-ray:** This procedure helps determine whether the cancer has spread to your lungs. Finding that your cancer has spread to your lungs is not a very hopeful sign, because it means the cancer has spread through your blood stream and has begun reestablishing itself in the lungs.

✔ **Bone scans:** This tool shows whether the cancer has spread to your bones and can indicate a spread of cancer to more distant sites of the body. Women with small-sized cancers and no evidence that it's spread to the nodes don't routinely need bone scans.

> ✔ **CAT scan or MRI:** You may need to have a *computer axial tomography scan* (CAT scan) or *magnetic resonance imaging* (MRI). These tests can look for the spread of cancer in other parts of your body, like your abdomen and pelvis.

To find out more about breast cancer treatments, check out Chapter 9.

Pathologic staging

Pathologic staging (done by a pathologist, who's an expert at looking at the cells under the microscope) is based on a review under the microscope of suspicious cells *after* the cancer in your breast is removed by lumpectomy or mastectomy, and the nodes under your arm are removed (see Chapter 5).

Because it's based on the actual breast tissue and lymph nodes that are removed during surgery, pathologic staging is the definitive staging, compared to the more preliminary staging based on the *biopsy* results (see Chapter 5). If your doctors are in the process of determining which stage your cancer is in, it means you have already been given a diagnosis of cancer, and now they're looking to see how extensive it is so that they can determine what treatment to give you.

The pathologist's findings provide much more detailed, specific, and, therefore, more accurate information about the cancer cells (see Chapter 6). For example, the pathologist can tell whether the cancer is moving out of (*infiltrating*) or remaining in (*in situ*) the area of the breast where it started.

Finally, by seeing whether the cancer cells are present in the lymph nodes, the pathology tests tell you whether the cancer has spread, which is one of the most important predictors of what treatment plan you need (Chapter 9) and what your prognosis (Chapter 8) is likely to be.

Step 2: Getting the lowdown on which stage you're in

After all the tests are complete and the reports are in, doctors put all the information together to calculate the stage of your cancer, more or less completing the puzzle. The puzzle can't be 100 percent complete because doctors examining your cancer don't have a way of knowing exactly where every cancer cell may be lurking, but after they review all the findings and calculate the stage of your cancer, they *can* tell you

> ✔ How extensive your cancer is.

> ✔ What your treatment options are. In Chapter 9, you can follow step-by-step exactly what treatment to expect for your particular stage of cancer.

> ✔ What doctors expect your prognosis to be according to the stage of your cancer, which we described in detail in Chapter 8? Your prognosis is only a forecast and not an absolute fact, but from it, you can at least begin having a more realistic idea of what you're facing.

When you first find out that you have cancer, thinking of the worst of possibilities is natural. But you really can't begin to tell how extensive your cancer is until you get the results of all your tests and find out what stage your cancer is in. The cancer often is much less extensive than you think.

What the doctors look for: TNM

The staging system also goes by another name: *TNM system.* That's because three important elements that go into calculating the stage of your cancer are the tumor (T), nodes (N), and metastasis (M). The TNM system is a two-step process, and the following subsections explain how it works.

Assigning scores

First, your tumor, nodes, and metastasis each are assigned their own individual scores. In all three cases, the lower the score, the better:

> ✔ **T score:** Your T score can range from 0 to 4. For example, when your score is T1, your tumor is 2 centimeters in diameter or less, but when it's T3, the tumor is more than 5 centimeters in diameter. Table 7-1 explains each T score in more detail. Figure 7-1 shows you various sizes of tumors.

Table 7-1	T Score Explanations
T score	*Explanation*
Tx	Primary tumor can't be assessed.
T0	No evidence of primary tumor.
Tis	Carcinoma in situ. Tis (DCIS) are ductal carcinoma in situ; Tis (LCIS) is lobular carcinoma in situ. Tis (Paget) is known as Paget's disease of the nipple with no associated tumor mass.
T1	Tumor 2 cm or less in greatest dimension.
T2	Tumor more than 2 cm but not more than 5 cm in greatest dimension.
T3	Tumor more than 5 cm in greatest dimension.
T4	Tumor of any size that's growing into the chest wall or into the skin, which is determined by your surgeon before or during surgery.

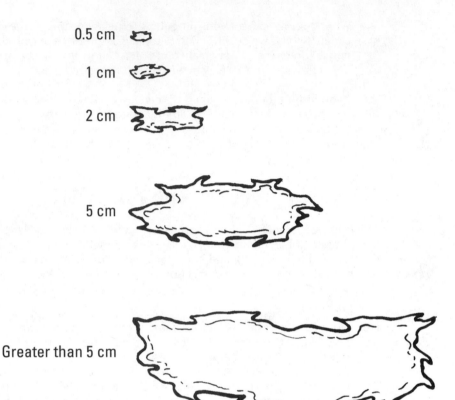

0.5 cm

1 cm

2 cm

5 cm

Greater than 5 cm

Figure 7-1:
Tumor sizes
to scale.

✔ **N score:** The lymph nodes under your arm are rated from 0 to 3 using a scoring system similar to the T score. Knowing whether particular lymph nodes have been affected is important, because if they are, it can indicate that cancer cells have spread to other parts of the body. (Chapter 2 explains more about the lymph nodes.) A score of N0 means that the cancer has not spread to the lymph nodes (and that's great news!). On the other hand, a score of N3 indicates that cancer has spread to internal mammary lymph node(s) beneath the breastbone.

There are two ways your N score is determined. The first, the clinical examination, is just a preliminary finding. Once the surgeon has actually gone in, taken out the node and sent it in for pathology review, you get the more accurate surgical N score.

• **Clinical N** is determined by whether you can feel the nodes.

• **Surgical N score** is determined by surgically removing the nodes and examining their pathology to determine whether the cancer has spread to the nodes, and if it has, to how many of the lymph nodes. A more recently developed procedure, called *sentinel-node biopsy,* has made the procedure so much easier by examining only the sentinel node, the first node to which the cancer cells travel, and the same determination about the presence and extent of cancer can be made. Find out all about sentinel-node biopsy in Chapter 10.

✓ **M score:** The final element is a determination of whether the cancer has spread to other parts of the body (metastasized) and is scored using a 0 or 1 score. A score of M0 means that the cancer hasn't metastasized to other parts of the body (very good news!), a score of M1 means that it has.

The M score is determined one step at a time as we explain in the "Putting the Pieces Together" section earlier in this chapter and in Chapter 5. For example, if a lump is found to be in situ (not spread), there's no reason to suspect a metastasis. However, if it's a large lump and has spread to the nodes, the previously described tests (blood tests, bone scan, chest X-ray) will be done depending on a logical order and based on your clinical symptoms. If you have a chronic cough that hasn't gone away, for instance, you'll probably have a chest X-ray.

Putting the scores together

After individual scores for each of these three elements are determined, they're combined to determine the stage of your cancer, as shown in Table 7-2. If you find it helpful, go ahead and highlight your particular stage. Many women want to understand exactly what their stage means and where it puts them on the scale. Others don't want to know the details. Do whatever feels more comfortable for you.

Table 7-2	Grouping Breast Cancer Stages		
Breast Cancer Stage	*T (Tumor)*	*N (Nodes)*	*M (Metastasis)*
Stage 0	Tis	N0	M0
Stage I	T1	N0	M0
Stage IIA	T0	N1	M0
	T1	N1	M0
	T2	N0	M0
Stage IIB	T2	N1	M0
	T3	N0	M0

(continued)

Table 7-2 *(continued)*

Breast Cancer Stage	T (Tumor)	N (Nodes)	M (Metastasis)
Stage IIIA	T0	N2	M0
	T1	N2	M0
	T2	N2	M0
	T3	N1	M0
	T3	N2	M0
Stage IIIB	T4	N0	M0
	T4	N1	M0
	T4	N2	M0
Stage IIIC	Any T	N3	M0
Stage IV	Any T	Any N	M1

Note: Stage designation may be changed if post-surgical studies find distant metastases.

Staging a Cell Coup

Breast cancer is grouped in five stages. You may have a friend with Stage IV, and you're terrified that you're going to have to go through the same treatment she did. However, if you've been diagnosed with Stage I breast cancer, your treatment options will be much different than hers. That's why knowing which stage of breast cancer you've been diagnosed with is so important.

A brief summary of each stage follows. Find the stage of breast cancer with which you've been diagnosed and see what it entails, and then you can turn to Chapter 9 to find out what your treatment options are and to Chapter 8 to find out how well you're likely to do. Your prognosis is only a prediction, not a fact written in stone.

Stage 0

Stage 0 includes two different types of cancer. Although both are cancers that have not spread beyond where they have started (which is great), they are, in fact, quite different from one another.

Lobular carcinoma in situ

Lobular carcinoma in situ (LCIS) refers to abnormal cells in the *lobules,* or the glands that produce milk, that has remained where it started. Most oncologists don't consider LCIS a true breast cancer but rather an abnormal growth of the cells in the lobules. These abnormal cells may indicate that you're at risk of developing breast cancer in the future, and although the risk is very low, continued and regular monitoring of your situation is important, so if it does develop into cancer, it can be caught early. You may also be prescribed *tamoxifen,* an antiestrogen drug that may lower your risk of developing cancer.

Ductal carcinoma in situ

The other localized cancer of the breast is *ductal carcinoma in situ (DCIS),* which is cancer in the *ducts,* or the milk passages that connect the lobules with the nipple, that has not spread. However, unlike LCIS, most women with DCIS will develop *invasive* (spreading) cancer at some time in the future if they aren't treated.

DCIS manifests itself in a variety of ways, which means that even though you and your neighbor are diagnosed with DCIS, your respective diagnoses, treatments, and prognoses may be different. Hers may progress to an invasive cancer, but yours may not, or vice versa.

In any event, you'll be sent for *magnification mammography,* where the picture or mammogram is magnified so doctors can see even the tiniest bits of calcium deposits. Your treatment options will vary, ranging from a *lumpectomy* (cutting out the cancerous tissue), a lumpectomy followed by radiation, or a *mastectomy* (where your whole breast is removed) with or without reconstructive surgery. You, your doctor, and members of your treatment team will discuss your treatment options and make the best decision for you.

The survival rate (which doctors measure in five- and ten-year blocks) for Stage 0 is 98 to 100 percent! Now, isn't that something to celebrate?

Stage 1

In Stage I, the tumor is very small, only about 2 centimeters or less in diameter (across), and it hasn't spread at all. In most cases, your treatment will be a lumpectomy (surgery to remove the lump in your breast and one or more nodes under your arm), which will be followed by radiation treatment (see Chapter 11). You may need endocrine (hormonal) treatment or chemotherapy. Because treatment options differ so much from one woman to the next, explaining exactly what your treatment journey will be like is difficult until you've had several more tests (for example, to see how fast or how slow your cancer is growing). After you know the results of these tests, you can find out what your treatment options are (Chapter 9).

If you've been diagnosed with Stage I breast cancer, your chances of survival are wonderful. They're 98 percent, which means that 98 percent of the women with this diagnosis have survived at least five years. Admit it, aren't you just a little bit relieved? I know the fear doesn't go away instantly, but at least you know that your odds of beating this disease are extremely high.

Stage II

As you can see in Table 7-2, Stage II breast cancer is further divided into Stage IIA and IIB because of the many possible ways in which your cancer can manifest itself. For example, if your cancer is scored *T1, N1,* your tumor is 2 centimeters or less across, and cancer was found in one or more lymph nodes (what doctors call an N1 or higher score *nodal involvement*) under your arm on the same side as the breast where the cancer was found. There's no evidence of any metastasis (M0). In other words, although the size of the cancer in your breast is very small, it has begun spreading to the nodes.

On the other hand, if your cancer is scored *T3, N0,* it means that the tumor in your breast is more than 5 centimeters across, but it has not spread to the nodes. This is one of the groupings in Stage IIB cancer.

In Stage IIB, the cancer is more extensive than in Stage IIA, which is why the survival rate among women with Stage IIB is not quite as high as women with Stage IIA. Eighty-eight percent of women with Stage IIA survive at least five years, but, by comparison, only 76 percent of women with Stage IIB survive at least five years. Why shouldn't you be one of them?

The treatment options for women with Stage II breast cancer are similar to women with Stage I in general, but as always, an individual woman's treatment options vary so much depending on a host of factors. We describe these options by stage in Chapter 9. General guidelines exist, but each woman is different, so talk to your doctor about your particular options.

Stage III

Stage III breast cancer also is subdivided based on how the cancer behaves. For example, if your cancer is scored *T2, N2,* your tumor is larger than 2 centimeters but less than 5 centimeters, it has spread to the lymph nodes under your arm, and the nodes are stuck to one another or to the chest wall, then your stage is IIIA. That isn't a good sign because it means cancerous cells are invading other cells and are tearing up the structure. Likewise, if they're stuck together or to the chest wall, removing the cancer alone is not possible, and that means the tissue to which the cancer is adhering also must be removed. You'll probably have chemotherapy to shrink the nodes to maximize the surgeon's ability to remove as many of the cancer cells as possible and limit the number of remaining lurking cancer cells.

When your cancer is scored *T4, N3,* the tumor has extended into the chest wall or to the skin of the chest and has spread to the lymph nodes that are under your breastbone, inside the chest, your stage is IIIB. That diagnosis can be disheartening because it means the cancer has spread farther than the breast and farther than the lymph glands under the arm. As a result, your treatment options will likely include chemotherapy and a mastectomy, which probably will be followed by radiation and possibly antihormonal medication.

About half the women with Stage III cancer (56 percent Stage IIIA and 49 percent Stage IIIB) survive at least five years, and go on to live full and meaningful lives. Think of yourself as a future member of this courageous sisterhood. Dealing with the difficult journey that lies ahead of you is going to be challenging, so we describe some strategies in Chapter 14 and 18 that other survivors have used to get through these trying times. Whenever you feel up to it, look at these two chapters and choose some of the strategies that you think will work for you.

The survival rate tells you what percentage of women with breast cancer live *at least* five years after being diagnosed; however, many of these women live much, much longer. The percentages are only projections, not absolutes, and many other factors can influence your individual prognosis. No one, not even your own doctor, can tell you for sure what your *exact* prognosis is.

Stage IV

What differentiates Stage IV from any of the other stages is that the cancer has spread beyond the breast and surrounding lymph nodes to other more distant organs, such as your bones or your lungs. Being diagnosed with Stage IV breast cancer is very hard to hear. It isn't going to be easy for you or your family. You need to think about the possibility of not surviving, and you need to begin making plans in case you don't.

The good news, however, is that very few women are diagnosed initially with Stage IV cancer today (because it's usually caught earlier), but if you or your loved one is diagnosed with Stage IV, the truth is that this is the worst kind of news you can hear. The statistics aren't in your favor. In Chapter 8, we share some of these figures with you. However, remember that these are predictions, not hard and fast rules. A small proportion of women with Stage IV breast cancer do live long and fruitful lives. Why shouldn't you be one of them?

Being diagnosed with Stage IV breast cancer doesn't mean that your death is imminent. And being diagnosed with Stage IV doesn't mean that you're without treatment options. Getting this news is a shock, and it's normal for your mind to freeze up for a moment when you hear this kind of news. Take your time, let it sink in, talk to your family and friends, and when you're ready, explore all the treatment options with your doctor. Only then can you make your decisions.

Chapter 8

Understanding Your Prognosis: Am I Going to Die?

*Y*ou've been told that you have cancer. Letting that information sink in is a good idea. You may feel like you need to act immediately, but *you don't*. Give yourself some time to think, come to an understanding of the situation, and then explore all your treatment options (which we discuss in detail in Chapter 9). If you're like most people, you're probably asking yourself, "Am I going to die?" In this chapter, we talk about this scary question.

You have the right to treatment information. Some women, however, don't want to know what to expect; they prefer putting their trust solely in the hands of their doctor. On the other hand, if you know what your options are, you can make a decision that's good for you and your family; when you know what to expect, you can plan for it.

Whether you choose to receive this information is completely up to you. If you don't want it, tell your doctor and simply skip this chapter. If you choose to review your prognosis, please remember that cancer doesn't have any hard and fast rules. You also need to keep in mind that most women do *not* die from breast cancer. Finally, recognize that your breast cancer journey won't be the same as anyone else's. Everyone's path is unique.

Prognosticating: Just a Prediction

Your prognosis is a forecast that's based on information gathered from thousands of women and reported in medical and scientific literature. However, it is only a *prediction* and not a fact set in stone. Your prognosis tells you how most women with findings similar to yours (tumor size, node spread, and metastasis) have done. You, however, may react very differently. Many individual factors, including your age, general health, and improvements in treatment, for example, can make your prognosis completely different from other women.

When giving you your *prognosis,* here's what your doctor is predicting:

- The likely course of your disease
- How you'll respond to treatment
- How likely you are to survive

So far, four factors have been proven to predict your prognosis. Those factors are discussed in the sections that follow.

The cancer's stage

The stage of your cancer indicates the extent of cancer spread (discussed in detail in Chapter 7). Because each stage of cancer affects your body differently, the stage in which your cancer is diagnosed has an impact on your predicted outcome. Generally speaking, the lower the stage, the less the spread and the higher the survival rate.

To devise a consistent way of understanding prognosis, doctors measure survival rates of women in five-year (and sometimes ten-year) intervals. Survival rates are merely predications based on information from large numbers of women with breast cancer. The rates refer to the percentage of women with cancer who live *at least* five years after being diagnosed, and yet many of these women live much, much longer.

A *five-year survival rate* is one way of measuring likelihood of survival. That rate reflects the percentage of people who live at least five years after their cancer has been diagnosed. Groups of people with cancer are followed, and many survive much, much longer than five years. *Five-year relative survival rates* are another way of measuring the likelihood of survival. In this more accurate measurement, anyone who dies from a disease other than cancer isn't included in the calculation.

So if your cancer is diagnosed at Stage 0, your five-year survival rate is 99 percent! The odds just don't get better than that, do they? Yes, it's true that the likelihood of surviving five-years gets lower with each stage, but the likelihood of surviving *at least* five years are very high in Stages 0, I, and II, and survival rates only begin to drop significantly at Stages III and IV.

You're better off thinking of yourself as being part of the group whose members do survive. Of course, being scared at first is natural. Who wouldn't be? But after the initial shock wears off (and it will), consider some of the strategies that can help improve your chances. We describe a whole range of them in Chapters 14 and 18 and invite you to choose the ones that work best for you.

After getting over your initial shock, take time to review your treatment options, explore them with your doctor, talk with your family, and ask your doctor many questions, before you come to any conclusions.

Giving nodes the nod

One of the most important predictors of the outcome of breast cancer is the number of *axillary* (under your arm) lymph nodes that contain cancerous cells.

The general rule is: The fewer the nodes to which the cancer has spread and the smaller the size of the tumor, the better the prognosis. If the cancer hasn't spread to any of the nodes, and the tumor is small, your chances for surviving five years are close to 100 percent! Here's something else really important to remember: If the cancer has spread to many of your nodes, it does *not* mean you're not going to make it. Far from it. Let me give you an example, even if more than four of your nodes have been found to have cancer cells *and* your tumor is large (for example, bigger than 5 centimeters in diameter) your likelihood of surviving *at least* 5 years is close to 50 percent. Why shouldn't you be one of those?

Gina C.

"To all you women out there who have just found out the news of breast cancer, I have a few words that may be of some help. My first thoughts of breast cancer were, 'How long do I have to live?' I had my own death report ready to fill out. But it's not that helpless. You will be scared because everything is new and you don't know what to expect. When you're scared, talk to God. Don't get me wrong, I'm not a Bible banger, but when you need the big guy, he's there for you. Live your everyday life to your fullest, and laugh a lot. It was my best medicine."

Grading a tumor: That's an automatic F!

The *grade* of a tumor refers to how much like a normal cell the cancer cell looks under the microscope. The grading system assigns a score shown in Table 8-1. You can see the grade of your tumor on your pathology report (see Chapter 6).

Grade is a much less important factor than lymph node involvement or tumor size in determining your outcome, but it plays a part in determining outcome. The general rule is the lower the grade, the better your prognosis. For example, if your cancer is staged at Stage I and your tumor grade is 1, your likelihood of surviving *at least* 10 years is 95 percent. It drops if it's at the same stage but the cancer is a grade 3 (83 percent).

Table 8-1		Grading a Tumor
Grade	*Also known as*	*What's happening*
1	Well differentiated	Looks the most like normal cells. Tends to be slow-growing and less likely to spread to the lymph nodes.
2	Moderately differentiated	Has some characteristics of normal cells. Doesn't grow as slowly as grade 1 but slower than grade 3 (intermediate).
3	Poorly differentiated	Looks least like your normal cells; tends to be fast-growing and likely to spread to the lymph nodes.

Explaining importance of hormone receptors

Your ovaries produce two hormones — estrogen and progesterone — which stimulate the growth of normal breast cells. However, these hormones also can stimulate the growth of some breast cancer cells.

Cancers that are stimulated by estrogen or progesterone can be identified by testing them for a *receptor*. A receptor is a connection that's on the inside of the cancer cell, to which hormones can bind. Think of a receptor like a key-hole into which the right key (hormones) fits perfectly. Cancer cells may have an estrogen receptor (ER), a progesterone receptor (PR), or both.

A much easier way to remember all this is simply to call them hormone receptor–negative (or positive).

- ✔ **ER-positive and PR-positive cells:** Cancer cells that have receptors (a key hole into which the key — hormones — can fit).

- ✔ **ER-negative and PR-negative cells:** Cells without these receptors don't allow hormones to enter the cells and make them grow. (It's like having a keyhole but the wrong key.)

Cancer cells that contain estrogen or progesterone receptors have a slightly better outcome than cells that don't, because they can be treated with hormone-related treatments such as tamoxifen. (You can read more about that drug in Chapter 13.) When your cancer cells are hormone receptor–negative, taking hormone-related medication won't help.

Your doctor can predict one more piece of important information from your hormone-receptor status. Studies show that women who are hormone receptor–positive have an increase in disease-free survival rates. This increase is about 10 percent at five years. Plus, when you're hormone receptor–positive, you have an even better overall chance of living. And that's no small chance in anyone's book!

Peeking at Other Predictors

In addition to the major predictors, researchers also are studying other factors that may turn out to be possible predictors. The sections that follow explain.

Faster than a speeding bullet? DNA replication rate

A cell's job is to replicate its entire genetic material and end up with two sets of paired (like identical twins) chromosomes. They do this by replicating their DNA (deoxyribonucleic acid — the code that has all the information about your body). Chapter 4 offers you more about the cancer cell.

The entire DNA replication process takes about six hours, and then the cells rest for about four more hours. (Hey, replicating their entire DNA strand is hard work. You try it!) The cell then goes into a mitosis phase during which it divides and becomes two separate cells.

Researchers have discovered that the rate at which the cancer cells replicate also predicts how fast- or slow-growing the cancer is. When the rate of replication is low, cancer cells are dividing slowly. When the rate of replication is high, cancer cells are dividing faster.

This method of prediction still remains a little controversial, mainly because it hasn't been standardized and hasn't been found able to predict survival on its own.

Tumor-suppressor gene

You know how you check to see whether the kids washed their hands or finished eating their breakfast, right? Well, dividing cells also must undergo a similar kind of scrutiny. Before they can begin replicating, they're examined to make sure that they're all correct — that is, to see whether they're in some way defective, or *mutated*.

Special *tumor-suppressor genes* are responsible for this examination. They tell the mutated cell to stop dividing because it's defective. One of these special genes is named p53.

But what if something goes wrong with the p53 gene? What if the very gene that suppresses tumor development becomes mutated? Well, in that case, it can't do its job, and defective genes begin to replicate. As a result, we now know that women who have a mutation in the p53 gene are more likely to develop breast cancer than women whose p53 genes are not mutated.

Although it seems logical that this mutation also influences how the cancer cell behaves (like how fast it grows), scientists still have no proof that's the case.

Oncogenes and HER-2

Your body has genes that make cells grow. They're called *proto-oncogenes*. They usually do their job just fine, but sometimes they become mutated into what are referred to as *oncogenes,* or genes that cause cancer.

One of the genes produces a receptor that helps the cells grow. It's called HER-2/*neu*, and it's an oncogene. In some breast cancer cells a genetic mutation occurs in the HER-2/neu gene (no one yet knows why this happens.) The HER-2 oncogene sends messages (like pulses of electricity) that cause the cell to grow and divide more rapidly (at 10 to 60 times their normal rate. Cells with too many such receptors appear to grow faster than other cells. Experts know that by looking at this factor in your cancer, they can tell whether you're going to respond to a treatment called Herceptin. This is a drug that can stop the uncontrolled growth, and it does this by binding (connecting) to the HER-2 oncogene.

Survival Statistics

No one wants to talk about death, let alone think about it, but the reality is that there are women who die from breast cancer every single year. Is it the number one cause of cancer-related deaths in women in the United States? No, lung cancer is. This information isn't helpful, however, if you have breast cancer and have never smoked in your life, but it is something to keep in mind.

Getting older

More than 40,000 women die every year in the United States alone from breast cancer. More than half of those who die are older than 70. Very few (around 1,000) are younger than 40, but if it's you or someone you love, who cares how low the number is?

Ethnicity makes a difference

Black women are more likely to die from breast cancer than White women. In fact, this group bears a disproportionate burden of deaths from many cancers. That's why the National Cancer Institute and The American Cancer Society are placing such emphasis on research to determine the causes, and to find solutions that decrease these disparities.

Incidence and death rates for women in other racial and ethnic groups (for example, Hispanic and Asian/Pacific Islander) generally are lower than in White and Black women.

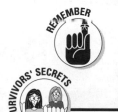

As researchers make new discoveries in diagnosis and treatment, the prognosis for women with breast cancer continues to improve. Although that may sound more like a patronizing, "Let's-just-make-her-feel-good" statement, it really isn't, because it's based on fact. Each new step in the right direction means a better chance for survival.

Nan R.

"My name is Nan, and I'm a three-year survivor of Stage 4 inflammatory breast cancer. I have no regrets about all that I've been through. It was an amazing, incredible journey. It puts life totally in the right places and makes you realize what's important. The day you hear the words, 'You have cancer,' your life changes and will never be the same again. From day one, I never said that I was dying from cancer. Instead, I said I was living with cancer. My doctors threw the kitchen sink at me. I bended a few times, but I never broke. If I can be of help to anyone going through this, it would be an honor."

Seeing into the future: Great hope abounds

You're probably frustrated (even angry) that medicine and research still can't predict exactly how your breast cancer will act. It isn't for a lack of researchers and doctors trying, but rather it's because many cancers have a combination of good and bad factors, and determining which factor predicts the cancer's behavior is impossible. For example, a small tumor that has spread to the nodes has good factors (small size) and bad ones (it's spread to the nodes). Knowing how much influence the good or the bad will have on you is difficult.

Researchers are tirelessly working to find new ways to better predict the prognosis for individual women with breast cancer, rather than for groups of women who may or may not exhibit factors similar to yours.

One of the more hopeful prospects is the study of *gene arrays*. A small piece of your cancer is put on a computer chip, which enables scientists to look at thousands of genes at once, rather than only one or two. Some of the early studies show that particular gene patterns may predict the outcome of a cancer better than even lymph node involvement. Although early results are very promising, doctors need many more studies and more time to follow up with women who are already participating before gene arrays can be used to determine treatment.

The reality is that most women do *not* die from breast cancer, and fewer women are dying from this disease than just a few years ago. The two main reasons that fewer women are dying from breast cancer today are

- ✔ Mammography (see Chapter 4). As doctors diagnose more women while cancer is *in situ* (localized) or in early stages of invasive cancer, fewer women will die. (Chapter 3 talks more in depth about types of cancer.)

- ✔ Improvements in breast cancer treatment. (Chapter 9 talks about treatments.)

Carol M.

"Breast cancer can build you up or tear you down, depending on how you perceive it. I feel breast cancer made me a better person. I eat better, exercise more, and truly appreciate each and every day I have. I have more strength and less fear than I ever had before. My faith in God has grown stronger, the sky is always bluer, and good times with my family and friends take precedent over having a clean house or making the perfect dessert. I would not trade the experience for anything. It took breast cancer to show me how to really live."

Chapter 9

You Mean I Have a Choice? Finding the Right Treatment for You

*Y*es, you have a choice of breast cancer treatments. In fact, you have many options: Your choices of doctors, treatment centers, and even the kinds of treatment all are up to you. By becoming a part of your own treatment team, knowing what treatment options are suitable for your particular form and stage of cancer, and understanding what to expect from each treatment option, you can make wise and informed decisions. Each member of your treatment team — and there are quite a few of them — is involved in your treatment in some way.

Together with your treatment team, your family, and other supporters, you can weigh the pros and cons of your options and make the right treatment decisions for you and your family. In this chapter, we walk you through this process step by step. Use this chapter as a map that shows you what to expect when, as a handbook of your treatment options, as a guide for questions to ask your doctor, and as a manual to understand your diagnosis and process of recovery. Chapters 10–16 describe each aspect of treatment in greater detail.

Going to Bat for You: The Treatment Team

Many people in addition to your primary doctor are involved in your care. Those people make up your *treatment team*. Each member is an expert in a respective field and each plays an important role at some stage of your journey. The team is dependent upon the facility in which you are treated and is created specifically for dealing with your case. In hospitals with more than one surgeon, medical oncologist, or radiation oncologist, you choose who you want.

Diagnosing

Several doctors may be involved in making the diagnosis of cancer, including your

- **Primary-care physician (PCP):** This doctor usually is the first that you encounter, probably has been looking after you for a while, and probably is the doctor who first feels the lump. When suspicious that the lump is cancer, your PCP refers you for a mammogram and/or further testing. Because your PCP isn't usually an expert in breast cancer, you probably won't be advised on the specifics of treatment. But your PCP can

  - Refer you to an expert in breast cancer treatment.

  - Advise your treating physicians (usually your oncologist and surgeon) about your general health and point out anything in your medical history that may affect your response to treatment.

- **Radiologist:** Radiologists specialize in the various tests used to detect cancer, including mammography, ultrasound, and other types of X-ray breast cancer screens. (See Chapter 5 for details about these tests.) The radiologist also performs a procedure known as a *needle biopsy,* which is the way most breast cancers today are diagnosed. The radiologist

  - Examines the results of the mammogram, ultrasound, and X-rays.

  - Interprets whether these tests indicate that your condition is likely to be cancer.

    These tests are used as the first screening. Other tests (such as a needle biopsy) may be needed to confirm the diagnosis.

  - Performs a needle biopsy whenever it's needed.

  - Sends the findings to your doctor (which may be the primary-care physician or surgeon).

- May share the findings with you. The radiologist may be the first doctor to tell you that you have an abnormal mammogram or that the cells that were extracted in the needle biopsy are cancerous.

✔ **Pathologist.** This doctor doesn't usually meet with patients. Instead, this doctor goes into action after surgery, looking at tissue samples removed during biopsy and other surgeries. The pathologist

  - Examines the cells extracted by needle biopsy under a microscope to determine whether they are cancerous.

  - Determines the type of the cancer cell.

  - Determines the stage of your cancer.

  - Sends reports (see Chapter 5 for more about these reports) directly to your treating physician, which is usually your surgeon.

Treating

Now that your diagnosis has been made, it's time to move on to treatment. Several doctors probably are involved in your care. The number depends on what kind of treatment you need? Why can't just one doctor be the one who diagnoses and treats you and stays with you throughout? Unfortunately, so much varied expertise is required for each of the specialties that can be a part of your treatment that no one doctor can possibly do it all, no matter how much he or she wants to. Because treatments for cancer vary so much, different types of oncologists have essentially become superspecialized in their respective fields of treatment. For example, a medical oncologist is an expert in drug treatments of cancer, a radiation oncologist specializes in X-ray treatments, and a surgical oncologist is in charge of the surgical aspects of your treatment. Depending on what kind of treatment you need, you may require one or all of the following oncologists:

✔ **Medical oncologist:** This doctor specializes in treating the medical aspects of your cancer and can

  - Describe the benefits and risks of each of your chemotherapy treatment options.

  - Give you the most updated information on the latest research.

  - Help you decide on the best course of action for you.

  - Prescribe your required chemotherapy or hormonal therapy (described later in this chapter) and take care of you during this part of the treatment.

  - Usually provide most of your follow-up care after your cancer treatment is complete.

✔ **Surgical oncologist (or general surgeon):** The surgeon is in charge of the surgical aspect of your treatment. Most surgeons who treat breast cancer are general surgeons, although some surgeons receive extra training in cancer surgery. Your surgical oncologist will

- Do the biopsy to determine the extent of your cancer. Several types range from simple needle biopsy (which can be done by the radiologist) to surgical types of biopsies (for full details see Chapter 5) that require the well-honed skills of the surgical oncologist.

- Give you the most updated information on the latest surgical research.

- Perform surgery to remove the tumor and other cancerous cells from your body.

- Tell you what to expect during the procedure, how long it takes to recuperate, how you can best prepare, and so on.

- Answer the questions you have about your surgery.

You may want to ask your primary-care doctor for a referral to a surgical oncologist rather than a general surgeon.

✔ **Radiation oncologist:** As an expert on various forms of X-ray treatment, this doctor specializes in treating patients who require radiation. (Chapter 11 talks about radiation therapy in depth.) The radiation oncologist

- Is in charge of your radiation treatments.

- Answers any questions you have about radiation treatment, including what to expect, possible long-term effects, and how radiation kills the cancer cells.

✔ **Anesthesiologist:** This doctor gives you the anesthetic that puts you to sleep for surgery and wakes you up again and makes sure that you're not in pain during and after surgery. The anesthesiologist speaks to you before your surgery and evaluates you carefully, making sure that you're comfortable and safe during and after the surgery.

✔ **Plastic surgeon/reconstructive surgeon:** This surgeon takes over during the reconstruction process. Reconstruction is done at the same time as the original surgery or later, as a separate surgical procedure. This surgeon works closely with the surgical and medical oncologists to make sure that your breast is reconstructed in the best possible way, taking into consideration your medical and surgical condition. (Reconstructive surgery is discussed in full in Chapter 15.)

Heading up the team

Having so many different doctors certainly seems overwhelming. Do you really need them all? Yes, ma'am, you do! Better yet, you want all of them on your team, and you want all of them to be experts.

But how do you know whom to talk to about what? Designating a *point person* (point doctor just doesn't sound good) to lead your team is best. Although this point person may change during the different phases of your journey, designating one of the doctors as the one who's in charge is important for you and everyone involved. The point person is the doctor who coordinates your treatment with other doctors, answers your questions, and helps you plan and decide your next steps.

There's no I in team

Here are some other members of your team who'll be incredibly important to you on your breast cancer journey:

✔ **Nurses:** The many nurses on your team assist with your care before, during, and after your treatment. The nursing field has different levels of certification; some nurses are registered nurses (R.N.s) who have academic degrees and are certified and registered by the nursing board. Licensed vocational nurses (LVNs) have training in nursing. Some R.N.s even receive additional specialty training in oncology (oncology-certified nurses). A nurse practitioner (who has a master's or doctoral degree) can actually diagnose and manage your care, conducting physical exams, providing follow-up care, and maybe even prescribing medication for you.

✔ **Social worker:** This person can help coordinate and provide your nonmedical care. A social worker can help you (and your family) deal with some of the overwhelming feelings that you may have, help you problem-solve, and refer you to other places or people who may be of additional help. The

social worker also can assist in helping you deal with what can sometimes be overwhelming insurance paperwork.

✔ **Physical therapist:** This health specialist assists you during the healing process after your surgery by showing you how to stretch and exercise correctly, so that you can become strong again.

✔ **Radiation therapy technologist:** This trained technician delivers the radiation therapy, making sure that you're positioned correctly and that you receive the correct dose of radiation.

✔ **Fellow:** If you're treated in an academic center, a fellow may be involved in your care. This is a doctor who is training to be an oncologist or a specialist in breast surgery. You'll often see a fellow accompanying your oncologist or surgeon. This doctor can be a very useful resource.

✔ **Resident:** You may see a resident while you're in the hospital or clinic. These doctors are training in medicine, surgery, or radiation.

You'll probably want to ask your medical oncologist or your primary-care doctor to serve as that person. But whomever you choose, make sure your point person lets the other members of your team know that he or she has been appointed. Knowing who's in charge reduces quite a bit of the confusion you can expect from having so many different kinds of doctors on one team.

You're the center of this team, even though you may feel as if everything is happening without you. However, whenever you do feel that way, stop, remind your doctor that your opinion is important, and explain that you need more information before you can make a decision. If you don't think you can do that, then ask your supporter to do it for you (see Chapter 20).

Turning the Tables and Testing the Doctor

If your primary-care doctor suspects that you have breast cancer, you're referred to a radiologist or surgeon for a definitive diagnosis. When they determine that you, in fact, have cancer, your primary-care doctor then refers you to a *surgeon* or *surgical oncologist* (cancer doctor) to begin planning your treatment. The surgeon plans the first part of the treatment during which the cancer is removed.

How do you know a good surgeon when you see one? Everyone needs a compassionate doctor who's familiar with the most up-to-date research, can tell you the truth, isn't condescending, and takes the time to explain your options carefully and patiently. Because this doctor monitors your health for several years after your treatment is over, you need to make sure that you're comfortable with him or her.

In these days of health maintenance organizations (HMOs), not everyone is lucky enough to be able to choose the perfect doctor. Still, it's a good goal to strive for. You can find a doctor with the medical qualifications and personal characteristics that help you the most. Of course, your medical insurance (Chapter 21) and where you live play big parts in this decision, but finding a doctor you're comfortable with is important. Shop around as much as you can!

Copping a 'tude? Back off, dude

Make an appointment with one or more surgeons so you can find the one with whom you feel more comfortable. You can find out whether your doctor is one of the best available in breast cancer treatment by asking questions like

- **Do you have experience with women with my particular kind of cancer?** If the doctor has treated only a few women with breast cancer, consider consulting an additional expert.

- **Are you board certified (trained in the specialty)?** Certification indicates that the doctor has had special training in this field. The more training the doctor has, the more knowledge the doctor has about the latest and most effective treatments.

- **Are you affiliated with a medical school or Comprehensive Cancer Center?** The answer to this question indicates whether the doctor is a leader in the field and is up to date with the latest research and treatments from around the world. The best treatments often are provided at the Comprehensive Cancer Centers (described in Chapter 23), all of which are affiliated with medical schools. Doctors who are affiliated with a Comprehensive Cancer Center have more expertise.

- **How many women with breast cancer do you treat every year?** No magic number of patients determines whether a doctor should be your surgeon, but doctors who treat many women with breast cancer have considerably more experience and expertise than those who treat only a few. That's definitely something to take into consideration.

- **What kind of surgical procedures do you perform? (More on surgery in Chapter 10.) How many per year?** Again, no magic number exists, but the more experience, the more expertise the doctor has.

- **Have you done any research in breast cancer?** Most medical doctors involved in education are involved in research that's aimed at making things better for patients. Research isn't essential in your surgeon, but it's an advantage.

- **In which hospitals do you have admitting privileges (meaning the hospitals to which the doctor can admit you for your surgery)?** This factor obviously affects your choice of hospitals. If you choose a particular doctor, you may not have a choice in the matter. Similarly, your choice may also be limited because of your insurance. If you find that you have a choice of hospitals, you may be able to choose one of the hospitals the surgeon can operate in.

- **Approximately how much time will I have with you during my regular visits?** No amount of time is specified, but the answer to this question may give you an indication of whether you'll be able to see the doctor long enough to ask questions and discuss concerns and issues. The amount of time obviously depends on the particular circumstances, such as when you're not feeling well or you're having a particular problem that you want to discuss with the doctor. In those circumstances, more time may be needed.

✔ **Will you be giving me my results, talking to my family, and answering our questions? If not, who will do those things?** Keeping you and your family informed is important, so that you can know what to expect (unlike the old days when doctors shared little information). If the doctor or the doctor's staff do not share any information or answer questions (which is very unlikely), leave the doctor's office!

✔ **How do you feel about working as a member of *my* treatment team?** Your team has many doctors, and each must be able to work together with others as a team, talking to each other, sharing their expertise, and doing these things in a way that makes life easier for you. If the doctor turns up a nose or rolls eyes at this question, again, leave the office!

You can tell a great deal about a doctor's personal characteristics by the way he or she treats you. How does the doctor handle questions? What is the doctor's personal attitude toward discussing your options with you? When a doctor is rude or disrespectful, regardless of how brilliant he or she may be, staying with that doctor usually isn't worth it (unless, of course, you have no other option). You can also gauge the atmosphere in the office by

✔ The appearance of the waiting room

✔ The attitudes displayed by receptionists and nurses and the manner by which they respond to your questions

✔ The promptness with which your calls are returned and you're informed about your lab results

If you need help in locating a highly recommended surgeon who specializes in and is an expert on breast cancer, you can contact any of the following organizations:

✔ **The American Cancer Society** (www.cancer.org)

✔ **The National Cancer Institute** (www.nci.nih.gov)

✔ **American College of Surgeons** (www.facs.org)

✔ **American Society of Clinical Oncology** (www.asco.org)

✔ **Association of Community Cancer Centers** (www.accc-cancer.org)

Jane P.

"When I found my lump, my doctor was very comforting and told me that I was almost surely fine. I went back to him, and I said, "I know you're most concerned about treating my breast, but you've got to treat my mind, too.""

You can also call cancer survivors' support groups, which will provide you with personal advice and guidance. (You'll find a list of these groups in Chapter 23.)

Evaluating a treatment center

When choosing your doctor you also need to assess the treatment center with which he or she is affiliated. The center must have one or more of the accreditations shown in Table 9-1.

Table 9-1	Accreditations and What They Mean to You	
Accrediting organization	*What it means to you*	*Is it a go?*
Commission on Cancer of the American College of Surgeons	The treatment center meets the very stringent criteria of the commission, and you'll receive total cancer care.	Go for it!
Joint Commission on Accreditation of Healthcare Organizations (JCAHO)	JCAHO assesses the overall quality of medical care provided by a hospital (cancer and other).	If your treatment facility doesn't have at least this accreditation, you seriously need to consider getting to an accredited hospital or cancer center, even if that means traveling to another city. Make sure that your insurance (see Chapter 17) covers the other facility.
National Cancer Institute. (Many centers call themselves Comprehensive Cancer Centers as a marketing tool, but only those designated as such by the NCI meet the stringent requirements. Currently 41 such centers are accredited in the U.S.)	These facilities specialize in the treatment of cancer, including conducting the latest up-to-date research, which is especially important when you've been told that you have a complicated form of cancer.	Go for it!

Buddying up

Remembering everything that the doctor told you on your first visit is nearly impossible, especially when it involves the word "cancer." Whenever you can, bring someone who's close to you with you to the appointment, and ask him or her to take notes. You can even ask your doctor for permission to tape your conversation. If the doctor says that's all right, bring a small recorder with you. If need be, you can make another appointment to review what was said, ask questions, and begin discussing your options.

Reviewing Treatment Options by Stage

You probably want to know what your treatment options are, so you can make wise and informed decisions. That's what this section sets out to do. It describes what you can expect at each stage of your treatment, beginning with evaluation and going through all the various parts of your treatment, including the long period of follow-up.

We've organized this section according to the stage of your cancer (see Chapter 7 for more on cancer stages). Stages of cancer tell you how extensive your cancer is, what your treatment options are, and what your *prognosis* (projected outcome) is likely to be. The five stages are numbered 0 through IV, with 0 being the least and IV being the most advanced. All you need to do is pick the stage with which you've been diagnosed and follow that section.

Here are some terms to keep in mind when you explore any kind of treatment:

- ✔ **Local therapy:** Surgery to remove the lump, either by a *lumpectomy* (surgery to remove the cancerous lump and surrounding tissue) or a *mastectomy* (removing the breast tissue). Radiation is also part of local therapy.

- ✔ **Systemic therapy:** Treatment directed toward the entire body that's used when cancer has spread or the tumor is of a certain size.

- ✔ **Relative risk and benefit:** The risk and benefit of one group compared with another group. For example, women older than 50 compared with women younger than 50.

- ✔ **Absolute risk and benefit:** The actual numerical risk (usually expressed as a percentage) of something happening to a group of women like you.

As with any medical treatment, cancer treatment isn't a simple, black or white, yes or no, either or kind of issue, because so many factors determine your treatment options. Some of those factors are

✔ Whether the tumor has metastasized

✔ If the tumor has metastasized, then to what parts of the body

✔ Whether you have a familial or genetic predisposition toward breast cancer

✔ Your age

✔ Your general health

✔ Other variables

What's more, women, as a group, present a conglomeration of factors (yup, we're complicated beings!), making the treatment options even more complex.

Treatment for each stage of cancer is divided into four phases:

✔ **Evaluation:** A range of tests determines what type of cancer you have, whether it has spread, and then where it has spread.

✔ **Treatment:** This phase may consist of a menu of treatment options. It may also feature initial treatment that occurs before the main treatment, which is kind of like a preparation for the main treatment. It's known as *neo-adjuvant treatment*.

✔ **Prevention:** You may also undergo treatment after the main treatment, which is known as *adjuvant treatment* and includes treatment to reduce the risk of the cancer recurring, or returning.

✔ **Follow-up:** Consists of regularly visiting with your oncologist, who monitors how you're doing and checks for recurrence. How many times a year you need to see your doctor varies from once a month to once a year. You may be following up for a few years all the way to your entire lifetime.

These treatment guidelines are based on the latest research and medical information in scientific and medical literature, including the National Institutes of Health Consensus Panel on the Treatment of Primary Breast Cancer, The St. Gallen International Consensus Conference, and the National Comprehensive Cancer Network. All these guidelines were developed by groups of all the top specialists from the leading cancer hospitals and organizations around the world. Two important words of caution before you begin reading about the treatment that's applicable to you:

✔ These guidelines are only guidelines, a set of recommendations for you to discuss with your doctor and medical team, and not a list of hard-and-fast rules for you to stick to.

✔ Research continues. New treatments will become available after this book is published. This immediacy is one of the most wonderfully exciting facts about breast cancer research, but it doesn't work well with publishing deadlines, so make sure that you ask your doctor whether anything new has come up during the last few months.

Stage 0: Lobular carcinoma in situ

Lobular carcinoma in situ (LCIS) refers to cancer in the lobes of the breasts that has remained where it started. The lobes are the glands in which the milk is produced. (Chapter 2 contains a great explanation about the parts of the breast, and Chapter 4 has more about what *in situ* means.)

LCIS is sometimes classified as *Stage 0 cancer.* Although it is called Stage 0, and its name sounds like cancer, oncologists today believe LCIS isn't cancer but rather an abnormal growth of cells in the lobules. These abnormal cells indicate that you have a risk of developing invasive breast cancer sometime in the future, but you don't have cancer right now. The treatment options for this stage and the advantages and disadvantages of each option are illustrated in Table 9-2.

Table 9-2	Treatment Guidelines for Stage 0 Lobular Carcinoma in Situ (LCIS)	
Treatment	*Advantage*	*Disadvantage*
Close Observation:		
Yearly Mammogram	Noninvasive treatment	Does nothing to reduce the risk; only helps to detect cancer early.
Physician exam 2–3 times/year	Many women with LCIS never get cancer so they've avoided a more invasive treatment	
Monthly BSE (breast self-exam)		
Tamoxifen:	Reduces the risk of developing cancer by 56%	May have side effects, including hot flashes, vaginal discharge or dryness, and irregular menses in women who are premenopausal. If you're postmenopausal, it may increase your risk of endometrial cancer.
Prophylactic mastectomy:	Maximum risk reduction	Major surgery (more radical than for treatment of cancer) for a disease you may never get.

Evaluation

You can't detect LCIS by breast self-examination, and the doctor can't pick it up on a physical exam. Not even a mammogram can tell you. The only time that these abnormal cells are detected is when you have breast tissue removed for some other reason, and the pathologist detects the LCIS while examining the tissue.

A pathology review (see Chapter 6) also is recommended, again to ensure that the cancer is, in fact, *in situ* and has not spread.

Treatment

Studies have found that women with LCIS are at a greater risk of developing invasive breast cancer in the future; however, that risk is only 1 percent per year. If you develop cancer, it may occur in either breast, not only the one in which the LCIS was found. Instead of remaining in the lobes, the cancer will be the kind that begins in the lobes or the ducts and then infiltrates out of the lobes or ducts.

Fortunately, your doctor will monitor and follow up with you very carefully. However, if you have a strong family history of breast cancer or are unwilling to take the chance of developing breast cancer, you can discuss with your doctor the possibility of having a bilateral (both sides) mastectomy with immediate reconstruction (discussed in full in Chapter 15). This surgery substantially reduces the risk of developing breast cancer; however, it won't reduce your risk to zero. Nothing does yet.

This kind of bilateral mastectomy has other risks (after all, it is a major surgery), not to mention the tremendous emotional significance to the women who have it done. You absolutely do not have to make the decision with any sense of urgency. In fact, we strongly recommend that you weigh the risks and benefits of such a major step with your doctor and close family members. Most women opt simply for careful life-long observation.

Because LCIS isn't really cancer but is instead a risk factor for developing cancer in the future, the key to treatment is prevention. You have several options that you can consider to lower your chances of developing cancer in the future.

Prevention

More recent research has found that taking tamoxifen, an antiestrogen drug that is described in detail in Chapter 11, lowers the risk of LCIS patients developing an invasive cancer in the future. Your doctor won't prescribe this drug if you chose to have a bilateral mastectomy.

Despite its incredible ability to prevent breast cancer, this antiestrogen drug, like any other medication, has its own risks. If you're postmenopausal, it may increase your risk of *endometrial cancer* (cancer of the lining of your uterus).

Follow-up

If you choose not to undergo any procedures, then you absolutely must follow a careful monitoring program. This program includes a history and physical every 6 to 12 months and an annual mammogram. What a precious gift you've been given! For the price of a few hours at the doctor's office twice a year, you can protect yourself against developing cancer. This program is even more vital than seeing your doctor for an annual pelvic exam. Surely, that's a small price to pay.

If you're taking tamoxifen and still have a uterus, you must have an annual pelvic exam, because tamoxifen increases the risk of endometrial cancer in women who are past menopause. If you still menstruate every month, your period gets rid of the lining of your uterus and any potential cancerous cells. If, on the other hand, you're past menopause and notice any unusual uterine bleeding, you must let your doctor know immediately.

Stage 0: Ductal carcinoma in situ

The other Stage 0 localized cancer of the breast is potentially more serious. This type of cancer starts in the ducts but hasn't spread, which is very good news. However, if it's not appropriately treated, there's a high likelihood that the cancer will return, and when it does, it has a 50 percent chance of being the kind of cancer that spreads (infiltrates). In fact, doctors believe that if it's left untreated, DCIS will progress to an invasive cancer in most women. How fast does it progress? It depends. That's why it's so important to have the right treatment, even though it may seem rather harsh for such a good-news kind of cancer.

DCIS manifests itself in a variety of ways, and each of these varieties grows in a different manner.

Evaluation

The first step in the evaluation is determining the extent of the tumor. A regular mammography (see Chapter 4) doesn't provide enough information in such cases, so your doctor will refer you for *magnification mammography*, which is a magnified view of the specific area in the breast where the cancer is located. Magnification mammography involves a very small extra dose of radiation, and shows only a small portion of the breast (the part the doctor's worried about) not the entire breast like regular mammography.

A magnification mammogram gives doctors a better chance of seeing the tiny calcium deposits that may indicate DCIS. The more precisely doctors can pinpoint these deposits, the better your surgeon can determine which treatment is appropriate for you and how much breast tissue needs to be removed.

The radiologist screens both breasts, so that your team can determine whether cancerous cells also are present in the other breast. You'll also have a pathology review to make sure that the cancer is, in fact, contained (*in situ*) and has not spread.

Treatment

Wouldn't developing a treatment plan that was specifically for your particular form of DCIS cells be great, taking into account all your needs? Yes, it would be great, but we're sorry to say that medical technology hasn't advanced that far. But guidelines that help your doctor and you decide which treatment option to consider and what the pros and cons of each are can be found in Table 9-3.

Table 9-3:	Treatment Guidelines for Patients with Stage 0 Ductal Carcinoma In Situ (DCIS)	
Treatment	*Advantages*	*Disadvantages*
Lumpectomy alone	Least invasive Fewest side effects	Highest risk of recurrence in the breast and having to deal with cancer again
Lumpectomy and Radiation Therapy	Adding radiation therapy reduces risks of cancer	Some cosmetic changes occur (in other words a change in the size of the breast or an indentation) from the combination of surgery and radiation therapy Six weeks of treatment (radiation therapy)
Mastectomy	Lowest risk of recurrence	Major surgery for a disease that isn't life-threatening You lose your breasts

Cancer treatments have, however, made some progress. In the past, all women with DCIS were treated in exactly the same way: mastectomy. Today, with more knowledge, you have a wider range of options. The problem is that because your doctor can't determine exactly how your particular cancer will behave, the best that he or she can do at the moment is offer you a menu of options, and then join you in choosing the treatment that's right for you.

So how can you make the best choice for you when doctors don't know your exact prognosis? You weigh your risk of developing invasive cancer and how extensive the DCIS is with the benefits that each of the treatment options provides in preventing the recurrence of cancer. You have three surgical treatment options (which are discussed in more detail in Chapter 10):

✔ A lumpectomy (cutting out the cancerous tissue)

✔ A lumpectomy followed by radiation therapy

✔ A total mastectomy (with or without reconstruction, as you choose)

Tamoxifen may be used with any of these surgical treatments.

Here are questions you may be asking yourself:

✔ **When is a mastectomy absolutely necessary?**

If the cancer cells involve more than a quarter of the breast (*a quadrant*), you really need to have a mastectomy. You can choose reconstruction, if you want, but conserving the breast really isn't feasible when more than a quarter of it contains cancer cells. (Please see Chapter 10 where we discuss all the aspects of a mastectomy, including the psychological ramifications. See Chapter 15 for more about reconstruction.)

This recommendation is not made lightly. Completely recognizing and understanding the importance of breasts, no one would choose to have a mastectomy if it wasn't necessary. But consider this: If the cancer in the ducts is extensive, that means it's likely to be in the other ducts but too small to be seen on an X-ray.

The risk of cancer recurring in the breast after a lumpectomy in this circumstance is quite high, and a recurrence of invasive cancer brings with it a possibility of death. We aren't saying this to frighten you; we just want to be completely truthful and help you choose the option that helps save your life.

If you have DCIS and choose a mastectomy, your chance for a total cure is 98 percent.

✔ **Can I have a lumpectomy and radiation and keep my breast?**

You have this option if all of the following are factors:

• The cancerous cells are present in less than a quarter of the breast.

• The size of the tumor in proportion to the size of your breast is small enough such that the cancer can be completely removed and leave you with a fairly regular-looking breast.

- During surgery, the surgeon is able to remove the cancer without cancer cells being present on the edges of the tissue that is removed, a condition otherwise known as *negative margins.*

Sometimes, the tumor is large in proportion to your breast. When that's the case, the surgeon can't cut it out without leaving a big dent in your breast or leaving behind only a little tissue. In such cases, we recommend a mastectomy.

✔ **Can I have just a lumpectomy?**

You can choose this option if all of the following are factors:

- The DCIS is small (usually less than 1.0 to 1.5 centimeters in diameter).

- The cancer is completely removed with a good rim of normal tissue on all sides of the excision (see Chapter 10 for more information on these details).

- The DCIS is *low grade,* which means the cells don't look badly abnormal under the microscope. For more information see Chapter 6.

Good results have been achieved with a lumpectomy alone in women whose cancer meets all three criteria. On the other hand, two recent studies have been conducted in which women with DCIS were randomly assigned to treatment with lumpectomy alone or to treatment with lumpectomy *and* radiation. Both studies found that *all* the women who had radiation along with the lumpectomy reduced their risk of cancer recurrence, but the absolute amount of benefit varied from group to group. Before deciding to forgo radiation, discuss the benefits of radiation with your surgeon and radiation oncologist.

If you're older than 85 and your doctor says that medically you can either conserve your breast or have a mastectomy, make sure you that you explore the risks and benefits of both options before making a decision. Doctors sometimes may assume that when you're older you don't care about your looks or your sex life, which may or may not be the case for you.

Prevention

Tamoxifen is an option for women with DCIS when the cancer cells contain estrogen or progesterone receptors. Tamoxifen can lower the risk of an invasive breast cancer or more DCIS developing after the cancer in the ducts has been removed. The benefits depend on

✔ Your type of surgery

✔ Whether one or two breasts are at risk

- Your own personal risk of recurrence
- Your age
- Your overall health

Follow-up

Regardless of what treatment option you choose, you need to see your doctor on a regular basis to make sure that the cancer hasn't returned. You need to schedule a history and physical exam every 6 to 12 months for five years and a mammogram every year. During the first year or two after treatment, when your breast is changing — the swelling goes down after surgery (see Chapter 10) and scar tissue that can occur after radiation and surgery develops — your doctor may want you to have mammograms of the breast that was treated twice a year. After the five-year period, and if all is well, you can cut your visits back to once a year and continue with the mammograms on an annual basis.

If you're taking tamoxifen *and* you're postmenopausal *and* you still have your uterus, you must have an annual pelvic exam, because, under those conditions, tamoxifen increases your risk of endometrial cancer. You can't let it slip the way you sometimes let your annual exam slip (come on, admit it, you know you do). If you still have a uterus and you notice any unusual uterine bleeding, you must let your doctor know immediately.

Stages 1 and 11

In Stage I, the tumor is about 2 centimeters or less in diameter and hasn't spread beyond the breast. In Stage II, the tumor is larger than 2 centimeters in diameter and/or has spread to the lymph nodes under the arm on the same side as the tumor; however, the lymph nodes aren't stuck to one another or to any surrounding tissue.

Julia W.

"After I found out that I did have cancer, it just kind of took the wind out of me. I had to stop for a few minutes and then regroup, and the physician was talking with me. We both decided living was better, even if that meant living without a breast or without a part of a breast as opposed to not living at all. I agreed with him because I enjoy life."

Scanning for friends

Friends may suggest that you have multiple scans or X-rays to see whether your breast cancer has spread. Of course, they say that because they read about it on the Internet or because someone else they know had it, and they do it out of love and concern for you. However, experts have studied these tests in thousands of women and found that scans for Stage I and Stage II cancers in women who have normal chemistry (normal blood test results) and no symptoms almost never find cancer. What these scans often find are things that you've probably had for years and that usually are completely normal, and then you end up having more tests to find out whether you have cancer. We've seen how this problem causes women a huge amount of anxiety, only to find out that they don't have cancer anywhere else at all. All that unnecessary worrying was for nothing. That's why we advise you not to have multiple scans when your doctor doesn't recommend them.

In Stage I and Stage II breast cancer, your overall treatment may include more than one treatment phase: the primary treatment, additional postsurgery treatment, and another treatment *before* your primary treatment.

Evaluation

Before you start any treatment, you must undergo many tests. The purpose of these tests is to give your medical team as much information as possible about all the various aspects of your cancer, which they need to be able to evaluate the treatment options that are best suited for your particular circumstances. Many of these tests are done on the cancer cells and are not something you have to do. Here's a list of the most common ones:

- **Mammography of both your breasts.** This test enables doctors to see precisely where the cancer is.

- **A pathology review.** The pathologist reviews tissues taken from the breast during biopsy and tests them in the following manner:

  - Evaluating S-phase or Ki-67 factors, which show how fast tumor cells are dividing (See Chapter 6), even though these tests are not always proven to be beneficial.

  - Checking for genes (HER-2/*neu* is one) that make the cells grow much faster than they should. Cells with too many HER-2/*neu* receptors grow very fast, but they also respond well to certain chemotherapy combinations (see Chapter 6).

- Determining the hormone-receptor level, which shows your team whether the tumor will be receptive to hormonal therapy. Again, see Chapter 6 for more info.

✔ **Chemical tests.** One example of a chemical test is a liver function test. This test is necessary because medications are processed by your liver, and your doctors need to make sure that your liver can handle it.

✔ **Blood tests.** The doctors need to know whether you are anemic or have any other blood abnormalities.

✔ **A bone scan.** This test may be done when blood test results indicate that the cancer may have spread to the bone. Enzymes from the bone are released into the blood. If these levels are high, a bone scan must be done. The bone scan suggests whether these abnormalities are caused by cancer, arthritis, or other bone disease.

Presurgery treatment

In some circumstances, women with Stage II and Stage III cancers can have chemotherapy before surgery. Huh? Isn't that putting the cart before the horse? Well, yes and no. Usually, chemotherapy is given after surgery to kill the cancer cells that remain in the body. Presurgery chemotherapy, however, shrinks the tumor to such an extent that, in some cases, a lumpectomy (which removes the tumor) rather than a mastectomy (which removes the breast) is possible.

Presurgery chemotherapy is a good option for you when you really want to keep your breast *and* you have a single tumor that is large relative to the size of your breast. To find out whether you're a candidate for lumpectomy, the surgeon must determine whether cutting out the tumor that remains after chemotherapy is possible. Bear in mind that the surgeons won't be able to make that determination until *after* you finish with your chemotherapy, so having presurgery chemo doesn't guarantee that you'll be able to keep your breast. (Chapter 10 talks more about mastectomy; Chapter 12 discusses chemo.)

Primary treatment

Your options depend on the various findings from your tests, including the size of the tumor, the spread of the cancer, and other factors.

Every woman with Stage I and Stage II usually, as a first step, has *local therapy* — treatment geared toward that particular area of the body. But treatment doesn't end there. Regardless of whether you have a lumpectomy or a mastectomy, you have one or most of the lymph glands under your arm removed. If you have a lumpectomy, radiation will be part of your treatment after surgery. The primary treatment options are presented in Table 9-4 and Table 9-5.

Table 9-4	Primary Treatment Options in Stage I and Stage II Cancers: For the Breast	
Treatment	*Advantage*	*Disadvantage*
Lumpectomy and Radiation Therapy	Allows you to keep the breast	You'll need 6 weeks of radiation therapy
	90% of women think it looks excellent or good	Small risk (less than 10%) of needing a mastectomy in the future if the cancer comes back
Mastectomy Alone	Radiation therapy usually not needed	Chest is numb
	No more mammograms on that side	Need to wear an external prosthesis (Chapter 15) if you don't have reconstruction
Mastectomy & Reconstruction	You don't have to wear an external prosthesis	Having reconstructive surgery may mean having more surgery
	Radiation therapy not usually needed	A reconstructed breast and nipple don't have normal sensation
	No more mammograms on that side	

Table 9-5	Primary Treatment Options in Stage I and Stage II Cancers: For the Underarm Lymph Nodes	
Treatment	*Advantage*	*Disadvantage*
Sentinel node biopsy is done only if:	Small operation with rapid recovery	Small risk (less than 5%) of needing further surgery if your nodes enlarge in the future
No clinical evidence exists that cancer is in the nodes	No drain tube after surgery	
	Very small risk of arm swelling (lymphedema)	

(continued)

Table 9-5 (continued)

Treatment	Advantage	Disadvantage
Axillary dissection is done if:	Gets rid of the cancer in the armpit area very effectively	Requires a drain tube after surgery
Clinical evidence exists that cancer is in the nodes	Very low risk (less than 3%) of cancer	Lifelong risk of arm swelling (lymphedema)
Sentinel node biopsy can't be done (in other words, if you're pregnant)		More painful than breast surgery
Your sentinel node can't be found		
Your sentinel node contains cancer		

Here are some questions you may be asking yourself:

✔ **Does a lumpectomy alter the shape of my breast?** A lumpectomy usually causes relatively small changes in shape and size of the breast. Most studies show that 90 percent of women themselves rate the cosmetic appearance of their breasts after a lumpectomy as excellent or good.

✔ **Is a mastectomy the only option?**

The five circumstances under which breast-conserving surgery absolutely *cannot* be considered are

- You have two or more primary tumors in separate parts of your breast.

- You've undergone several surgical attempts to remove the cancerous lump, but each time, the margin of the removed tissue has had cancerous cells.

- You're in your first or second trimester of pregnancy. Radiation treatment can harm your unborn child.

- You've previously had radiation treatments on your breast.

- You have many calcifications in your breast that appear malignant.

In addition to these five circumstances, conserving your breast may be difficult when your symptoms include any of the following:

- A history of an autoimmune disease, such as *scleroderma* (a disease of the connective tissue) or *systemic lupus erythematosus* (SLE).

Radiation may worsen your disease. You may have severe shrinkage of the breast or develop skin problems, if you have radiation.

- A very large tumor and small breast. A lumpectomy cannot be done in a way that's cosmetically appealing. However, chemotherapy to shrink the cancer may make a lumpectomy possible.

- A very large breast, so that radiation can't be given in a uniform way to the entire breast. If you have an experienced radiation oncologist, however, this problem is rare.

Even after meeting all the criteria for a lumpectomy, some women nevertheless choose to have a mastectomy instead. They do so because they believe that if they just remove the breast, the cancer won't come back. The reality, however, is that if you have Stage I or Stage II breast cancer and have a mastectomy or lumpectomy with radiation, your chances of surviving are exactly the same.

✔ **Do you treat the nodes, too?**

Axillary dissection, or removal of the lymph nodes under the arm, is very effective in getting rid of cancer cells in the armpit (see Figure 9-1). However, if no cancer cells are present in those nodes, removing them doesn't benefit the woman at all. In fact, it is accompanied by an unpleasant side effect called *lymphedema,* or swelling of the entire arm, which means women may be required to wear an elasticized stocking on the affected arm. The thing is, the only sure way that the surgeon can tell whether cancer cells are present in the underarm lymph nodes is by removing them and examining them under the microscope.

Sentinel node biopsy is a tool that was recently developed for reliably finding out whether the lymph nodes contain cancerous cells (see Figure 9-2). The procedure involves removing only one or two of the nodes that are the first ones into which the cancer drains — thus the name "sentinel." Your surgeon finds it by injecting radioactive particles, blue dye, or a combination of both into your breast on the day of surgery. The lymph node that turns blue or radioactive first is the sentinel node. If the sentinel node doesn't contain cancer cells, none of the other nodes are likely to contain them, either.

You may not be able to have a sentinel node biopsy for the following reasons:

- You have an abnormal or worrisome node, which can be felt in your armpit. Those kinds of nodes have to be removed, so sentinel node biopsy doesn't provide any useful information.

- You're pregnant or nursing. The radioactivity and the blue dye used to find the sentinel node aren't safe for pregnant or nursing women.

- You've had previous surgery in your armpit, which may change the way cancer cells spread in the armpit thus rendering sentinel node biopsy much less accurate.

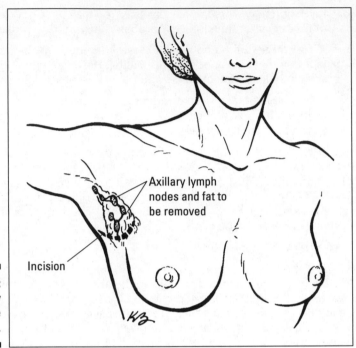

Figure 9-1:
Axillary
node
dissection.

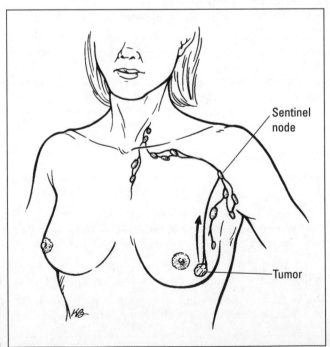

Figure 9-2:
Sentinel
node biopsy.

Postsurgery treatment

You've completed your primary treatment. Why should you have more of what is known as *adjuvant therapy*? Minute cancer cells may have spread. In fact, some chance of this happening exists whenever your tumor was larger than one centimeter in diameter (See Chapters 6 and 7 for implications of size), even if your surgery was deemed a success.

Several factors determine whether you're through with treatment after surgery or whether you need additional treatment after surgery. Tables 9-6 and 9-7 illustrate these factors.

Table 9-6	Post-treatment Necessity and Route You're Likely to Take	
The factor	*Do you need further treatment?*	*What treatment?*
Lymph nodes did not contain cancer cells and the tumor is less than or equal to 1 centimeter in diameter	No, but if tumor had hormone receptors, tamoxifen can be considered for prevention of new cancers in the opposite breast.	Tamoxifen
Lymph nodes contain cancer cells	Yes	With negative hormone-receptor results you'll receive chemotherapy. With positive hormone-receptor results, you'll receive chemotherapy and endocrine therapy. If you're hormone receptor–positive and older, you may receive endocrine therapy only.
Tumor measures greater than 1 centimeter in diameter and the lymph nodes do not have cancer cells	Yes	When you're hormone receptor–negative, and pre- or postmenopausal, you'll receive chemotherapy. When you're hormone receptor–positive and premenopausal, you'll receive tamoxifen plus chemotherapy. When you're hormone receptor–positive and postmenopausal, you'll receive antihormonal drugs or treatment that prevents the body from creating hormones (aromatase inhibitors) and possibly chemotherapy depending on your level of risk.

Table 9-7		Will You need Radiation After Surgery?
Stage	*After a Lumpectomy*	*After a Mastectomy*
Stage I	Always	Almost never
Stage II	Always	If more than four nodes have cancer cells, Yes
		If 1–3 nodes have cancer cells, maybe
		If no cancer cells are found in any of the nodes, rarely

All this information is a lot to remember. Here's a suggestion: Take this book to your next appointment, turn to this chapter, and ask your doctor to highlight the areas that pertain to you.

Treatment after surgery

Regardless of whether you have a lumpectomy or a mastectomy, you may have a course of chemotherapy after the surgery. If your cancer is hormone-positive, you'll also be prescribed an antihormone drug. In addition, you may undergo more treatment, depending on the type of surgery you have:

- **Lumpectomy:** You need radiation therapy, which usually is given after you complete chemotherapy.

- **Mastectomy with more than four cancerous lymph nodes:** You need radiation therapy. When fewer than four lymph nodes are involved, the benefits of radiation are controversial.

- **Mastectomy with none of the nodes involved:** Radiation therapy rarely is needed.

Follow-up

Guidelines for Stage I, Stage II, and Stage III breast cancers are similar.

- If your cancer was *invasive* (spread beyond the cells where it started), you need to see your doctor every few months for two years. If all's well after, then the rate of visits drops off.

- If you had a lumpectomy, you need a mammogram six months after you complete your radiation therapy, and then a yearly mammogram.

- If you had a mastectomy you need a mammogram of the other breast every year after surgery.

- If you're on tamoxifen and still have your uterus, you must have an annual pelvic exam. Report any abnormal uterine bleeding to your doctor immediately.

Stage III

If Stage III is your diagnosis, it can mean several different things. Either your tumor is larger than 5 centimeters in diameter and has spread to the lymph nodes, or the tumor is any size, has spread to the lymph nodes, and they're attached to one another or to surrounding tissue. Or perhaps your cancer has spread to the skin or chest wall or the internal mammary nodes under your breastbone.

Inflammatory breast cancer (a rare form of breast cancer described in Chapter 2) also is grouped in Stage III.

Not everyone with Stage III breast cancer has the same extent of the disease. In fact, Stage III is further divided up into Stages IIIA and IIIB, which are dependent upon the size and other characteristics of the tumor and the number of nodes involved. That's why your treatment options vary depending on whether you're diagnosed with Stage IIIA (see Table 9-8) or Stage III B cancer, (see Table 9-9).

Evaluation

Many of the tests for Stage III cancer are the same as for women with Stage I and Stage II forms of the disease, which are described in detail earlier in this chapter. However, if your blood-test results indicate that the cancer is in other parts of your body, or if you have any other symptoms of spreading cancer (See Chapter 16), you may also need a few additional tests, including a bone scan and an MRI or CAT scan of your abdomen.

Table 9-8	Surgical Options in Stage IIIA Breast Cancer	
Procedure	*Advantages*	*Disadvantages*
Modified Radical Mastectomy with or without radiation	Immediate pathology information to guide your postoperative treatment	You lose your breast You have to wear an external prosthesis (if you don't choose reconstructive surgery) Your chest will be numb
Chemotherapy before Surgery and Try to Have A Lumpectomy (Instead of a Mastectomy)	May allow you to keep the breast Tells you if your cancer is sensitive to (will be killed by) the particular chemotherapy used	You don't have the complete pathology before your treatment. Doesn't always result in being able to have a lumpectomy, but you needed chemo anyway.

(continued)

Table 9-8 *(continued)*

Procedure	Advantages	Disadvantages
Modified Radical Mastectomy and Reconstruction (with or without Radiation Therapy)	You'll have a new breast	Having reconstructive surgery means having additional surgery Your reconstructed breast and nipple won't have the sense of feeling of your natural breast If you need radiation therapy, it may alter the appearance of the reconstruction

Table 9-9 Surgical Options in Stage IIIB Breast Cancer

Options	Treatment must include
No options are available.	Presurgery: Chemotherapy first to shrink the cancer so that it can be removed surgically Surgery: Modified radical mastectomy (your choice whether you want a reconstruction), which includes removing the lymph glands under your arm. After surgery: 1. Radiation therapy 2. More chemotherapy possible and 3. If the tumor is hormone receptor–positive, you may have hormonal treatment.

Treatment

All the treatment options that your doctor can offer you are described in great detail in the various cancer treatment options listed in the "Stage II" section earlier in this chapter, so we only describe them briefly here.

Stage IIIA

If your tumor is larger than 5 centimeters and has spread to nodes under your arm, but the nodes are not stuck together or to any other surrounding tissue, you have two options for treatment:

> ✔ **Modified radical mastectomy.** In this surgery, the surgeon removes your breast and underarm lymph nodes. You can choose to have reconstructive surgery, either immediately or later.
>
> ✔ **Chemotherapy before surgery followed by a lumpectomy.** A lumpectomy allows the breast to be saved, provided the tumor shrinks enough to make this type of surgery possible.

If your cancer has been diagnosed as Stage IIIA, but the nodes under your arm are stuck together or stuck to the tissue around them, you're then reclassified as a IIIB and your treatment guidelines are like the ones listed for Stage IIIB in the section that follows.

Table 9-10 tells you what your post-treatment options are for Stage IIIA.

Table 9-10	Stage IIIA: Post-treatment Necessity and Treatment You'll Need	
The factor	*Do you need further treatment?*	*What treatment?*
Mastectomy and the tumor is hormone receptor–negative	Yes	Chemotherapy after surgery Usually radiation to chest walls and nodes
Positive hormone-receptor status	Yes	Chemotherapy after surgery Usually radiation to chest wall and nodes Hormonal treatment after chemotherapy
Lumpectomy (you had chemotherapy presurgery) and positive hormone-receptor status	Yes	Hormonal treatment if cancer is hormone receptor–positive Probably more chemotherapy Radiation to breasts in addition to lymph nodes

Stage IIIB

Treatment for women with Stage IIIB breast cancer starts with chemotherapy to help shrink the tumor to a state where it can be operated on. If the chemotherapy is successful and the tumor shrinks enough, you'll have surgery: modified radical mastectomy, which includes removing the lymph glands under your arm. This treatment may be followed by more chemotherapy. Reconstruction, if you choose it, is usually not done during the mastectomy but rather at a later date.

After surgery, you'll have radiation therapy to the chest, the nodes above your collarbone, and the nodes that are inside your chest wall. If the tumor is hormone receptor–positive or unknown you'll receive an antihormonal drug.

When chemotherapy isn't successful and the tumor remains too large to operate on, you may have to have radiation treatment before surgery. Radiation usually reduces the tumor sufficiently for the surgeon to operate. If, however, it doesn't shrink enough (rare), there's no effective standard treatment. You and your doctor will have to decide on an individual plan of treatment that suits you and your family.

Follow-up

Guidelines for Stage I, Stage II, and Stage IIIA breast cancers are similar:

✔ When your cancer is invasive (spread beyond the cells where it started), you need to see your doctor every few months for two years, and then the rate of visits will drop off.

✔ If you had a lumpectomy, you need a mammogram six months after you complete your radiation therapy, and then a yearly mammogram.

✔ If you had a mastectomy, you need a mammogram of the other breast every year after surgery.

✔ If you're on tamoxifen and still have your uterus, you must have an annual pelvic exam. Report any abnormal uterine bleeding to your doctor immediately.

Stage IV

Fortunately today, few women are initially diagnosed with Stage IV breast cancer — that is, cancer that has spread to distant parts of the body.

If you've been diagnosed with Stage IV breast cancer, you need to know that not all Stage IV cancer is the same. In some women, the cancer has metastasized to the bone and stayed there, while in others, it has spread more widely throughout the body. In some women, the cancer grows slowly (which results in a better prognosis), but in others, the cancer is very aggressive, spreading quickly and making treatment much more difficult.

Because of the variations in cancer — how fast it spreads, where it spreads to and several other factors — defining exactly what your treatment and prognosis will be is difficult.

If you've been diagnosed with Stage IV breast cancer, your treatment has two goals:

- ✔ Improving or maintaining the quality of your life
- ✔ Prolonging your life

Your doctors should give you treatment that doesn't leave you toxic, nauseous, and miserable. If your quality of life is awful, your remaining years will be difficult. Yes, we said it: your remaining years. How long you have to live depends. Very few women with Stage IV disease die soon after they're diagnosed. The average time alive is two to three years, but the variability is great.

More recently, studies have shown that with the right treatment (such as with hormonal treatments, chemotherapy, and combinations of chemotherapy and Herceptin, (a drug that acts against tumors with the gene HER-2, a gene that spurs the cancer cells to grow faster), the lives of women with Stage IV cancer can be extended.

In determining the right treatment for you, your doctors must determine whether the cancer has spread beyond the *supraclavicular* lymph nodes (the ones above your clavicle). If it hasn't, you'll receive the same treatment as women with Stage IIIB breast cancer. If it has, several other important decisions must be made before you decide on treatment. Table 9-11 presents those decisions.

Table 9-11	Treatment for Stage IV Cancer That's Spread Beyond Supraclavicular Lymph Nodes
The factor	**What treatment?**
Hormone receptor–positive, spread of the disease affects only bone or soft tissue (in other words, chest or abdomen lymph nodes)	Tamoxifen or if you are postmenopausal, aromatase inhibitors (which prevent estrogen from being made).
Hormone receptor–negative	Chemotherapy.
Cancer has spread to one or more internal organs (for example, your liver) and hormone–receptor positive	Chemotherapy is a possibility, plus hormonal treatment.

You may want to consider asking your doctor about participating in a clinical trial. These studies of promising new treatments that are not yet widely available are investigated to determine whether they're safe and effective. As such, they often offer hope after regular, more well-established treatments have not.

Being Pregnant: Special Considerations

Unfortunately, more women are being diagnosed with breast cancer during pregnancy than was the case in previous years. This increase probably can be attributed to the fact that more women are delaying pregnancies until they reach their late 30s and early 40s, ages at which breast cancer is more common than when they were in their 20s. Because your breasts change during pregnancy, and you're probably thinking more about your baby than you are about cancer, breast cancer can end up being detected at a later stage of the disease in women who are pregnant (in other words, when the disease has progressed further).

The most difficult part of facing breast cancer when you're pregnant is making a decision about treatment. The general approach is: "Abort the cancer, not the baby," but ultimately you and your family make that decision. How far along you are in the pregnancy is an important factor in deciding what you need to do.

Pregnant women who have breast cancer are more likely to end up having a mastectomy, not because they have bigger tumors but because radiation therapy to the breast area is not safe for an unborn child. Once the pregnancy has progressed to the second trimester, certain chemotherapy agents are safe and can be used without affecting the unborn child. Tamoxifen, one of the more successful hormonal treatments, cannot be given to pregnant women because its effects on the fetus are not known.

Women of childbearing ages obviously have certain other considerations to deal with when facing breast cancer. The issue of fertility is an important one, and you need to discuss it thoroughly with your oncologist, because chemotherapy can induce premature menopause, especially in women older than 40. You may also want to talk with a reproductive endocrinologist before starting chemotherapy.

Rolling Hot Off the Presses: Recent Developments

Medicine and research move in steps, sometimes more slowly than we'd like, but they do progress. Here are a few of the most recent developments in breast cancer research:

- Prophylactic (preventive) mastectomy reduces the risk of breast cancer by about 90 percent in women who are at high risk for developing breast cancer (family history of breast cancer).

- A sentinel node (first node with cancer) can be identified in more than 90 percent of women with breast cancer. The false-negative rate is less than 5 percent.

- New endocrine treatments have increased treatment options for women with metastatic cancer that is hormone sensitive. As more studies are completed, researchers may find that these treatments can be used as the treatment after surgery or even as a method of prevention.

Part III:
Buckling Up — Traveling Through Treatment

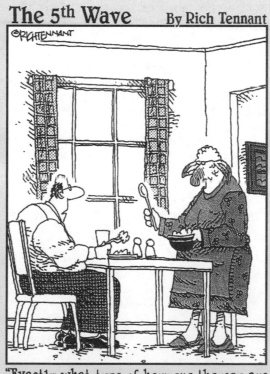

The 5th Wave   By Rich Tennant

"Exactly what type of hormone therapy are you taking?"

In this part . . .

Your choice of treatment options depends on many factors that you explore when participating in and making decisions about your course of treatment. This part describes the nuts and bolts of what to expect from surgery (Chapter 10), radiation (Chapter 11), chemotherapy (Chapter 12) and/or hormonal therapy (Chapter 13), and strategies for evaluating and deciding on the most up-to-date treatments available. Ways of coping with the unpleasant and arduous side effects of therapy are suggested in this part, including the devastation of losing one or both of your breasts. Chapter 15 explains reconstructive surgery alternatives, and Chapter 14 provides information about deciding on complementary and alternative methods used by cancer survivors. If the cancer returns (a recurrence), Chapter 16 provides you with what you need to face that challenge and come out a winner. The realities of life with breast cancer are covered in Chapter 17, where we familiarize you with insurance benefits and legal rights.

Chapter 10

Knowing What to Expect from Surgery

Almost every woman who's diagnosed with breast cancer requires some form of surgery as part of treatment, be it lumpectomy or mastectomy. This chapter describes the various surgical treatments you may have, and what to expect from them.

In addition to providing an overview of the surgeries, which is only part of your treatment, we give you an idea of what you can expect before your operation, during it, immediately after surgery, and after you're back home. (Your full treatment plan varies, depending on a host of factors that we discuss in detail in Chapter 9.) We also provide you with a list of questions to ask your surgeon so that you can find out more helpful information about each of these phases.

Note: The terms *doctor* and *surgeon* are interchangeable in this chapter.

Studying the Surgeries

The primary purpose of surgery is to get rid of as much of the cancer as possible in an attempt to prevent its *recurrence,* or return. Since the discovery of breast cancer treatment more than a hundred years ago, the medical world has completely revamped its thinking. When treatment first was described, medical experts thought that a cure was most likely when they removed the entire tumor, the rest of the breast, the muscle on the chest, and the lymph glands. However, when clinical experience didn't show a better prognosis for women who had this radical mastectomy, less radical forms of surgery were found to be successful. Today women even have the option of choosing between the following two types of surgery:

- **Breast-conserving surgery.** In the most common type of breast cancer surgery today, surgeons remove (or *excise*) the cancer in a surgery called a *lumpectomy* (or lump removal), all the while making every attempt to preserve as much of the shape and size of the breast as possible.

- **Mastectomy.** Preserving your breast isn't always possible (see Chapter 9 for reasons why). When your breast cancer falls into that category, you'll have a *mastectomy,* which is the surgical removal of all the visible part of your breast (see the "Mastering mastectomies" section later in this chapter). It differs from the old-fashioned radical mastectomy — the chest muscle is now saved.

In Chapter 9, we discuss your various treatment options, including surgery, in detail. Take your time to review these options and discuss them with your doctor. Make sure that all your questions are answered. Don't feel too embarrassed to ask anything, and together with your family and your doctor, you can come to a decision about what surgery and treatments you're going to have.

Conserving your breast

Whenever doctors are able to do so, they try to conserve your breast by removing only the cancerous lump rather than the entire breast.

Here's the dilemma: On one hand, the surgeon's goal is the removal of all the cancer, which means making sure that the *margins* (the outer edges) of the breast tissue that is removed are free of cancer. (More about lumps can be found in Chapter 4.) To do that, the surgeon must take out even more tissue than is cancerous. On the other hand, the surgeon wants to make your breast look as good as possible and doesn't want to remove more than is necessary. Sounds like an impossible task, doesn't it? Fortunately it isn't.

Surgeons like Dr. Monica Morrow, a coauthor of this book, and others have developed guidelines for professionals in their field regarding who should and shouldn't have breast-conserving surgery. The guidelines are based on the latest research. For example, when a *magnification mammogram* (a mammogram that offers an enlarged view of the cancer in your breast) shows that the cancer is localized, the surgeon can safely perform breast-conserving surgery.

Are you ready for some really encouraging news? Breast-conserving surgery has very few complications. In fact, it's usually done as an outpatient surgery or with an overnight stay.

Surgeons perform two different types of breast-conserving surgery that are defined by the size of the cut and how much skin and breast tissue has to be removed:

- ✔ *Lumpectomy,* **wide local excision:** Most people know this type of surgery simply as a *lumpectomy.* Doctors, however, include the additional descriptor, "wide local excision," which defines the surgery a little more specifically. An incision is made in the skin to reach the tumor, but skin is not removed unless the tumor's stuck to it. The tumor and a small margin of the surrounding (cancer-free) breast tissue are then removed, as shown in Figure 10-1.

- ✔ *Quadrantectomy:* This fancy-sounding name simply means, "removing a quarter (fourth)." This type of surgery is usually performed on women whose primary tumor is so large that a small lumpectomy isn't possible. In this surgery (illustrated in Figure 10-2), in addition to the tumor, a larger area of the breast surrounding it, from the nipple all the way to the top edge of the breast, is removed. The amount of breast tissue that's removed is wider and deeper than in a simple lumpectomy, and the skin that covers the tumor sometimes is also removed.

When a larger amount of breast tissue and skin are removed, it stands to reason that a larger dent will remain in your breast. If your breasts are small, and you need a large amount of breast tissue removed, your surgeon probably will not recommend a quadrantectomy but rather a mastectomy with reconstruction. Despite surgeons' careful attempts to achieve as normal looking a breast as possible, it isn't always possible. Other aspects that affect cosmetic outcome include swelling and retraction after radiation treatment (which usually stops three years after you complete radiation treatment).

Lumpectomy leader

For many, many years, mastectomy was considered the only way to treat breast cancer surgically. In the 1980s, an Israeli president's wife decided that she wasn't going to have a mastectomy, choosing, instead, to have a *lumpectomy.* This decision caused such a furor in Israel that you would've thought she was inciting women to rise up in rebellion against all that was decent and good in the world. Fortunately, for all women, medical research has come a long way since then.

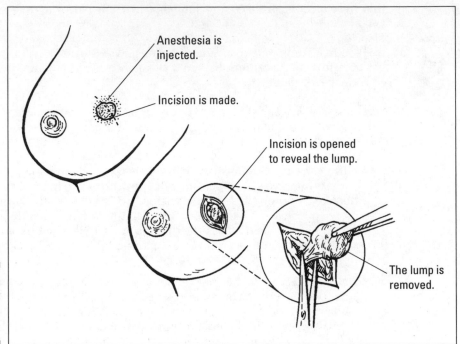

Figure 10-1:
Lumpectomy,
wide local
excision.

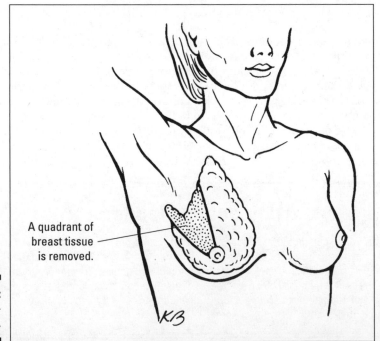

Figure 10-2:
Quadran-
tectomy.

Under certain circumstances, a lumpectomy absolutely is not an option. For example, if you've been diagnosed with DCIS or invasive cancer, and the cancer cells have spread to more than a quarter of your breast, a mastectomy with or without immediate reconstruction is strongly recommended. These circumstances are listed by the stage of your cancer.

Many women who are eligible for breast-conserving treatment often are not offered that option.

Be sure to ask your doctor, "Am I eligible for breast-conserving therapy?"

- ✔ If the answer is no, you can then ask your doctor to explain the medical reasons why you aren't eligible.
- ✔ If the answer is yes, you can then ask your doctor to discuss this treatment option with you. You may decide not to choose the breast-conserving option, but at least you've explored it.

Mastering mastectomies

Twenty-five years ago a mastectomy meant that a woman had her entire breast, including the chest muscles and lymph nodes under her arm, removed. This surgery was known as a *radical mastectomy,* and it certainly was *radical.* Fortunately, here's another area in which medicine has made progress. (Although we agree with you that it sometimes feels like it just isn't moving fast enough.)

Women don't have to have radical surgery anymore. If you're told that you need a radical mastectomy, get a second opinion.

Getting a second opinion

A recent study found that more than half of all cancer patients sought a second opinion. Guess what? Women with breast cancer were the group who sought a second opinion the most. Almost three-quarters of them did. Dr. Monica Morrow's recently published study of women who sought second opinions found that the reason most women who were eligible for breast-conserving surgery but didn't have it was that the doctor hadn't told them about their options. (Dr. Morrow is a coauthor of this book.)

When treatment team members reviewed the treatment plans for these patients, a different treatment was recommended for almost a fourth of them. If getting a second opinion is an option that your insurance carrier permits, go ahead and do it. Even when your insurance doesn't cover it, you may want to pay for a second opinion yourself, because it's that important. Although you may get the same recommendation, you nevertheless have explored your options.

Nowadays, surgeons perform two kinds of mastectomies:

✔ **Modified radical mastectomy:** Although we use one term, modified radical mastectomy (see Figure 10-3), it nevertheless refers to a few different surgical procedures, depending on what's done to the *pectoral muscles* (muscles attached to the front of the chest wall and upper arms). These muscles usually can remain intact, but there are occasions when the smaller, deeper *pectoralis minor muscle* is cut out partially or entirely, depending on the spread of cancer.

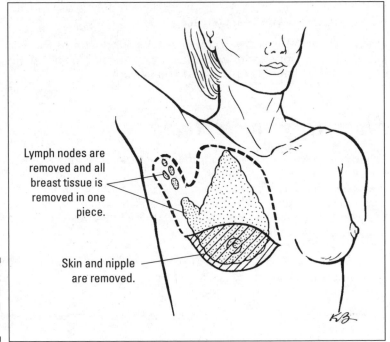

Lymph nodes are removed and all breast tissue is removed in one piece.

Skin and nipple are removed.

Figure 10-3:
Modified radical mastectomy.

In all types of modified radical mastectomies, all the breast tissue, the *fascia* (covering) of the pectoral muscle, and some of the axillary lymph glands are removed, as are the nipple and areola. If you had an open biopsy (a diagnostic surgical procedure described in Chapter 4), your surgeon will remove that scar on the skin as part of your new incision. Sometimes the skin and fascia that don't have to be removed can be preserved for reconstruction.

After all the breast tissue is removed, the surgeon inserts drains under the skin flap and the wound is sewn up. (See the "Healing wounds: Draining is a pain" section later in this chapter.)

Jen H.

"I decided, with my husband, to have both breasts removed because of my past history with fibroid adenomas. I couldn't imagine a future overcome with anxiety as I worried whether the lumps in my remaining breast (the other one had to be removed because of the cancer) were cancerous. No doubt existed that I'd always have more lumps, and for my piece of mind, I needed to get rid of both breasts forever. This decision was not a hard one for me, but we wondered whether insurance would cover the removal of the noncancerous breast or whether we'd be paying for it on our own. It was coming off, no matter what the cost. The insurance came through and I had immediate reconstruction."

✔ **Total or simple mastectomy:** This procedure is the same as a modified radical mastectomy, except that the pectoral muscles and the axillary nodes are kept intact. Removing the lymph nodes can cause *lymphedema* (a swelling of the arm that can become a permanent, uncomfortable condition, we describe it in the "Lymphedema" section toward the end of this chapter.) Simple mastectomy is becoming the most common form of surgery performed today, now that sentinel node biopsy is available.

✔ **Skin-sparing mastectomy:** If you're having reconstructive surgery, instead of removing the skin, the excess skin of the breast is preserved, and the covering of the pectoral muscles can also be safely preserved if it makes reconstruction easier. This type of procedure can be done with either a modified radical mastectomy or a simple mastectomy. (Check out Chapter 15 to find out how this skin is then used in rebuilding your breast.)

Women with DCIS, Stage I, Stage II, or Stage IIIA breast cancer, and women who have a prophylactic mastectomy are eligible for this process. As you can imagine, this type of procedure requires much more technical expertise, but it's being done more and more frequently, and women who have it are most appreciative of the results.

✔ **Prophylactic mastectomy:** Women who are at high risk for breast cancer (see Chapter 3 to find out whether you are) may choose to have a mastectomy to reduce the risk of getting breast cancer. The decision to undergo this procedure obviously is not one you jump into, but as we explain in Chapter 3, it's something you discuss at great length with a genetic counselor, your doctor, and your loved ones.

Joanne B.

Advantages of a double mastectomy (partial list):

✔ "I will develop some expertise in prosthesis (also known as falsies) and may rely on them whenever a party gets boring.

✔ "Men have to admire me for my mind.

✔ "When I spill food (as I do often) it lands on my jeans now. Not so noticeable.

✔ "I know what I'm talking about when I call someone a 'useless tit.'

✔ "My confused 91-year-old Mom is even more certain that I'm my dad or the son she never had."

Disadvantages of a double mastectomy (partial list):

✔ "I don't have the shelf that holds a few cookies while I'm working on a row of knitting.

✔ "I'll have to put my pasties and tassels in my hope chest.

✔ "I'll never win a wet T-shirt contest — maybe runner-up or booby prize.

✔ "I won't ever be able to be a topless waitress. Perhaps, if I'd had a single mastectomy, I could have obtained part-time work."

Lillie S.

"My husband told me, 'You're not losing part or all of your breast. Your surgeons' mission is to transform you from a victim into a survivor and sail you up that survival curve today.' I tell that to every woman I meet whose been diagnosed with breast cancer. You're exchanging your breast for another chance at life, and that's a fair trade, I think."

Easing into Presurgery

Some women prefer going into surgery with no knowledge of the procedure; others prefer reading every book, article, and Internet site on the topic. Each of these extremes can be a little dangerous. Not knowing anything prevents you from being properly prepared for the experience, including knowing what questions to ask your doctor. On the opposite side of the coin, knowing about *everything* can have you so freaked out that you may not want to go through with the surgery at all.

No matter what your natural inclination is, experts agree that having some information (not necessarily every piece of info ever documented), having your questions answered, and knowing what to expect can help you go through surgery with greater ease.

Meeting with your surgeon

Meeting with your surgeon is a good first step in this process. See Chapter 9 for a full description of your treatment team. During your meeting you need to be able to do the following:

✔ **Become familiar with your surgeon.** I'd feel very uncomfortable if someone I didn't know, no matter how great the surgeon is reputed to be, was going to operate on me before I had the chance to become acquainted with that person. This is your opportunity to ask:

- **What's your experience with women with breast cancer? How many women with breast cancer do you treat every year? What kind of surgical procedures do you perform?** The answers to these questions give you an idea of the extent of the surgeon's experience with women in similar situations. If the surgeon has little experience and you have a choice, keep looking for a surgeon you're comfortable with.

- **Are you board certified?** This means the surgeon's been trained in a specialty. You should only see a surgeon who's board certified in general surgery or board eligible (waiting to take the exam.)

- **Are you affiliated with a medical school?** This indicates the surgeon's active in this field and up-to-date with the latest research and findings. Although this affiliation is not a necessity, it can be a real plus.

- **What's your perspective on my surgery? What are my options?** Explaining whether you have options, what they are, the pros and cons of each, and specifying why one or other procedure is being recommended indicates that the surgeon isn't performing surgeries in cookie-cutter fashion. Including you and your family in the decision-making indicates the surgeon's respect of each patient as a unique individual.

- **What is your perspective on nodal surgery? Will you perform a** *sentinel-node biopsy* (examination of first lymph node under the arm, described in full in Chapter 9)? This indicates whether the surgeon is able to perform the more up-to-date form of testing for cancer in the nodes under your arm.

- **What can I expect from my surgery? How long is the healing period? What side effects, if any, can I expect? Will you be following me up in the hospital? How long will I be there?** This gives you an overview of how the surgeon expects your surgery and recovery to be.

   Do you feel as though you're being railroaded into a particular treatment or that your questions aren't being answered? If your insurance coverage (or your pocketbook) permits, seek a second opinion. In fact, second opinions are encouraged. (Chapter 9 explains this in greater detail.)

✔ **Help your surgeon become familiar with you.** This includes

   - Providing a full medical history.

   - Making sure that the medical information your surgeon has about you is accurate, including whatever medications you're currently taking. Your list of meds needs to include prescription drugs, over-the-counter medications, vitamins, and supplements. Some may increase your risk of bleeding and have an effect on how you heal after surgery.

✔ **Discuss your decisions.** Discussing your decision is especially important when you have to make choices about whether you're having a mastectomy or breast-conserving surgery, whether you're having reconstruction, and so on. A good doctor listens to your opinions and guides you with advice, without forcing an opinion on you.

Here are a few questions that you may want to ask your doctor:

✔ **Will I have the surgery outpatient or inpatient?** A mastectomy is usually done inpatient, but many breast-conserving surgeries can be conducted as outpatient surgery. Ask what your doctor suggests.

✔ **What are the risks of my getting an infection after the surgery?**

✔ **What are the risks of my getting _lymphedema_ (swelling of the arm, explained later in this chapter), and what can be done to prevent it?**

✔ **What do I need to do to prepare for the surgery?**

✔ **What can I expect when I go home?**

✔ **What can I do to prepare for when I get home?**

Although the biopsy shows that you have breast cancer, the extent of your cancer won't be known until you receive the results of the pathology tests after the surgery (discussed in Chapter 6). These findings determine what additional treatment you need to have after surgery. You may want to discuss these treatment options with your surgeon. That way, you'll know what your treatment options are and what possibilities to expect after surgery.

Breast cancer surgery for men

For men who have breast cancer, preserving the breast is difficult because their breasts are small and the primary tumor is usually located in the center of the breast. The usual treatment for men with breast cancer is a mastectomy. If the tumor isn't stuck to the pectoral muscle, a modified radical mastectomy is usually performed. If the cancer has spread widely in the pectoral muscle, a radical mastectomy may be necessary, although men, like some women, can be treated with chemotherapy before surgery to shrink the tumor (see Chapter 12 for more details on this treatment).

Giving consent, getting instructions

A *consent form* explains the procedure you're about to undergo, including other procedures that may happen in an emergency. The consent form is the contract between you and the surgeon: what you expect the surgeon to do and what the surgeon indicates will be done. It requires your agreement and signature to allow the surgeon to perform the operation.

You can ask for this form to be mailed to you in advance so that you can read it in detail and prepare your questions before you meet with the doctor. Most doctors and hospitals comply with this request. When you don't understand something, don't be shy about asking. It's your body and your life, and having an understanding before you sign for what procedure you're going to have and all that entails is really important.

You may be presented with three kinds of consent forms:

- ✔ **Surgery:** This form, which includes a description of the particular surgery you'll be having, gives the surgeon permission to operate on you. It also includes consent for general care during the operation, and often for blood transfusion, if it's needed during surgery.

- ✔ **Anesthesia:** A separate consent form gives permission for the anesthesiologist to administer drugs to put you to sleep (general anesthesia) or make you drowsy during surgery.

- ✔ **Research:** Sometimes the hospital is participating in a research study and may ask you to be a part of it. The study and its purpose and all the potential benefits to others will be described in this consent form. Even though the study may not directly benefit you, it may help many other women in the future. (A *clinical trial* is one specific type of research described in Chapter 9.) Participating in research is purely voluntary and it's your choice whether to participate.

In addition to the consent form, you may be asked to do some things before surgery:

✔ **Stop taking any medication (including aspirin) that will prevent your blood from clotting, for about a week or two before surgery.** Ask for a list of these drugs and check *all* your medications against it.

✔ **Donate blood in case you need a blood transfusion.** You probably won't need it (few women do, and even then, it's only in cases of certain major reconstructive surgery), but just in case, it'll be ready for you.

✔ **Avoid eating or drinking anything for a certain time period before surgery.** This is especially important if you're going to have *general anesthesia* (described later in this chapter).

Heading in to Surgery

Today is the day you go into surgery; you may come out with a breast very different from the one you have now. You may feel relief that the cancer is being taken out of your body or horrified at the thought of what you are about to go through. You may be anxious about the surgery or impatient about getting it over with. You may feel all of these things. One thing you can be sure of. You will be going through several steps and knowing what to anticipate at each step along the way helps make the process much easier.

Talking with the anesthe-zzzz-iologist

At some point in time before the surgery, you meet with the anesthesiologist. That meeting may be the day before surgery or the morning of, depending on the circumstances. In that meeting, the anesthesiologist asks you questions about your medical history and your current state.

When the anesthesiologist asks you questions, be honest. Not revealing everything or giving half-truths can hurt you. If you're taking illicit drugs, tell the anesthesiologist. If you ate before the surgery, even though you weren't supposed to, tell the anesthesiologist. Your meeting with the anesthesiologist is a time to be honest and precise, because the anesthesiologist can't do a proper job without accurate information from you. Believe us, the anesthesiolgist isn't there to judge you. You won't shock him. He's heard it all before!

Finally, the anesthesiologist talks to you about your anesthesia options. Because breast surgery is extremely safe, even when you have certain medical conditions that preclude you from having a general anesthesia, other anesthetic options are available that you can safely have.

Your own personal bridge over troubled waters

Regardless of whether you have inpatient or outpatient surgery, make sure that someone you care about comes with you. Having this person with you is about more than just having a ride home; you're going to need moral support. After all, this isn't just your toe that's being operated on.

On the other hand, what if everyone in your large family wants to come with you, leaving you overwhelmed and exhausted? Just remember that you're the one who's going through the surgery, so feel free to ask as many or as few people to be present as you're comfortable with. The rest of the clan can come see you when you're feeling better.

Most people consider the anesthesiologist to be the doctor who keeps them asleep during surgery. Although that's true, in fact, the anesthesiologist is also the doctor who makes sure that you

✔ **Get hooked up to an intravenous line (IV) through which your medication is administered.**

✔ **Stay alive during and wake up after the operation.** The anesthesiologist does this by administering a combination of drugs based on your body's unique metabolism. (The risk of dying during breast surgery is less than the risk of being struck by lightning!) The anesthesiologist's other responsibility is to keep you pain-free, both during the surgery, and immediately after it. (More on pain later in this chapter.)

✔ **Can breathe during the surgery.** Some of the anesthetic drugs paralyze you, so that you don't cough or move during the operation. Therefore, a tube is placed down your windpipe and connected to a breathing machine. The anesthesiologist also makes sure that when the tube is removed, you're ready and able to breathe on your own.

✔ **Do (or don't) need a pre-med.** A *pre-med* is a light anesthetic that helps calm you before you're given the main anesthetic. Whether you receive a pre-med is usually determined by a combination of factors, including anxiety, the surgery, and the preference of the particular anesthesiologist. Talk to your anesthesiologist about this option. (Once, after getting a lovely dose of pre-meds, I was greeting and waving to everyone in the hospital corridors as though they were all my long-lost best friends.)

Sashaying in to the operating room

It's time to get in costume — hospital gown, paper cap, and warming socks (Don't forget to ask for the warming socks!) — and hit the operating room

(O.R.). The nurse helps you get settled into bed. The orderly, a doctor, or a nurse wheels you into the operating room. The particular type of surgery you have (see "Studying the Surgeries" section earlier in this chapter) determines the amount of time that you're in the O.R. You usually aren't in there for more than a few hours.

The entire O.R. team is present for surgery, although they may not all be there when you're first wheeled in. The team includes your surgeon, the nurse (or two), the anesthesiologist, and perhaps one or two additional assistants.

You're well monitored during surgery. In addition to the anesthesiologist making sure that you're unconscious and receiving oxygen, your blood pressure and heart rate are also monitored.

After the surgeon completes the surgery, inserts the drain (if you need one), and sews up the wound, the nurse bandages it. The breast tissue that's removed is sent to the laboratory for testing. The anesthesiologist removes the breathing tube and makes sure that you can breathe on your own. You're all done. Now you're wheeled into the *recovery room,* where you join other patients who are recuperating after outpatient surgery. Nurses and other staff monitor you there.

Morning, sleepyhead

Don't expect to open your eyes and be ready to jump out of bed. General anesthesia takes time to work its way out of your body. You'll probably feel groggy for a little while, so just rest. This day isn't for conquering the world; you can always tackle that one later, if you insist! Your body's been through plenty, but you made it. Close your eyes and rest for a while.

When you wake up you may

- ✔ **Feel cold and shivery.** You'll be covered with blankets, but don't hesitate to ask for more.

- ✔ **Throw up.** It won't last long. Ask your nurse for a bucket and a wet cloth. (A bedpan or trash bin will do, too.) Ask your nurse or family member to wipe your forehead and mouth with a clean wet cloth, and you'll soon be feeling much better. (I have a friend who's been with me through all my surgeries, and somehow or other, I've always managed to throw up on her. Poor girl!)

- ✔ **Not feel much pain.** Of course, in the beginning, this lack of pain is because of the anesthetic. However, even after it wears off, you probably won't experience much pain. If you do, tell the nurse and ask for some pain medicine.

✔ **Be bandaged.** You won't be able to see your wound for a while.

✔ **Have drains.** In that case, you'll see them protruding from under the bandage (as shown in Figure 10-4). You don't have to do anything to them immediately, so don't worry about them now.

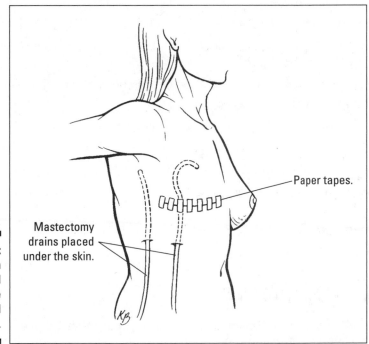

Paper tapes.

Mastectomy drains placed under the skin.

Figure 10-4: Wound with wound closure strips and drain.

When you're staying in the hospital for 24 hours or more, you may have a visit from someone from Reach to Recovery or a similar program. The woman who visits you has gone through breast cancer surgery in the past. Her job is letting you know how to access services that you may need in the future and giving you a temporary prosthesis (more on this in Chapter 15) to take home as a starting point. She's also there as a living witness that a meaningful and healthy life is not only a possibility but also a reality after breast cancer surgery.

Getting the heck outta Dodge

Your surgeon or the recovery room nurse will give you a sheet of instructions and go over with you how best to care for yourself when you get home. You'll probably be groggy, so ask the surgeon to go over it with the family member or friend who brought you in. If you have questions the next day, call the nurse at your surgeon's office.

Make sure that you have the following questions answered before you leave:

- How do I take care of my wound?
- What do I have to do to take care of the drains?
- How will I recognize whether I have an infection?
- What do I do if I have pain?
- When should I begin using my arm? How? Are there movements I shouldn't do? Should do?
- Should I exercise or not? If so, what kind of exercise?
- When can I wear a bra again?
- When can I begin wearing the prosthesis?
- What can I eat, or should I not eat?
- How do I make an appointment with a Reach to Recovery volunteer?
- How do I know what I should call you or your nurse about and what's normal?
- When is my next appointment with you?

You're Going Home

Depending on the type of surgery you have, you'll either be an outpatient or be discharged within a day or two. Most women want to go home, where they feel more comfortable. You may be concerned about how to take care of your wound and drains, but after you read this section, you'll be able to manage with little difficulty.

If you can't do it yourself, make sure that you ask a friend or family member to help. If you have no one you can count on, ask the social worker at the hospital to find you someone who can assist you.

Feeling pooped

You'll be tired when you get home. That's to be expected and completely normal. After all, apart from the physical trauma your body has experienced, you have to consider the emotional and psychological aspects of losing a breast. Respect your body's need for rest.

Ruth R.

"I noticed a difference between my two periods of recovery. I was out of work for ten days with the lumpectomy and nodal surgery, but went back sooner after the mastectomy because I felt fine. My surgeon assured me that the second surgery was indeed more invasive. The only explanation I could figure was that I had become a mom five and a half years after the lumpectomy — I had adopted a school-aged son. My world was different now. I think just having him around me made me feel better quicker."

If you haven't already done so, start becoming aware of your needs and expressing them to others. If your friends want to visit, and you're not too tired, let them come. If you need to rest, ask them to wait until you're awake or just sit beside you quietly. It's completely up to you. Friends and family often are unsure what to do, and they'll have to take their cues from you (see more about friends and family in Chapter 20.)

Friends may want to help but don't always know how. Ask them to do things for you that you can't do at the moment: Ask a friend who loves your children to take them to a movie, and another who lives near you to do your grocery shopping. A friend who's a great cook can bring over all the food she wants to cook; even if you don't feel like eating it now, your family and visitors will certainly appreciate it.

Preventing pain

Most women who have breast cancer surgery don't experience much pain, and if they do, it's only for a short time.

Your surgeon will prescribe pain medication pills for the first few days after surgery. Take them only as your doctor prescribes them. In fact, you'll probably discover that you won't need them for as long a period of time as the doctor prescribes. Although people sometimes tell you to put hot or cold pads on for pain, avoid putting anything on your incisions unless directed to do so by your doctor. Your skin at the incision is numb, and you could burn it.

Most pain pills can cause constipation, so if that happens to you, eat fruit, dried fruit, or other roughage.

Nan R.

"I have to say, being an expert on surgeries (after having many of them for all kinds of ailments), this was by far the easiest one I ever had."

Handling severe pain

Experiencing any of the following is a rare occurrence, so if it happens to you, be sure that you call your doctor.

- New severe pain.
- No relief from existing pain, despite taking the medications.
- Nausea, confusion.
- An inability to walk, eat, or urinate.

Feeling phantom pain

Have you ever heard of a soldier whose amputated leg itched or hurt? That's called *phantom pain*. The same thing can happen with some women who have a mastectomy. Some women experience sensations that the breast is still there, even in a breast that's been removed for weeks, months, and, in rare circumstances, several years after the mastectomy.

Healing wounds: Draining is a pain

Your wound may be covered with a bandage so that you can't really see your chest for a few days. Under the bandage, the wound is probably taped with wound closure strips (sterile tape strips that hold a wound closed really well). You don't need to worry if the wound closure strips come off; the stitches are buried under the skin.

Once you leave the hospital you're responsible for caring for your wound and changing the dressing. Your surgeon will tell you how to take care of all this until your next visit. At that time, the surgeon looks at how well it's healing and advises you on the next steps.

If you have a mastectomy or an axillary dissection, you may also have one or two drains — one from your breast and the other from under your arm —

taped down onto your chest (as shown previously in Figure 10-4). These drains are plastic or rubber tubes open on one end in the wound with a plastic bulb on the other end that collects the fluid. The drain helps direct fluid that accumulates in the wound.

Your doctor or nurse shows you how to empty the drains every day into a measuring cylinder that you get from the hospital before leaving after surgery. When you empty the drains, you record the amount of fluid that comes out so your surgeon can monitor when it's okay to remove the drain. It's easy to do: Open the bulb and the fluid pours out. Although you're likely used to handling your own body fluids, this process can make you a little queasy. The drains are removed as soon as drainage drops to a level where the surgeon thinks it's safe to remove them, usually less than an ounce per day. The removal, although not painful, produces a weird pulling feeling. Drains usually stay in for a week or two.

Going back to bra-sics

Comfort is of utmost importance considering your return to wearing a bra. If you had a lumpectomy, you probably need some type of chest-area support. An older bra that's a little loose and doesn't have underwire usually is best.

After a mastectomy, the hospital may give you a special surgical bra. Sometimes, the doctor may not want you to wear a bra while the drains are in.

When that's the case, you can get a mastectomy bra after your drains are out. The bra, which is designed especially for women who've had this kind of surgery, gives you the support you need on your shoulders and under your breast without cutting into or pushing on the area of your breast that's been operated on. Wearing this kind of bra also helps you avoid needing to raise your arms or struggling to control awkward straps. You can get these bras at department stores, mastectomy boutiques, or online. (Try www.tlccatalog.com.) See Chapter 24 for tips about how to find these specialty stores in your area or online.

Reviewing side effects and complications

After surgery, you may experience one or more of the side effects described in the subsections that follow; however, most are rare.

Pulling, pushing, and pain

You may experience

- ✔ Uncomfortable tightness
- ✔ Pulling, especially under your arm
- ✔ Bruising
- ✔ Pain

Exercise is the best way to get rid of these problems. Your surgeon usually provides you with instructions about when you can start stretching and what movements to do. Whenever necessary, you may also receive a referral to a physical therapist.

Numbness

After a mastectomy, the skin of the chest area is numb. This numbness is unavoidable because of the severing of the tiny nerves that ran between the breast and the skin. After a year or two, most women get some feeling back, and many get lots of feeling back.

Eventually, you'll get to know how and where you want your breast and scar touched or not touched. After you find out, you need to make your intimate partner aware, too. Chapter 19 can help you get there.

Infections

Some women may develop infections after breast-conserving surgery or mastectomy. Examples include an *abscess* (boil) or *cellulitis* (inflammation of the tissues). These infections usually occur within 5 to 14 days after surgery, and cause

- ✔ Pain that is usually mild at first but can increase in severity.
- ✔ Redness that spreads away from the incision. A small ¼-inch area of redness around the incision and drain is normal.
- ✔ Swelling that's more than was present during the first day or two after surgery.
- ✔ Fever that's in excess of 100 degrees Fahrenheit (F).

If you're one of the few people who develops these symptoms, let your doctor know. If, for example, you spike a high fever in the middle of the night, call your doctor's answering service to find out whether you need to go the emergency room or pick up prescribed antibiotics.

Continued fluid buildup

In some women, fluid continues accumulating even after the drains have been removed. This problem is called a *seroma*. Seroma usually occurs in women who are obese, who've had an open biopsy followed by a mastectomy, or whose cancer has spread to many nodes.

If this buildup happens to you, you must return to the doctor's office, so the fluid can be drained.

A fluid buildup may result in an infection and a delay in the healing of your wound. If fluid continues to build up after drains are removed, tell your doctor. This is more of an inconvenience than an emergency, but the best way to get rid of the fluid is to drain it off.

Lymphedema

Lymphedema, a swelling of the arm caused by a buildup of lymph fluid, is a word that's dreaded by any woman who's had breast cancer surgery that involved removal or radiation to the axillary lymph nodes. Lymphedema is different than a *seroma* where fluid is in a space left by surgery. With lymphedema, the fluid is in the tissue itself. One in five women who've had their lymph nodes removed, or who've had radiation to their nodes, is at risk for developing some amount of lymphedema; however, in most women, lymphedema is mild. (We describe the lymph nodes and their relationship to breast cancer in Chapter 3.)

If you have lymphedema

- The skin of your arm feels tight.
- Your wrist and/or hand feel like they can't move much.
- Your arm feels full or heavy.
- You can't fit into your regular shirts or wear your rings or watch even though you haven't put on any weight.

Doctors are hopeful that as *sentinel node biops*y (described in Chapter 4) becomes more commonplace, the risk of lymphedema will decrease. However, women whose cancer has spread to the lymph nodes and who, therefore, have to have them removed, continue to face the risk of lymphedema. The other real bummer is that it can develop at any time after the surgery — even many (10 or even 20) years later.

To minimize the risks of infection and of lymphedema developing in months and even years after surgery, you need to take proper care of yourself. The American Cancer Society recommends that you do your best to avoid infection, because no infection means a lower risk of developing lymphedema. Here are some of the ACS's proper-care recommendations:

✔ Whenever you have to have blood drawn, an IV, or an injection, get it in the arm opposite where you had your surgery.

✔ Wear protective gloves when you do housework or gardening, and wear insect repellant outdoors.

✔ If you shave your legs and underarms, use an electric razor. It's less likely to cause cuts or graze your skin.

✔ Keep your nails and cuticles moist with cream, and don't use scissors to cut loose skin.

✔ If you sew, use a thimble.

✔ If you do get a cut on your hand or arm, wash it, smear it with antibiotic cream, and cover it with a small bandage.

✔ Avoid sunburn. Use sunscreen and stay out of the sun.

✔ Use oven mitts when you cook and don't stand too close to oil in pans to avoid getting burned.

✔ Avoid excessive heat, such as from hot tubs or saunas.

The ACS also recommends that you avoid constricting your arm by

✔ Not wearing tight clothing or jewelry.

✔ Not using shoulder straps for your heavy purses or briefcase.

✔ Wearing a bra that doesn't dig into your shoulders.

Call your doctor's office if you notice swelling (regardless of whether it's painful) that lasts for a week or two. This may be a sign of lymphedema.

Confronting Surgery's Emotional Consequences

So far, we've discussed the physical aspects of your surgery. However, you obviously must factor in some psychological consequences, too. What these consequences entail and their extent differ from one woman to another.

However, several emotional aspects with which all women who undergo breast cancer surgery must contend include getting acquainted with your altered body, recognizing the possible effect that surgery can have on your own image and your intimate relationships, and waiting for the results of your pathology report. (In Chapters 18 and 19, we discuss some of the common feelings you may experience, and some of the ways to help you cope.)

Carol M.

"Having a mastectomy is devastating to a woman. Just look around you and see why. Breasts have been the focus of female anatomy as perfect pecs are to males. Well, if you lose a breast, and even if you have reconstruction, you won't be exactly the same as you were before the surgery. I had to learn to come to terms with my new body."

Getting to know your new body

When to look at your newly defined breast is entirely up to you. Some women want to do it immediately; others want to wait until they feel stronger. Some prefer to be alone when they look at the wound; others want a loved one present. Don't feel pressured either way.

Don't be too concerned when you're scared to look at your new body; take whatever time you need. Some women rip open their pajamas to get the first look over with, others do it more slowly. Some women take one quick glance and never look again. How you confront your new appearance is entirely up to you. You may choose to do it when you're alone in your room or to have your partner standing beside you. It's an individual choice.

No emotion is the wrong one when you see your new body. You may scream or burst into tears, you may silently cry, or you may simply be silent. If you burst into hysterical laughter that turns into a wail of tears, it's okay. If you scream so loudly that you alert the neighbors, too bad for them. And if you make no sound at all, except the crying in your heart, it's your choice. There is no right or wrong way.

You may even be surprised that it doesn't look as bad as you'd imagined or feared, especially after a lumpectomy.

In time, and with support from other survivors, your loved ones, and your friends, you'll love and embrace your body and learn to love who you are. In the words of my friend Cyndi: "There's more to life than my left breast."

Coping with it between the sheets

Intimacy also is often a concern. You may worry that your sexual partner may not find you appealing anymore. If you don't have a partner, you may worry that no one will find you attractive. The issue of sexual pleasure also is a concern. If you no longer have a nipple, you may be concerned about not being able to feel, even when you get a newly constructed breast. You may also have a concern because any touch to your breast is no longer pleasurable and may even be uncomfortable.

All these concerns are completely natural but from a medical perspective, you can have sex whenever you want to. In Chapter 19, we describe the many ways you can rekindle intimacy after your mastectomy.

Waiting for the other shoe to drop

You can't know for sure what the next step will be until you receive your pathology results. Chapter 5 decodes that bugger for you.

You can predict some things, though. For example, if you had breast-conserving surgery, you will have radiation. However, you may also require additional surgery if the margins of the breast tissue that was removed had cancerous cells, because that means not all the cancer was removed.

Waiting isn't easy under any circumstances, and especially when you're waiting for the possibility of more bad news. When you've just had surgery and you feel weak, stiff, and vulnerable, it's even more difficult.

Know one thing: You aren't alone on this journey. In Chapter 16, we give you suggestions for looking after yourself, and in Chapter 14, we describe several methods for helping you get through this trying time. In these chapters, you'll be able to find some things that can help you move on as soon as you know what the next phase of your treatment involves.

Carol M.

"The first four or five times I had sex with my husband after my surgery, I cried and cried in his arms because I felt so ugly. He, being the saint that he is, convinced me that I was a beautiful person and that the body didn't mean that much to him. I had to realize that my body never would be the same again, that the reconstruction I had wasn't that great, and that I'd always be lopsided and missing a nipple, until I decide to undergo more surgery, which I had decided against. Every day of my life I am reminded of my breast cancer and that this is it. And, after considering the alternative (death), having one good breast isn't all that bad."

Chapter 11

Knowing What to Expect from Radiation Therapy

• •

In This Chapter:

▶ Destroying hidden cancer cells

▶ Evaluating the effectiveness of radiation therapy

▶ Regarding the risk of radiation therapy

▶ Understanding what to expect before and during treatment

▶ Surviving the side effects

• •

Regardless of what kind of surgery you have to remove your cancer, you can never be sure that all the cancer has been removed. Cancerous cells may be lurking about, and you know what those cancer cells do when they're left undestroyed? They multiply. Some of the crafty little devils even find ways to spread to other parts of the body, growing and causing havoc on their journey. (See Chapter 4 for a description of how breast cancer cells do this.)

When cancer cells are lurking around after surgery, they can be found in three types of places: local, regional (spread to nearby lymph nodes), or systemic (spread into the bloodstream). What can you do about these criminals? Call the police, of course. The police probably can chase away the *local* hooligans and arrest the *regional* thugs. They can scare them enough that the thugs and hooligans never return. However, the police definitely have a much harder time reaching all those *systemic* gangsters, and may have to call in a larger, more powerful organization, like the FBI, to help with a systematic way of dealing with this widespread scourge.

Think of *radiation therapy* as police force sharpshooters. In the same way that crack sharpshooters are extraordinarily accurate in pinpointing their targets, able to shoot just the criminal and no one else, radiation therapy works in a similar way. *Radiation therapy,* which is when radiation (think X-ray) is beamed directly at the regional cancer cells, is discussed in this chapter. We also explain about its risks and benefits and focus on what you can expect during this form of breast cancer treatment.

Opening Fire via Radiation

Directing a stream of high-energy particles or waves, such as *X-rays* or *gamma rays*, at cancer cells damages their DNA. The damage prevents the cells from dividing and reproducing themselves, and as a result, the cancer can't grow. (See Chapter 4 to meet these little fellows known as cancer cells.) Radiation can be directed very accurately at a specific part of your body. When it is, the radiation destroys cancer cells in

- ✔ The skin of the chest wall where your breast was removed (the *local area*)
- ✔ The lymph nodes under your arm (the *regional area*)
- ✔ The remaining breast tissue if you've had a *lumpectomy* (removal of the cancerous lump and some surrounding tissue)

However, if cancer has spread to other parts of the body, radiation therapy *cannot* destroy it. You'll have to have *systemic* treatment, which is achieved through chemotherapy (described in Chapter 12) or hormonal therapy (see Chapter 13). That's why radiation therapy always may be considered only a part of your larger treatment plan and not the entire treatment.

Giving Radiation a Thumbs Up: Effectiveness

Removal of the cancer through surgery always is a part of your treatment, but radiation therapy may or may not be a part of it. Whether you have radiation treatment depends on a combination of factors like the type of cancer you have, how aggressive it is, how far it has spread, and several other variables (see Chapter 9 for a full list). For example

- ✔ If you have a lumpectomy for *invasive cancer* (or cancer that has spread beyond the cells where it started), radiation to the breast always will be a part of your therapy.
- ✔ If you have a lumpectomy for *ductal carcinoma in situ* (cancer that has started in the ducts of the breast that has not spread, also called DCIS), radiation often but not always is used.
- ✔ If you have a mastectomy for invasive cancer, you may receive radiation depending on your level of risk of having a recurrence.

✔ If you have a mastectomy for DCIS, radiation is almost never given because the cancer cells have not moved beyond the ducts (that's what *in situ* means) and the ducts have been removed in the mastectomy.

After breast-conserving surgery

In breast-conserving surgery, the risk of cancer cells remaining, lurking or hiding close by always is a threat, even when the surgeon does an immaculate job of carefully removing them. That's why radiation is so important if you have breast-conserving surgery. It zaps those cancer cells that may be lurking behind and reduces the risk of recurrence significantly. For example:

✔ In one large study of women with invasive cancer who received radiation treatment, radiation reduced the risk overall by 75 percent. To the individual woman, the absolute benefit was a reduction from 35 percent likelihood of recurrence to 10 percent likelihood.

✔ In another study of women with DCIS who were given radiation therapy, the absolute benefit was a reduction from 14 percent likelihood of recurrence to only a 4 percent likelihood.

However, your particular benefit may be greater or lesser, depending on the characteristics of your particular cancer, so you need to talk to your doctor.

Surveying survival

The only way of knowing whether a treatment improves a woman's chance of survival is by conducting a clinical trial in which some women receive radiation therapy and some don't. Researchers then follow both groups of women for many years to determine whether the women in one group survive longer than the women in the other.

Several of these studies were conducted many years ago, in the 1970s and 1980s. In fact, those clinical trials were among the first to be done. So what's the problem? Well, the way radiation therapy was delivered in those decades is much different than radiation treatments used today. In the past, radiation therapy could cause damage to the heart. In fact, many of the studies found that radiation therapy reduced deaths from breast cancer but increased deaths from heart damage.

More recently, a *review study* was completed. That's the kind of study in which researchers review *all* the studies ever done on a subject and reanalyze the data. I'm glad I'm not doing it, because it involves tons of really complicated statistics! Anyway, the researchers concluded that as long as doctors can find ways of avoiding damage to the heart, which newer techniques seem to do, radiation therapy adds a small survival benefit.

The results of these large studies are clear. If you're eligible for and have breast-conserving surgery, and you follow it up with radiation, you substantially reduce the rate of local recurrence.

After mastectomy

Two important reasons for having radiation therapy after you've had a mastectomy are

- ✔ To reduce the risk of local and regional recurrence. This is a proven benefit.

- ✔ To improve your chances for survival by killing the lurking local and regional cancer cells that may be resistant to chemotherapy. Yes, some of them may not be affected by chemotherapy but can be killed by radiation therapy.

Even though your breast has been removed through a mastectomy (see Chapter 10 for a full discussion of this surgery), a very real risk of local recurrence exists. The risk varies depending on the number of lymph nodes to which the cancer has spread. It

- ✔ Is low (2 percent to 10 percent) for women whose cancer hasn't spread to the lymph nodes

- ✔ Rises to as high as 30 percent in women whose cancer has spread to the nodes. The risk increases proportionally to the number of nodes to which the cancer has spread. In short, the more nodes involved, the more likely the cancer is to return to the area where the breast used to be.

Once cancer returns, it can be controlled only in half of the women in whom it returns.

So, if you've had a mastectomy, check out Table 11-1 to see how much radiation reduces your risk of recurrence.

Table 11-1	So You Had a Mastectomy. Now What?	
The cancer	*Will you have radiation?*	*Recurrence rates?*
You're considered at high risk if the cancer has spread to at least 4 lymph nodes and/or the tumor was very large.	Yes.	Radiation therapy has been shown to significantly reduce the risk of local recurrence (by at least two-thirds) in women who've had a mastectomy and who are at high risk for recurrence.

The cancer	Will you have radiation?	Recurrence rates?
Has spread to 1 to 3 nodes.	Maybe.	A large clinical trial currently is testing this situation. While awaiting results, your doctor will consider the size of your tumor, the amount of cancer in the nodes, and other factors that affect the risk of local recurrence.

The results are very clear. When you've had a mastectomy, and you're at high risk for recurrence, adding radiation to your treatment substantially lowers the likelihood of having a local recurrence.

Knowing Nearly Every Pro and Con

Just like any other treatments, radiation therapy has its pros and cons. In the treatment of breast cancer, it fortunately has many more pros than cons.

Pros

Because of incredible advances in technology, radiation therapy is much safer now than it was in the early days of its use. The result is an ability to treat breast cancer with radiation at a considerable reduction in risk by

- ✔ **Delivering the radiation at an angle:** The machine that delivers radiation is so precise now that it delivers radiation at an angle that bypasses the heart and lungs. This system is called *tangential radiation,* because the radiation is delivered at a tangent to the breast rather than directly at the patient's body.

- ✔ **Precisely calculating radiation angles:** Radiation oncologists are able to calculate the *precise angles* at which the rays need to be directed, or focused, toward your breast so that they reach the particular area where the cancer is (see "Measuring for Treatment" later in this chapter).

- ✔ **Precisely calculating radiation dosages:** Amounts of radiation can be calculated so precisely that each part of the breast gets the same amount of treatment. Look down at your breasts. Their curves aren't perfectly symmetrical. So if they're irregular, how can you be sure that each part of the breast gets the same amount of radiation? Scientists have found ways of measuring the *precise dose* that needs to be delivered to a particular part of the breast and ways of checking to ensure that the exact amount was delivered to the correct spot.

Combining these factors ensures that you receive only the exact amount of radiation needed at precisely the correct spots with minimal risks to the rest of your body.

Cons

Telling you that radiation carries absolutely no risk whatsoever would be wrong; it does have risks. But thanks to advances in technology, these risks affect less than 1 percent of women treated with radiation. What can you encounter?

- ✔ **Developing other cancers:** Radiation therapy increases the risks of getting other cancers, but the risk is small, less than 1 percent over ten years. The kinds of cancers with which this small risk is associated include lung cancer in smokers and *sarcomas,* or cancer of the soft tissue or bone. No evidence points to any increases in the risk of breast cancer in your other breast being caused by radiation.

- ✔ **Being hard on your heart:** Radiation therapy can cause some heart damage including the risk of heart attack seen more than ten years after radiation therapy primarily in women older than 60. Most of the studies conducted were done with older radiation therapy methods before newly instituted safeguards described in the previous section were put in place. The risk, however, may be (studies don't all agree on this) greater when the cancer is in your left breast, because it's so much closer to where your heart is located.

Most women are extremely concerned about the risk of radiation, especially with regard to developing other cancers. These concerns are very understandable, and you'd be right to worry, if it were 50 years ago. Fortunately, thanks to research, medicine has come a very long way from the old days of radiation. Telling you that radiation carries absolutely no risk would be wrong; it does. But today, thanks to advances in technology, these risks affect less than 1 percent of women treated with radiation. Your doctors monitor the treatment dosage and you very carefully.

Preparing Yourself for Treatment

You won't begin radiation treatment until a few weeks after your surgery, when you're healed and feeling stronger. If, however, your treatment also includes chemotherapy, you'll have completed that too, so it may be as long as four to eight months after surgery before you begin receiving radiation therapy. (See Chapter 12 for more information about chemotherapy.)

Think of it this way: Radiation therapy kills the leftover cancer cells that are lurking in your body, just waiting for the next opportunity to strike. With radiation, you get them before they can get you!

Women who are pregnant *cannot* be treated with radiation therapy during their pregnancies because of the potential deleterious effects radiotherapy can have on a developing fetus. Let your doctor know immediately if you suspect that you may be pregnant. More important, take precautions during your treatment so that pregnancy doesn't become an issue.

Calling a team meeting

You won't be alone on your journey through radiation treatment. Your radiation therapy team is a group of highly trained experts that will be right by your side. The team actually numbers quite a few, and each member has a distinct role to play in your treatment:

- ✔ *Radiation oncologist:* This doctor designs your treatment, precisely writing out exact guidelines about how radiation is to be delivered and monitoring you weekly during your treatment. The radiation oncologist will be glad to answer all your questions, so you can go through treatment knowing what to expect.

- ✔ *Radiation therapist:* This technician receives specialized training in delivering radiation in precise doses to specific spots. Did you think the technician just pressed a button and the machine did the work? The technician also is in charge of keeping detailed notes about each of your treatments and recording exactly how you respond each time that you have treatment. Your radiation oncologist reviews these reports and then modifies and adapts your treatment as needed.

- ✔ *Radiation nurses:* These registered nurses have additional training in radiation therapy and can help you cope with your treatment and any of its side effects. They're often the ones who have answers to questions that can arise after you begin treatment.

You can read more about your team's starters and bench players in Chapter 9.

Pulling out the measuring tape

Before you begin the actual radiation therapy, you have two appointments:

- ✔ **Your first visit** is a consultation with the radiation oncologist, who discusses the risks and benefits of radiation therapy with you. The radiation oncologist will probably provide you with a sheet of information explaining treatment, its benefits, possible side effects, and how to take care of yourself before, during, and after your treatment. Nevertheless, having a list of questions is helpful in ensuring that you leave no stone unturned.

Here are some questions to get you started with your radiation oncologist:

- What will my particular radiation treatment involve?

- When will it begin? How long do you anticipate the treatment will last?

- Can you review in detail the benefits versus the risks of my treatment?

- What side effects am I likely to have? I read that these (pull out your handy list, which you copied from this book) side effects are possible. Because I can't prevent them, what can I do to take care of them?

- How long after my treatment ends do the side effects last?

- What are the chances of radiation affecting my heart and/or lungs?

- What are my chances of getting other cancers from the treatment?

✔ **Your second visit** is called a *simulation*. Think of it as being measured for the perfect fit. A series of accurate measurements are taken so that the radiation oncologist can determine which spots to irradiate. The detail, accuracy, and perfection that are required in taking these measurements are why you can expect this visit to be the longest; count on at least a few hours.

Here's what you can expect to go through when you're measured on your second visit. You will

- Lie on your back on a machine with your arm raised above your head. You can see an example in Figure 11-1. The machine looks just like the one that delivers the radiation therapy, but it is a simulator that takes pictures of you from different angles. All this information is fed into a special computer that calculates exactly where your ribs, heart, lung, and breast are.

- Have a few additional measurements taken with other machines. These studies may include an X-ray or CAT (computerized axial tomography) scan, which are used in case additional information is needed to complete the simulation.

- Perhaps have a cradle made to hold your upper body. The cradle, made of plaster, is designed so that every time you lie in it, you're in exactly the same spot and positioned at exactly the same angle. Because making a cradle can take a few hours, it may be prepared during a separate visit. Not everyone has to have a cradle made, even though everyone has to stay in one position during the treatment.

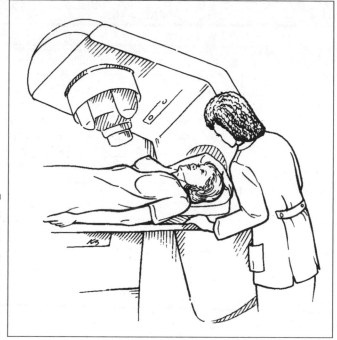

Figure 11-1:
Nothing like
some cold
machinery
to put you
right to
sleep, is
there?

- Have your breast, chest, collarbone, and under your arms marked by your doctor with indelible (or permanent) ink that looks like little blue dots. These marks are made so your doctor can zap the exact spot that needs to be targeted each time you come in. This may be a teeny bit painful, so talk to your doctor about ways of not feeling the discomfort.

  If you're Jewish you may feel uncomfortable having a tattoo. If you're an Orthodox Jew and tattooing is not allowed, ask your Rabbi for a special medical dispensation.

After your second visit, your radiation oncologist then compiles all your information, including the measurements, your mammograms from before and after surgery, your pathology report, and every other piece of information.

Caring for your skin

Before going in for radiation treatment, and even during it, you need to make a few changes to your normal routine. Table 11-2 gives some of the do's and don'ts that will affect your routine.

Table 11-2	Sensitive You	
Avoid	*Why*	*Try instead*
Perfumed products including deodorant, perfume, talcum powder, deodorizing body soaps, and any perfumed lotion.	Some of the ingredients (like aluminum) in perfumed body products may interfere with radiation.	Mild fragrance-free soap. For your armpits: cornstarch or a deodorant crystal (which looks like a stone and can be purchased at most health-food stores). Ask your doctor about approved lotions.
Tough bathing habits including very hot or very cold water and scrubbing.	Your skin will be extremely sensitive, requiring careful coddling.	Washing very gently with lukewarm water. A sponge bath is good, too.
Using a razor.	Your skin needs love; sharp metal doesn't provide it.	An electric razor, provided you use it very gently.
Sun, wind, cold, and any other harsh elements.	They can burn or tear fragile skin.	Covering the area being irradiated.
Sunscreen during treatment (After treatment you'll have to use sunscreen.)	Radiation may burn your skin.	Hats, gloves, scarves, long sleeves, pants.
Icepacks or hot water bottles on the areas being treated.	They can burn.	Clean wet cloths that you soak in ice water.
Scratching your skin.	Doing so may cause an infection.	Talk to your doctor about a lotion to help because most itching is caused by dryness.

They Don't Call It a Regimen Because It's Easy

Your radiation oncologist determines the type and dosage of radiation therapy you're scheduled to receive. Theses factors vary slightly from person to person and facility to facility.

Nan R.

"The thing with radiation is that you don't feel anything (just tired), but it's like getting a bad sunburn, and sometimes your skin can break down in blisters. My treatment started with chemo November 6, 1999, and was followed by mastectomy surgery February 20, 2000, my last chemo May 24, 2000, and my last cycle of radiation August 16, 2000. When you're going through all this, you think, 'Is there light at the end of the tunnel?' I walked out of the radiation clinic, kissed the ground, and yelled to God, 'Thank you,' for I'd made it to the top of the mountain."

An overview

Your radiation therapy is comprised of one or two types of treatment.

- **Treatment:** You can usually expect to receive radiation therapy once a day for five consecutive days (Monday through Friday) for a total of five to six weeks. The treatment itself lasts only a few minutes.

- **Boost:** After the five- to six-week treatment regimen is complete, you may require an extra dose of radiation called a *boost dose,* where an electron beam is directed at the spot where the tumor was. Because the former location of the tumor is the area where the risk of recurrence is the highest, it gets the highest dose of radiation therapy.

Experiencing a typical treatment day

Wondering what your typical treatment day looks and feels like? You can expect to go through the following seven steps and more every day that you have radiation treatment. The one, or two, or three 30-second bursts of radiation treatment you receive will seem like a cakewalk compared to all the preparations you have to go through to get to them.

1. **Getting into your gown.**

   You'll be asked to take off jewelry from your neck and ears.

   Wear something loose fitting and comfortable to help you slip in and out of it quickly; it *will* be more comfortable if your breasts swell or become sensitive.

2. **Waiting.**

Then you wait to be called (and wait some more). If you can, bring something that you enjoy doing with you, like your book, music, or paper for writing letters. While you're waiting is a great time to catch up on stuff you never have time for (like that gorgeous sweater you started knitting last winter but never finished the sleeves.)

3. **Being placed by your technician into position on the table under the machine that delivers the radiation.**

This may include your technician placing you comfortably in your plaster cradle and placing the cradle on the adjustable table under the machine that delivers radiation.

4. **Removing your gown and covering you with a sheet.**

The technician does these things for you.

5. **Fine-tuning the way you're positioned so that you're in precisely the spot you need to be in.**

The technician spends quite a few minutes getting you properly situated for treatment.

6. **Positioning the machine.**

The technician also properly aligns the machine with the way you're positioned on the table.

As you may have guessed, Steps 3 through 6 can take quite a few minutes.

7. **Being left all alone.**

The technician leaves the room but still can see you, because only a glass wall separates the two of you. You'll also be able to speak with each other through an intercom.

8. **Receiving the treatment.** It takes only 30 seconds and feels like lying out in the sun (minus the sun block cream).

9. **Repositioning.**

After administering the actual treatment, the technician returns to you and readjusts the machine to the next angle of treatment.

Judy V.

"During each shot of radiation, count "Mississippi", it makes the time go faster. Counting one-potato, two-potato isn't accurate. If you're counting potatoes you'll get done too fast and you'll panic and think they left the machine on too long. Only "one-Mississippi, two-Mississippi." does it accurately.

SURVIVORS' SECRETS

Amanda C: 11 years old

"After the chemo was finished, Mom had to have radiation. That's when they aim powerful beams at the cancer spots to make sure they're all gone. I remember when we went to the radiation doctor's office, and I was waiting for my mom to finish her treatment. I liked to watch "The Price Is Right" in the waiting room and eat brownies. My mom had a special gown that she wore, and she left me in the waiting room for just a few minutes. It didn't take very long, and she said it didn't hurt at all. I met some of her new friends while we waited. She went every day, but I went only a few times and each time I wanted to stay longer to watch more TV."

From: Amanda and the big "C" unpublished manuscript sent to me by Amanda.

10. **Delivering more treatment.**

   The technician steps out again to deliver the next 30-second treatment. The number of treatments depends on whether only the breast, chest wall, or supraclavical nodes, or the internal mammary nodes are being treated. Usually one to three treatments are administered.

In addition to the treatment, you may have blood drawn once a week or so, so that your doctor has an indication of how high your blood count (platelets and red and white blood cells) is. However, because the radiation that's delivered to your bone marrow (which is where the blood cells and platelets are made) is limited, checking your blood isn't always necessary.

TIP

Try to take your radiation treatments at a facility close to where you live or work. That way, you can schedule your treatments at times that don't cut into your day. If you're working, you can come during your lunchtime and pop back into the office afterward. Living or working farther away from the facility can make the travel to your appointments seem like such a time drain, and most women find that factor the most frustrating and difficult part of radiation treatment. (Check out Chapters 16 and 17 where we describe techniques to help you get through the bad times.)

Sticking It Out During Symptoms

As is true of virtually any treatment, radiation therapy can be accompanied by possible complications, risks, and side effects. The most common side effects include

- ✔ **Fatigue:** You'll probably start feeling tired after a few weeks of radiation therapy, and the fatigue increases as treatment continues. Give in to it and rest. You'll start feeling stronger and more energized in time after your treatment has ended.

  If you feel so exhausted that you're quite debilitated, let your doctor know.

- ✔ **Redness in the treated breast:** Your breast will become redder just as if you were lying out in the sun. This effect may turn your skin a shade darker, just like a suntan. The changes in skin color usually fade in six months to a year.

- ✔ **Skin changes:** All over your body, your skin may become either increasingly sensitive or you may experience a decrease in feeling. The skin and the fatty tissue of your breast may feel thicker and firmer than before, and your pores may become larger and more apparent.

  Consult your doctor or nurse whenever your skin gets very rough, red, and painful, a cut becomes infected, or severe itching lasts more than a few days.

- ✔ **Change in breast size:** Most women's breasts get larger from fluid buildup during treatment. The enlargement eventually goes away after treatment, but it may take as long as three years for your breast to reach its final size.

- ✔ **Loss of appetite:** Losing your appetite as a result of radiation therapy happens only rarely, but if it does, it's really important that you try to eat.

- ✔ **Lowered sexual drive:** You may experience a lowering of your sexual drive during treatment, but in time it will return. See Chapter 19 for some ways to rekindle intimacy after treatment.

Chapter 12

Knowing What to Expect from Chemotherapy

In This Chapter

▶ Considering chemotherapy as the ultimate weapon

▶ Weighing the benefits and risks of chemotherapy

▶ Knowing what to expect from chemotherapy treatment

▶ Coping with temporary side effects and long-term risks

*W*hat's the first thought that comes to your mind when you hear the word "chemotherapy?" If you're like most people, you're probably thinking about losing your hair, experiencing nausea or exhaustion, and enduring the incessant intravenous drip. What all these have in common is that they are some of the negative aspects of chemotherapy. Although they're totally valid concerns, rarely does someone who's just learned she must undergo chemotherapy think of it as her hope for a longer life.

In this chapter, we discuss how and why chemotherapy is so effective in destroying cancer. We also look at its risks and side effects and examine the question of whether it can help *you*. Finally, we cover what you can expect from your treatment and how to cope with some of the side effects while keeping your eye on the goal.

Opening Fire via Chemo

Maybe you'll need chemotherapy, but again, maybe you won't, and Chapter 9 helps clarify just what treatment is in store for you. If you don't need it, don't even worry about it, enjoy! If you do need chemotherapy, then the chapter you're reading is the one for you. You probably have many questions about chemo, like what kind of chemo you'll get, for how long, whether there will be needles, and so on. Many different factors (like the type of your cancer, how far it has spread, your age, your general health, and so on) determine the what and how and when of your chemotherapy. By the time you've read this chapter, your questions will be answered.

Treating the whole system

By the time your cancer has been detected, breast cancer cells may have spread to other parts of your body. Sometimes, they're easily found. Sometimes, they're not. Because doctors have no exact ways of accurately predicting where breast cancer cells will be found, they sometimes treat your entire body. This type of treatment is known as *systemic treatment,* which means a treatment that's geared toward the entire body rather than to one specific organ or site. No matter where the cancer cells are, the chemotherapy (often referred to as "chemo") destroys them. *Hormonal therapy*, which we tackle in Chapter 13, is another form of systemic treatment that may be used (but only under specific conditions).

Simply put, chemotherapy refers to drugs (usually a combination of drugs) that are given with the following two major goals in mind:

  ✔ **Preventing the cancer cells from returning.** (Chapter 16 has recurrence information.)

  ✔ **Increasing your chances of survival.** Chemotherapy's job is to kill those lurking cells. Chemotherapy and hormonal therapy are the only treatments that reach *all* parts of the body, so they are the only way to kill cells that escape the breast and lymph nodes after surgery and radiation therapy. Killing those lurking cells is how chemo and hormonal therapies increase survival.

Killing cancerous cells with chemotherapy may be done when

  ✔ The cancerous tumor has been removed but doctors suspect cancer cells remain elsewhere in the body. Doctors call this treatment *adjuvant treatment* — treatment after surgery (read all about this in Chapter 9.)

  ✔ Your cancer is known to have spread outside the breast to other parts of your body. In medical terminology, this is called *treating metastatic disease*.

Halting cancer cell replication

Chemotherapy drugs attack the ability of cancer cells to replicate (which is described in Chapter 4). Each type of chemotherapy drug does so differently:

   ✔ Some drugs damage the part of the cell that helps the cell divide.

   ✔ Some drugs damage parts of the cell after it's copied itself and is ready to divide.

   ✔ Some drugs damage the cell's duplicating system. *Duplication* needs to happen before the cell can divide and make more cancer cells.

As a result, the cells can't divide, copy, or duplicate themselves, no matter how hard they try. So, when the cell dies, no other cells take its place (tough luck, buddy). The cells become more vulnerable during chemotherapy, and so they succumb easily to the drugs.

Friendly fire: Hurting the good guys

Because chemo extends throughout your entire body, it also affects cells other than the cancerous ones, including the cells in your

   ✔ Hair follicles

   ✔ Bone marrow

   ✔ Mucous membranes of your mouth, vagina, and intestines

That's why your hair falls out, your immune system suffers, your mouth develops sores, and your vagina gets dry. These are some of the really awful aspects of treatment (more about side effects and how to cope with them in the "Dealing with your new 'do: Temporary side effects" and "Looking at scarier stuff: Long-term side effects" sections later in this chapter).

Researchers continuously are working to develop new treatments that are just as effective (if not more so) but without the side effects. Other researchers are working to find ways of targeting and killing *only* the cancer cells, without harming any of your regular cells at all.

Giving Chemo a Thumbs Up: The Good News

By destroying cancer cells and preventing them from multiplying, chemotherapy not only increases your likelihood of surviving but also decreases the risk of recurrence.

Peg I.

"On the tenth day of my chemotherapy, I spiked a low-grade fever. I was hospitalized, and the staff and all my visitors were isolated from me through gowns and gloves and masks. It was a horrible time, because I felt like I was in prison. No one could touch me with their hands without wearing gloves. I didn't have any human physical contact for three days. You don't know how much human touch means until you don't have it anymore."

Reducing risk of recurrence

A few years ago, a seminal study was published that had an enormous influence on current adjuvant chemotherapy treatments. In it, researchers analyzed combined data from 69 earlier clinical trials of adjuvant therapies in which close to 30,000 women participated. The study contains huge amounts of data. In research, the larger the sample size, the more accurate your findings and conclusions can be. In addition, because some women in these studies were treated with chemotherapy at least 15 years ago, it was possible to follow their cases for many years to determine whether adjuvant chemotherapy reduced the likelihood of *recurrence* (cancer returning) and prolonged their lives.

The findings were extremely encouraging in terms of preventing recurrence and increasing the likelihood of surviving. Chemotherapy significantly reduced

- ✔ The likelihood of recurrence of cancer by 25 percent. This reduction in risk was greatest during the first five years after chemotherapy, although a reduction (albeit smaller) also was noted after the first five years, too.

- ✔ The annual odds of death by 15 percent. This reduction in risk occurred during the first five years after treatment and persisted during the next five years. (However, some women had a recurrence of cancer after the first five years, and some died as a result.)

- ✔ The significant reductions in recurrence and death were apparent in:

  - Women whose cancer hadn't spread to the lymph nodes *and* in those where it had.

  - Premenopausal *and* menopausal women.

  - All age groups, although the benefit was greatest for younger women.

Translating the findings into figures that have meaning for you

These findings are encouraging, but I bet you want to know what they mean for *you*. Most studies report on the decrease in the likelihood of cancer returning or the increase in the likelihood of recurrence or survival in percentages. However, these percentages are proportional for the group as a whole, when compared with groups who didn't receive chemotherapy. Here's the thing: There is *no* way to calculate an individual person's risk. The closest researchers can come is looking at the risk for a group of women just like you, which is known as *absolute risk. Relative risk,* on the other hand, is the amount of proportional risk reduction derived from treatment.

Calculating how much chemotherapy reduces your risk of recurrence

Findings from hundreds of studies clearly demonstrate that chemotherapy reduces the risk of recurrence by at least one-fourth to one-third. Most studies report on the decrease in the likelihood of cancer returning or the increase in the likelihood of recurrence. Findings from the seminal study are encouraging, but what do they mean to you?

First and foremost, knowing your individual level of risk of the cancer coming back is essential for calculating your specific personal benefit from chemotherapy. You can find out your personal level of risk by checking out Chapter 16, where we discuss recurrence, or you can ask your oncologist.

In general terms, if you are at high risk of recurrence, say 66 percent, and you were part of a group of 100 women who have the exact same cancer in the same stage (and with all other factors being the same including the same chemotherapy for those receiving it), that means

- ✔ **Without chemotherapy,** 66 of the 100 women in your group (66 percent) will have a recurrence.

- ✔ **With chemotherapy,** 44 (one-third fewer) to 50 (one-fourth fewer) of the 100 women in your group will have a recurrence after having chemotherapy. The absolute benefit is 22 percent; the relative risk reduction is one-third.

Does that show that chemotherapy is good? You're darn tootin' it does. When you compare 66 recurrences without chemotherapy to 44 to 50 with chemotherapy, that means 16 to 22 women will be spared the anguish of recurrence if they're treated with chemotherapy. Another way of looking at it is that it decreases the risk of cancer recurring by one-third. Bring it on!

Likewise, if you are at low risk of recurrence, say 10 percent, and you were part of a group of 100 with the same cancer, same stage, and essentially all the same factors, that means

✔ **Without chemotherapy,** ten of the 100 women in your group (10 percent) will have a recurrence.

✔ **With chemotherapy,** seven (roughly one-third fewer) to eight (roughly one-fourth fewer) of the 100 women in your group will have a recurrence. The absolute benefit is 3 percent, but the relative risk reduction is still one-third.

Is that good? Of course it is. When you compare 10 recurrences without chemotherapy to seven or eight with chemotherapy, that means two or three women, who are at low risk anyway, will be saved the anguish of recurrence. Every single life saved is, of course, precious. Again, another way of looking at it is that it decreases the risk of cancer recurring by one-third.

On the other hand, if you're at low risk, you may be weighing two or three chances in 10 with what you're facing by undergoing chemotherapy (that's coming up in the sections that follow), which can be harrowing at best. Who's to say what risk is high and what risk is low in that case? When you're considering your personal level of risk in deciding whether chemotherapy will be of benefit to you, only you (and your loved ones) can know for sure what's best.

Complicating your matters is the fact that your individual risk of recurrence can fall anywhere within a broad range of between 2 percent and 90 percent, not to mention all the other factors that can effect your outcome and thus come into play when you decide on your treatment (see Chapter 9).

Living longer

Even more significant than knowing whether chemotherapy reduces the risk of the cancer returning is knowing whether chemotherapy helps you live longer. Two very important factors have been found that predict outcome in women with breast cancer (see Chapter 7). These factors are

✔ The number of nodes to which the cancer has spread (the fewer the nodes, the better the prognosis)

✔ The size of the cancer

Knowing whether chemotherapy *will* extend your life can help you make a wiser decision about whether adding it to your treatment regimen is worth it for you.

Your projected likelihood of surviving at least 10 years depends on the size of your tumor, whether it has spread to the nodes, and your age.

Adding chemo when you're younger than 50

If you're younger than 50 years old, and your cancer hasn't spread to the nodes, and you choose not to have chemo, the average chance for surviving at least 10 years is already quite good (the range is 70 percent to 90 percent, depending on the size of the cancer.) If you opt for chemotherapy, your likelihood of surviving increases by another 3 percent to 7 percent on average. The specifics of your cancer may change these numbers.

Do these statistics warrant your going through chemotherapy? Only you can say.

On the other hand, if your cancer has spread to the lymph nodes, the average chances for surviving 10 years without chemotherapy is 42 percent (that's for all women, including those with the entire range of node involvement and tumor sizes.) It's higher for some women (for example, those with a small tumor, 1 node involved) and lower for other women (for example with a big tumor and 10 nodes involved.) Having chemo increases your likelihood of surviving by an additional 11 percent, which is a substantial increase in anybody's book. Thus the decision can be much easier. No matter what, the decision is yours. (By the way, these figures are extrapolated for only a 10-year time frame, because that's the longest period from which researchers conducting the study were able to gather accurate information.)

Adding chemo when you're older than 50

What if you're older than 50? If your cancer hasn't spread to the nodes, the average chances of your living at least 10 years are 67 percent without chemo, and having chemo increases your chances by only 2 percent. If your cancer has spread to the nodes, the average chance of surviving 10 years is 46 percent without chemo, and having chemo increases your chances by 3 percent. So having chemotherapy, *in this case,* doesn't really improve your likelihood of surviving by that much. Survival increases by only 2 percent when your cancer hasn't spread to the nodes and by only 3 percent when it has spread to the nodes. Again, these are only averages. Based on the specifics of your cancer, you can get more or less benefit.

SURVIVORS' SECRETS

Sonia's savvy

I (Ronit Elk, a coauthor of this book) remember once sitting in my friend's Sonia's living room, while she chatted and laughed with her visitors. The fact that she was in the middle of a chemotherapy cycle and, at that point, completely bald didn't faze her at all. The visiting nurse arrived with the day's chemotherapy in a little plastic bag, and the conversation stopped, but only for a moment. The nurse checked Sonia's portacath, took her temperature, and fiddled with the tubes. When she discovered there was no stand from which to hang the chemotherapy bag, she effortlessly rigged it up to a painting on the wall. After opening the valve at the top of the tubing and feeling satisfied that the solution was dripping at the correct speed, the nurse waved goodbye and the party continued with Sonia sitting cross-legged in front of the already dramatic abstract painting that was made even more so with the long infusion drip becoming an integral part of its imagery.

Predicting outcome by using genetics

A study published in December of 2002 reported on a brand-new, more accurate way of predicting outcome, which is based on genetic profiling of the cancer itself. Although very promising, it still hasn't been proven. Perhaps, sometime in the future, this approach may result in a much more accurate way of determining who will benefit from adjuvant therapy, and who won't, which, of course, will prevent women being under- or overtreated. Stay tuned!

The relatively small increase in survival that chemo can provide is why you must consult with and seek advice from your doctor and loved ones so that you determine whether adding chemo to your treatment regimen is worthwhile based on your specific cancer details.

For people with breast cancer who are ages 50 to 69, breast cancer is overwhelmingly the primary cause of death!

Deciding Whether Chemo Is Right for You

After you find out how much chemotherapy will increase your chances for survival, you can weigh those benefits with side effects and risks (described later in this chapter). But before you decide whether chemo's the treatment that you want, you need to gain a complete understanding of the specific benefits, side effects, and risks of the particular form of chemotherapy *regimen* you're facing. Suffice to say, chemotherapy can be extremely grueling, and that's why in this section we carefully explain all the factors you need to known when making an informed decision about undergoing chemotherapy.

Reviewing recommended guidelines

Treatment guidelines (recommendations for treatment) have been developed (and are described in full in Chapter 9) for how to treat you based on the stage of your cancer (Chapter 7) and, in particular, whether it has spread to the lymph nodes or beyond. These factors definitely help you determine what treatment, including chemotherapy, you need to have.

These guidelines may be modified on the basis of whether your tumor is made up of cells that contain hormone receptors. Many (but not all) cancer cells have *hormone receptors* for estrogen. Hormone receptors are the part of the cancer cell to which estrogen sticks. When estrogen binds with cancer cell hormone receptors, it stimulates the cancer cells to multiply. Cancer cells with these receptors are called *hormone receptor–positive.* Similarly, cancer cells that don't have receptors are called *hormone receptor–negative.* The great news is that if your cancer cells are hormone receptor–positive, a drug known as tamoxifen halts cancer cells from multiplying, thus ensuring you a better prognosis.

Treatment guidelines and nodal involvement

Chemotherapy is recommended when

- ✔ The cancer has spread to your lymph nodes.
- ✔ The cancer has not spread to your lymph nodes, but the tumor is large or shows other unfavorable characteristics that make it possible that the cancer has spread beyond the breast.

One of the most important predictors of outcome in breast cancer is the number of *axillary* (underarm) *lymph nodes* that contain cancerous cells. Finding cancer cells in these nodes indicates that the cancer hasn't stayed in the area where it began. Instead, it shows the cancer has begun to travel through the lymph nodes to other parts of the body. Chapter 4 talks in depth about how cancer spreads through the lymph system and beyond.

Treatment guidelines and metastatic cancer

When the cancer already has metastasized, or spread to other parts of the body, chemotherapy can extend the amount of time you have left, even if it's only by a few months. Today, most women with metastatic breast cancer receive some form of systemic therapy, either chemotherapy or hormonal therapy.

Because hormonal therapy is the most effective treatment when the cancer has the estrogen receptor (although not without risks described in Chapter 13), doctors strongly recommend that women with hormone receptor—positive tumors, without extensive metastases, receive hormonal therapy. Chapter 13 also describes hormone therapy in depth.

Pat C.

"Chemotherapy was the hardest thing for me to go through. I felt like I was getting a lethal injection every time I went. But you know, my nurses made it so easy for me. They are very comforting and reassuring. My oncologist is also wonderful. He told me straight up what everything was and why. He continues to be a very good person as I go through my checkups."

Peggy B.

"The first treatment brought about my hair loss in exactly two weeks. The nurses told me it would probably happen on Day 18. I had that day circled on my calendar and was convinced it wouldn't come out before then. That was the worst time for me emotionally, because I had a beautiful full head of soft, thick, curly hair. A few days before it started coming out in handfuls in the shower, I had a headache and a very sore, tender scalp. I had no idea these symptoms were a precursor to the fallout. I thought I had prepared myself for this eventuality by cutting my hair real short and trying on my wig. But, believe, me, nothing ever prepares you for complete hair loss. It took a little more than a full week for all of the hair on my head to come out. I cried for days. Shortly after that, I lost my pubic hair, and to me, I looked like an alien. I lost my eyebrows and eyelashes about two to three weeks later. By the last of my treatments my hair started to grow back. It first grew back curly with my original color of brown, but it's very fine and soft, like baby hair. All my body hair is back, too, which is really nice."

Women with cancer that has spread to other parts of the body may also be treated with chemotherapy. Recent clinical trials have shown that more effective therapies (including chemo) have been able to prolong the lives of women with metastatic breast cancer, and with continued research, it is hoped that these improvements can be increased.

Making a decision

After you find out the stage of your cancer and understand the recommended treatment guidelines, you need to make your decision. Guiding you through your decision-making process will be a good medical oncologist (Chapter 9 explains how to find one, and Chapter 23 cites many resources for you to start with).

Meeting with a medical oncologist

If your surgeon thinks you can benefit from chemotherapy (and even if not), you need to meet with a *medical oncologist,* a doctor who specializes in treating cancer through medication. The medical oncologist not only is an expert in determining which treatment works best for particular types of cancers but also is knowledgeable about how to minimize chemotherapy's long- and short-term side effects.

On your initial visit to your medical oncologist, you need to ask for your *absolute rate* of cancer recurrence and the *absolute benefit* of chemotherapy. Your absolute rates will tell you the likelihood of your

✔ Cancer returning without chemotherapy

✔ Cancer returning with chemotherapy

✔ Surviving at least 10 years without chemotherapy

✔ Surviving at least 10 years with chemotherapy

Another important question to ask on your initial visit is whether your oncologist *recommends* chemotherapy. In addition to this question, be sure to ask

✔ What are your qualifications, expertise, and experience?

✔ Which types of chemotherapy/hormonal therapy am I eligible for?

✔ What is my prognosis with and without chemotherapy?

✔ Which of these regimens do you recommend and why?

✔ Please can you tell me everything about the chemotherapy/hormone therapy regimen you recommend? What are its benefits, short-term side effects, and risks?

✔ How will you monitor my progress and potential side effects during treatment?

Checking with your doctor about the benefits of chemotherapy for you

Many doctors recommend that you have chemo no matter what the likelihood of it improving your chances. Others recognize that the attitudes each woman has toward small benefits vary considerably, and if chemo won't increase your chance for surviving by much, they'll tell you so, although they'll probably leave the decision whether to undergo chemo up to you and your loved ones.

Getting a second opinion; making comparisons

Getting another doctor's opinion is neither unethical nor rude; in fact, most doctors recommend that you get a second opinion. You may find that another oncologist recommends a different regimen or may even recommend chemotherapy when the first doctor advised against it. These differing opinions can be confusing and even alarming to many women, but opinions differ because no hard-and-fast rules about chemo exist, only guidelines and projections.

Considering both oncologists' opinions is important. When comparing the two oncologists' opinions, list the points on which they agree and disagree. If they essentially agree with each other, your decision is much easier. If they don't agree, consider the reasons each one gives you for their respective opinions. If necessary, you can ask for another consultation with the oncologist from whom you most want to hear.

Susan K.

"I learned how healing laughter can be, and I continued to use laughter to help me and my friends and loved ones get through the tough times. For example, during my chemo, one of the lawyers in the law office where I worked teased me good-naturedly that he was glad he wasn't the only bald person in the office. After I was finished with my chemo and radiation, my co-workers hung a banner in my office that read, 'You've been through an ordeal that would defeat many, but you made it through, and you look great, and you have more hair than Pete.'"

Putting it all together to make the best decision for you

Write down all the information you've gathered from your doctor and oncologists on a sheet or two of paper that you've divided into two columns. In one column, write the reasons for chemotherapy, and in the other, write the reasons against it. Your decision boils down to a battle between the following two factors:

- ✔ **The benefits.** List all your personal factors and the numbers. What's the likelihood that chemo will increase your life span? What's the likelihood that it will reduce the risk of the cancer returning?

- ✔ **The risks.** List all the side effects, which, although they're usually temporary, may cause you considerable difficulty. Don't forget to jot down the long-term risks. You can't predict in advance which ones you'll experience, or to what degree, but you need to consider them all carefully.

Don't make your decision alone. It's too difficult. Talk with your oncologist. Talk with your loved ones as well; you know that they care. If you don't have anyone you trust, or if they all live too far away, ask to speak with a cancer survivor or a social worker at the hospital. Chapter 24 provides survivor group information.

Calling Up the Regimen (t) to Wage War on Cancer Cells

Okay: You've decided to go through chemotherapy. Now it's time to find out what it involves. A good way of thinking of chemo is like a tough program, more like a regimen, which you're going to go through for a time. Remember when you had a newborn baby who kept you up every night for months on end? That was a regimen you experienced and made it through. And what about the time you had to work overtime for weeks at a time, with no weekends off, because of a looming deadline? You got through that time, too, right? You'll get through the regimen of chemotherapy, too.

Something else that you need to remember at this point is that many women have been on this journey before you, and most of them have made it to the other side and are now leading full lives. What's more, they'll be there for you and welcome you into their exclusive club of breast cancer survivors. No one ever wants to volunteer to join, but once you're a member, you'll receive so much support, advice, and comfort, that few leave it.

Every journey is unique, but all have many common threads. The following subsections reveal those threads.

Pedaling through cycles, doses, and methods

The type of chemotherapy, the specific dose, the number of doses you receive, and the entire length of time you're taking the drugs are known as the *regimen.* Chemotherapy regimens almost always are administered in *cycles,* which means that you receive doses of chemotherapy several days in a row and then the daily doses stop for a while to give your body time to regroup, and then you receive more doses for another several days and then it stops, and so on. (Examples of cycles are demonstrated in the "Creating a cocktail: Combining drugs" section later in this chapter)

Cycling through

Your doctor prescribes chemotherapy, just like your doctor prescribes antibiotics but obviously not for the same reasons! Chemotherapy drugs are administered just like antibiotics, either intravenously or by pill. Chemotherapy comes in different varieties and dosages, as do antibiotics. And those doses are given to you over a specific period of time, just like antibiotics.

SURVIVORS' SECRETS

Amanda C.: 11 years old

"The first time I saw Mom after her hair was shaved, she had a hat on and took it off for me. It shocked me and made me so sad. It made me sad because most women have hair. I had only seen pictures of ladies without hair. I wanted her to look the way she did before cancer. I was afraid for other boys and girls to see her without a hat. I wished this never happened to us. But my *Oma* (grandmother) helped me by saying that no matter what she looks like on the outside, she is still the same person on the inside."
From *Amanda and the Big "C"*

Roberta H.

"There were funny moments like the look on the cat's face when she tried to lick my bristly head during a moment of catnip-induced feline dementia, ending up with an unexpected hairball on her tongue."

However, when you're prescribed an antibiotic, your doctor always tells you to take all the pills as scheduled, a certain number of times per day, until they're all gone. That way, the empty pill bottle tells you that you're done with your antibiotics.

Undergoing chemotherapy, however, is not as cut-and-dried as taking a round of antibiotics. Because of how powerful chemotherapy drugs are and how toxic they can make you, you need to take them for a while and then not take them for a while, in other words in an on-again, off-again *cycle*. The two reasons that follow are among several important ones that explain why administering chemotherapy in cycles is so important. The cycles

✔ **Give your normal cells a rest.** Keep in mind that in addition to attacking the cancer cells, your normal cells also are being bombarded. Thus, not taking chemotherapy drugs for a short spell enables normal cells the chance to regroup. In other words, the toxic effects of the treatment subside, so that the cells can regenerate. This rest is especially important for the cells in your bone marrow where your blood cells are made.

If too many normal cells are knocked out at once, your immune system becomes compromised. Sometimes, very high doses of chemotherapy are given. Such high doses of chemotherapy damage the *stem cells* (cells that produce blood cells) in your bone marrow, which, in turn, lowers your *white cell count* (white cells protect you against infections) and results in a shortage of *platelets* (which stop your bleeding). You then become extremely vulnerable to serious infections, your blood doesn't coagulate, and you're at risk for life-threatening complications.

✔ **Cause more of the cancer cells to be affected than if chemo were administered all at one time.** All cells (including cancer cells) go through cycles in which they replicate, divide, split, and so on. Different kinds of cells do that at different times, thus when the chemo is given at different times it catches different cancer cells in the act (when the time is ripe).

Each treatment combination has its own schedule, depending on the particular chemotherapy drug and the time it takes for its toxic effects to leave the system. For example, one of the more common chemotherapy treatments, Adriamycin (doxorubicin in generic form, described later in this chapter), includes four cycles that are given over the course of every three weeks. The total treatment lasts about three and a half months. Most treatments last from three to six months, although some extend longer, and most are given with a break of three weeks between cycles — the amount of time it takes for the bone marrow to recover.

Homing in on dosage

Unlike antibiotic therapy, where your doctor may tell you that you're going to take 500 mg twice a day, the dose of chemotherapy that you receive is calculated by your doctor on the basis of your height and weight.

Putting the paper boy to shame: Delivery method

Almost all treatments can be given at a treatment center on an outpatient basis. Sometimes, they can even be administered at home.

Chemotherapeutic drugs can be delivered in the following ways:

- Intravenously, which is also called an *infusion* and is the most common way to give chemotherapy
- Orally via pill

Your oncologist determines which of these methods is the best way for you to get your chemotherapy, depending on the type of drug you need, the particular way each drug needs to be administered, and your health. (See why you need a great oncologist? This is complicated stuff!) Of course most of us would prefer popping a pill (or many pills) to having to have medication delivered intravenously. Maybe one day that will be the case, but for now, it unfortunately isn't. Most chemotherapeutic drugs cannot be given orally and must be delivered intravenously. That's because the only way any drug works — chemo, antibiotics, heart medications included — is by getting it into the blood stream, which, in turn, delivers it to the rest of the body. The only drugs given as pills are those that can be absorbed from the stomach and are not made inactive by the acid in your stomach.

Expecting to get poked with those darned needles

Chemotherapy drugs are introduced into your bloodstream through a needle placed into your vein. They can be delivered intravenously in three different ways:

- **Regular intravenous.** Ever had a blood test? What about receiving medication intravenously when you were sick? It's the same with chemotherapy. First the needle is inserted in your vein, and then a tube is attached to a bag of the liquid medication. At the end of that session, the needle is taken out. The next time the same process is repeated, and the time after, and the time after. That's why more permanent and convenient and less painful ways exist. They're described next.

✔ **Indwelling catheter (also known as permanent IV):** A narrow tube is surgically inserted under the skin through a small cut at the top of your chest, near your collarbone. It leads directly into a blood vessel. The small cut is stitched up, and the protruding end is sealed with a plug and covered with a dressing when not in use. An indwelling catheter like this provides care providers with easy access to a vein, instead of having to stick you every time you undergo treatment.

✔ **Portacath:** A portacath also can be surgically inserted under the skin on your chest. It's completely buried under the chest skin; nothing sticks out, but using one still requires a needle stick; however, a portacath is easier to find than a vein (you don't need to worry about caretakers digging around to find one), hurts less than a regular IV, and is less likely to get infected than the indwelling catheter.

Catheters and portacaths are merely hybrids of regular intravenous delivery of medications, serving as accommodations for the frequency with which IV meds are administered in chemotherapy. They benefit patient as well as caretaker.

The advantage of receiving treatment through an indwelling catheter is that you don't have to be continually stuck with needles. The disadvantage, however, is that the IV needs to be flushed out regularly (weekly or every two weeks) to prevent clotting. On rare occasions, you may have an infection around the portacath or indwelling catheter that can be extremely uncomfortable. Let your doctor know if you notice swelling and redness around it.

Whenever your veins are bad (nurses always seem to be mumbling, "Where *is* that darn vein?" as they struggle for the third time, leaving you black and blue) or you're assured of having a long chemotherapy regimen, you'll be advised to consider the portacath or indwelling catheter instead of having an IV inserted every single time you receive a treatment. Which method will your doctor advise? Well, it depends on how long you'll be receiving chemo, what your veins look like, and other practicalities. That's why it's so important that you are treated as an individual, unique patient, rather than in some cookie-cutter fashion.

Pulling in for a fill-up: Receiving the chemo

Most hospitals have a chemotherapy treatment center or a separate room or area where chemotherapy is routinely administered.

Here's the usual chemotherapy drill:

1. **You're given a comfortable chair to sit in.**

   The chair's usually the kind that you can lie back in. It's sort of like a recliner, but bigger and sturdier.

2. **An oncology nurse puts a needle into a vein on your arm (the arm opposite the breast with cancer).**

3. **The nurse hooks the needle up to a tube attached to a plastic bag filled with chemotherapy medicine that begins dripping into your vein.**

4. **You sit and wait until all of the solution has gone into your vein.**

   This can take from half an hour to a few hours.

5. **The nurse disconnects you, and you're on your way.**

Some women arrive carrying briefcases filled with paperwork, some do their knitting, others read a good book, and then they even drive themselves home after a treatment. Of course, the same woman can be as weak as a feather and require someone to wheel her out to the car or even require hospitalization at some time during her treatment. How you react to chemo depends on

✔ The particular chemotherapy used

✔ The stage of the cycle (how far along you are in the process)

✔ Your body's response (Some women can eat a cheeseburger right after, others vomit at the smell of food.)

Creating a cocktail: Combining drugs

An important large study has shown that using a combination of drugs significantly improves the outcome in women with breast cancer. On average, the annual odds of recurrence were reduced by approximately 25 percent, and the odds of death were reduced by approximately 15 percent.

Peg I.

"I got permission to leave on a flight to New Orleans two days from dismissal. I wore a mask to protect myself from germs on the flight, and I rode in a wheelchair most of the time. By this time, I had no hair anywhere — no eyelashes, no eyebrows, no hair. It felt so strange to be seen that way. And I felt like even less of a human being in that wheelchair. I wore hats, but I had awful hot flashes that turned me beet red, with sweat pouring down from everywhere. It was not pretty. I got so I didn't look at my hairless head in the mirror; I didn't really pay attention to it.. It's like when I don't notice all the freckles on my face. It just became a normal part of me in my new body."

Jen H.

"Another thank you needs to be expressed for the new antinausea medicines that are available today, because they work miracles! I was sick throughout my treatment, yet it didn't get bad or keep me in bed until my final treatment."

The most common combinations of drugs used in treatment are briefly explained in the listing that follows. Bear in mind a couple of things. First, as new research information becomes available, these combinations may become outdated, and second, each of these treatment regimens works in a different way, but in any event, launches a multipronged attack on cancer cells.

CMF

For a long time, the most common treatment combination was cyclophosphamide (Cytoxan), methotrexate, and 5-fluorouracil (5-U), CMF for short. The group of women that is more likely to benefit from this treatment includes women who are at lower risk for recurrence and those who cannot tolerate anthracyclines (see "Anthracyclines" next). Cytoxan is administered either intravenously or orally, while methotrexate and 5-flourouracil are administered intravenously. This regimen lasts for six months.

Anthracyclines

Chemotherapy usually includes a type of drug called *anthracycline,* which produces better results than nonanthracycline chemotherapy, a finding that has been confirmed by several studies. The anthracyclines in use are doxorubicin (most common) and epirubicin. Since the results of those studies became known, treatment regimens that include anthracyclines have become the standard of care for most women whose cancer has spread to more than one lymph node *(node-positive)* and for many women whose cancer hasn't spread to the nodes *(node-negative).*

Some of the several treatment regimens that include anthracyclines are

- ✔ **CAF:** This regimen combines cyclosphosphamide, doxorubicin (Adriamycin), and fluorouracil and is prescribed for women with node-negative and node-positive types of breast cancer. It is administered intravenously in four to six cycles.

- ✔ **AC:** This regimen combines doxorubicin (Adriamycin) and cyclophosphamide and is prescribed regardless of whether the patient's cancer has spread to the nodes. It is administered intravenously in four to six cycles every three weeks. AC often has fewer side effects than CMF;

however, whether four cycles of AC is equivalent to one of the longer anthracycline-containing regimens still is not known.

✔ **AC paclitaxel or docetaxel:** This regimen adds paclitaxel or docetaxel to the AC regimen listed in the previous item and is commonly prescribed for women whose cancer has spread to the nodes. It is administered intravenously by following four cycles of the Adriamycin and cyclophosphamide with four cycles of paclitaxel (Taxol) or docetaxel (Taxotere).

✔ **CEF:** This regimen combines cyclophosphamide (Cytoxan), epirubicin, and 5-fluorouracil and is prescribed for node-positive and node-negative cancers. It is usually administered intravenously for six cycles. A clinical trial comparing CMF with CEF, a combination that includes epirubicin (known as a sister drug of adriamycin) indicated that patients who received CEF had a much better outcome, including an improved survival rate.

Despite all that researchers have learned about chemotherapy for early stage breast cancer, several questions persist. For example, are there better chemotherapy drugs than currently are in use? How many cycles of chemotherapy should be given?

Clinical trials throughout the U.S., and around the world, for that matter, are addressing these questions. Your oncologist may talk to you about a clinical trial. If that happens, your oncologist will provide you with a very detailed consent form, explaining why the trial is being done and outlining the possible side effects of the drugs being used in the trial. The consent forms can be a little scary, so be sure and read them carefully and discuss them in detail with your oncologist and the members of your treatment team. These trials are extremely important. Without them, doctors wouldn't know what they know now. Your participation in a trial may help not only you but also many other women in the future.

SURVIVORS' SECRETS

Barb L.

"I had four cycles of Adriamycin cytoxan. After my first cycle of chemo, I thought it was a piece of cake. I was just a little queasy. The first thing I did after my first chemo was cut off my hair. It was going to fall out anyway, and doing so made accepting hair loss easier. After the second cycle is when I really hit the wall. I have never felt so sick and tired in all my life. Everything changed. You just try to find anything to eat and drink that won't make you sick. I have to say that I survived on mashed potatoes every day, and on pizza, pasta, pretzels, and peanut butter. Some people lose weight from chemo; others gain weight. I lost a total of 50 pounds. In between cycles of chemo, you learn to live with being tired every day. For me, I was sick for four days after chemo, and by the fifth day I started to feel a little better. By the time I felt as good as it's going to get, it was time for chemo again."

Peggy B.

"My greatest fear with chemo was losing my energy. My oncologist told me that patients who exercise do the best on chemo. I was always a great believer in exercise and an avid walker. I maintained a constant regime of walking, Pilates, hand weights, and riding my bike, and I basically sailed through chemo with no problems."

In a clinical trial, the standard therapy is compared to a new therapy that is thought to be more effective or to have fewer side effects, based on early study results. By participating in a clinical trial, you get the best available treatment or something that may even be better.

Chemotherapy plus other treatments

Chemotherapy won't be the only form of treatment you'll undergo in your battle with breast cancer. Instead, it forms a part of a more extensive regimen that's tailored to the particular characteristics of your cancer, such as the stage and grade of the cancer, the size of the tumor, and whether it's spread to the nodes under your arms or even metastasized to more distant parts of the body. All the various treatment regimens, including the one you're most likely to receive, are described in detail in Chapter 9.

Chemo 'n' surgery

Most women begin chemotherapy after they've recovered from lumpectomy or mastectomy surgery (described in Chapter 10).

However, in some circumstances, chemotherapy also is given before surgery. The purpose of this *neoadjuvant chemotherapy treatment* is to shrink the tumor to such an extent that instead of having to have a mastectomy, you may be able to have a lumpectomy, or to make your tumor small enough that it can be removed by surgery.

No evidence shows that having chemotherapy before surgery improves survival. Studies have shown your survival is the same regardless of whether you have chemotherapy before or after surgery, but it helps doctors find out whether more chemotherapy is needed and whether you'll respond to a certain drug. With that information in hand when it's time for chemotherapy after surgery, your oncologist has a better idea about which drugs you respond to.

Chemo 'n' radiation

Radiation therapy, which we describe in Chapter 11, destroys cancer cells in your breast tissue, in the skin of your chest wall, and in the lymph nodes under your arm, but it cannot destroy cancer cells that have spread to other parts of the body. That's where chemotherapy comes in.

After a lumpectomy, radiation is routine. After a mastectomy, although adding radiation to chemotherapy can reduce the risk of recurrence in the area of the surgery, its effect on survival is uncertain. Recently, a panel of experts recommended that after mastectomy, women whose cancer had spread to four or more lymph nodes *should* receive a combination of radiation therapy and chemotherapy. Whether women whose cancer has spread to one to three nodes and who receive this combination have a better outcome is unclear. Discuss the specifics of your circumstances with your doctor.

Chemo 'n' hormonal therapy

Finally, chemotherapy may also be combined with *hormonal therapy* (usually tamoxifen) a treatment that blocks the effects of estrogen (see Chapter 13). This combination of treatments is equally effective in reducing the risk of recurrence in pre- and postmenopausal women who have positive hormone receptors. By depriving the cell of its hormonal stimulation, hormonal therapy slows or even halts the growth of cancer cells. Hormone therapy is given after chemo. New research shows that giving them both at the same time is not as effective as giving them sequentially.

Reviewing the recommendations for combined therapy

Guidelines recommend how to use adjuvant therapy; however, these are not hard and fast rules, they're simply recommendations (see Table 12-1). For example, if your cancer hasn't spread to the lymph nodes, and your tumor is 1 cm in diameter or smaller, you won't need chemo, but you will be prescribed tamoxifen if your cancer cells have a hormone receptor (Chapter 13.) On the other hand, if your cancer has spread to the lymph nodes, you're premenopausal, and your cancer cells are hormone receptor–positive, you'll get chemo and tamoxifen. (See Chapter 9 for more about this therapy.)

Table 12-1	Recommendations for Adjuvant Therapy		
Cancer Size	*Lymph Nodes*	*Estrogen Receptor*	*Recommended Treatment*
Less than 1 cm (diameter)	Negative (no spread to lymph nodes)	Positive (cancer cell has an estrogen receptor)	Consider tamoxifen for prevention and therapy.

(continued)

Table 12-1 *(continued)*

Cancer Size	Lymph Nodes	Estrogen Receptor	Recommended Treatment
Less than 1 cm (diameter)	Negative (no spread to lymph node)	Negative (cancer cell doesn't have an estrogen receptor)	Chemotherapy is not routine because of the very small benefit, although some women choose to have it.
Greater than 1 cm (diameter)	Negative (no spread to lymph nodes)	Positive (cancer cell has an estrogen receptor)	Tamoxifen and chemotherapy. The benefit of adding chemotherapy varies with tumor size and the woman's age.
Greater than 1 cm (diameter)	Negative (no spread to lymph nodes)	Negative (cancer cell doesn't have an estrogen receptor)	Chemotherapy.
Any size	Positive (the cancer has spread to 1 or more lymph nodes)	Positive (cancer cell has an estrogen receptor)	Tamoxifen and chemotherapy. In women with significant other health problems, chemo may be omitted.
Any size	Positive (the cancer has spread to 1 or more lymph nodes	Negative (cancer cell doesn't have an estrogen receptor	Chemotherapy.

Sticking It Out during Symptoms

Most side effects improve after a while, but they can be difficult to live with when you're experiencing them. Other side effects have serious long-term consequences. Doctors will tell you how much better things are now than they used to be, and that's all true. But how does that information help you when your hair has fallen out and you're too sick to take care of the kids? Frankly, it doesn't.

Fortunately, medications are available that can help you deal with some of the more debilitating side effects: Some meds help the bone marrow recover after chemotherapy, and some reduce nausea. You may be able to continue living your life, albeit it at a reduced rate. In this section, we cover the possible side effects you may experience and discuss strategies for getting through them.

Side effects of chemotherapy vary greatly and depend on a variety of factors, including you and your treatment. Symptoms can depend on the treatment itself, including

- Type of drug
- Dosage
- Other medications you're taking
- The time of day you receive the drug
- How long you're on the drug
- Current stage of treatment you're going through

You play a role in managing your symptoms. You're an active recipient. Check out Table 12-2 for some tips about how to minimize your symptoms.

Table 12-2	Chemo Cause and Effect
If you . . .	*Then you'll . . .*
Go into treatment well prepared and knowing what to expect (reading this book helps tremendously)	Cope better with treatment.
Have a medical team that prepares you well for treatment (explaining everything and reassuring you that they'll be there for you), and treats your symptoms *as soon as* they occur	Be likely to have fewer symptoms. This case is especially true with regard to *anticipatory vomiting* (when you vomit before you're given medications), which can be prevented either through medication or various behavioral techniques. (See Chapter 14 for descriptions of alternative methods.)
Eat the right foods and avoid the others (very spicy, fatty, sweet, or salty foods)	Help control nausea.
Eat small meals (rather than heavy ones) and bland food and drinks served at room temperature	Help prevent nausea.

(continued)

Table 12-2 *(continued)*

If you . . .	Then you'll . . .
Find your own ways to cope with treatment	Cope better. Some women choose spirituality or religion, while others cope by reading. Some prefer relaxation and guided imagery, and others write in their journals. Still others prefer relaxation and hypnosis. (Chapter 14 offers suggestions.)
Exercise during chemotherapy	Have fewer side effects than women who don't. That's a no-brainer. If you can't do anything strenuous, then don't, but take a few minutes to walk around the park or in the house.
Have support (discussed in depth in Chapters 20 and 22)	Navigate your journey through breast cancer with far greater ease.
Anticipate nausea	Likely feel nauseated. (This is called *anticipatory nausea and vomiting*.)
Feel anxious before your treatment	Not likely tolerate the treatment as well as when you're relaxed.
Have a history of chronic and heavy drinking	Experience fewer symptoms with some chemotherapy drugs. (Sorry, this isn't a good enough reason to become an alcoholic!)

Dealing with your new 'do: Temporary side effects

Some of the temporary side effects of chemotherapy may include hair loss, mouth sores, and vaginal dryness. Your hair will grow back a short time after you finish your treatment, the mouth sores will go away, and unless you begin menopause, your vagina will resume its normal moisture. You may also experience a change in your menstrual cycle, which may be temporary or permanent. At certain times, you'll also be susceptible to infections, bleeding, or bruising. During the time when your immune system is most vulnerable, you may be asked to stay away from crowds or to wear a mask to protect you from picking up an infection that will be hard for you to fend off.

Hair loss

Losing hair is probably the most upsetting side effect. It happens with certain drugs like doxorubicin (where hair loss happens soon after beginning treatment) and CMF (where half of the women lose their hair, and half have thinning of the hair).

When you lose your hair, it isn't like it all falls out at one time, but rather it often comes out in clumps in your hand or you find your whole pillow covered in hair. Not only do you usually lose the hair on your head, but you also lose it from the rest of your body, including your eyebrows, eyelashes, and pubic area. It can leave you feeling vulnerable and unprotected, which is understandable.

Most cancer survivors recommend that you cut off your hair before it falls out, so that your experience is less traumatic. Until your hair grows back, you have several options: You can wear a wig, a scarf, or choose between many of the other glamorous (and ordinary, if you prefer) head coverings that are available. Some women prefer going bald. It's up to you. Sonia (who was mentioned in a sidebar earlier in this chapter) had the most glamorous photos taken of her in a dramatic outfit, her face perfectly made up, and her head as bald as a bowling ball. They line her entrance hall all these years later as a reminder of her days of courage.

Although it won't happen immediately, your hair will grow back. The new growth usually starts with a little peach fuzz, and then the hair grows back in. It may even grow back in a different color (often darker) and texture (often curlier) than before. But when did women ever let their natural hair color limit their looks?

Nausea and vomiting

Many factors contribute to nausea and vomiting, including the medication (some cause it, some don't) and how you react to it. However, there's really no reason for you to feel miserable:

- ✔ If you feel nauseated, tell your treatment team and work together to find what works for you. Your doctor may prescribe some antianxiety medication for you.

- ✔ Take medication that controls nausea and vomiting before you start treatment and continue as prescribed after it. Doing so sometimes helps.

  You'll be given a number of drugs to help to prevent nausea and vomiting. You'll be given antisickness drugs in the vein prior to chemotherapy, and antisickness pills to take at home. Your nurse will explain to you how to take the pills at home. Some are taken each day for two or three days after chemo and others are taken only when you feel nauseous.

✔ If you do vomit, ask your doctor for a suppository form of antinausea medication. If you find that you vomit over a few days, you can become dehydrated, so you need to let your doctor know whenever you have small, dark amounts of urine (some medications cause dark urine, too), dizziness, and a very dry mouth.

Appetite loss and weight gain

Did you know you that can lose your appetite and yet gain weight? Sounds like the worst of both worlds, doesn't it? Treatment can change your body's nutritional needs and impair how much you eat, how you digest food, and how your body uses it.

The average weight gain is eight pounds, so don't worry about obesity. Sometimes, you gain weight because you eat food that's higher in calories because everything else looks so unappealing. And sometimes you gain because you may not be moving around as much as you usually do.

Some of the weight gain can be the result of fluid retention; tell your doctor if you suddenly happen to put on weight (like five pounds overnight), if your ankles or feet feel and look very swollen, or if you have shortness of breath. Some drugs (anthracyclines) may cause heart problems that result in fluid retention, but this is rare. Most of the time, the fluid retention is a temporary minor situation, which is not caused by your heart. Your doctor will check you to see if there is anything to worry about.

When you're up to it, you can try to do some aerobic exercises. Not only will doing so help with the weight, it can stimulate your digestion, prevent constipation, and help you maintain your energy level. Not only that, it can also help you feel good (what a concept!). You may also want to try some of the special recipes (such as the one's you can get through the National Cancer Institute or the American Cancer Society) for dishes especially intended for people going through chemotherapy.

Mouth soreness

Some chemotherapy drugs may cause the membranes that line your mouth, throat, and digestive tracts to become irritated and sensitive. They may become red and inflamed.

Avoid spicy foods (don't worry, you can go back to the hot sauce after chemo), acidic fruit (those pineapples will have to wait until next season), and very hot drinks. Use a soft toothbrush, so your gums don't bleed and rinse often with the mouthwash recommend by your oncologist. If your gums bleed, your platelet count may be low, so be sure to let your doctor know. Keep a good lip balm nearby (nothing works as well as good old petroleum jelly) so you can keep your lips well moistened.

Peg I.

"When I started chemo, I was an intelligent woman about whom others in my school district thought highly. Several teachers came to me for advice on how to help children with reading. I was a Title I reading specialist, but now I can hardly finish a statement. I have a hard time thinking of words. I can picture what I want to say, but I'm unable to come up with the correct words. I have to write everything down or it's gone from my memory. It was worse while going through chemo and has gradually gotten better over time."

Fatigue

Just what you needed, something else to make you feel exhausted! As if your life's regular demands weren't enough, now there's chemo. Sometimes, fatigue is caused by the effects of the drugs and usually builds up after you've been undergoing treatment for a while.

When your blood cell count is down, and you're producing fewer red blood cells (the kind that carry oxygen to your body), feeling tired and even dizzy is natural. If your blood count is too low, your doctor may prescribe iron supplements, medications that speed red blood production, or even a red blood cell transfusion.

Give yourself permission to rest when you need it. You'll probably need to take naps during the day and may have to cut down on what you usually do. (I know you have so much you have to do, kids to take care of and so on, but now is the time to ask your loved ones to help. If you can, cuddle up with your favorite blanket and/or partner and read a book or watch a funny movie. Humor is a much-neglected medication that can work wonders. (See Chapters 18 and 20 for more suggestions on how to do this.)

Susceptibility to infection

A low white cell count makes you vulnerable to infection. Whenever your white cell count is low, avoid crowds and anyone you know who's sick. If you feel like you may be getting sick, let your doctor know sooner rather than later, especially if you spike a fever.

Chemobrain

If you've ever heard the term "chemobrain," understand that it wasn't coined by doctors, but rather by survivors. *Chemobrain* only recently is attracting attention. Some women complain that their memory and concentration just aren't what they were before chemotherapy treatment. In some women, this fogginess clears up with time, but in others, it lasts longer. The causes of chemobrain aren't clear yet.

Karen D.

"I hated every aspect of chemo. It was a silent hate. A private, silent war. I hated the colors of the chairs, I hated seeing a woman puking in a garbage can as she got her chemo, I hated waiting for the meds to come up from the lab, I hated the smell of the cancer ward. I hated seeing the really sick people wheeled in on their beds to get treatment. But along the way I met some really courageous women who had a lot more problems than I did. I learned to keep cheerful."

Keep a notepad or an electronic organizer with you and write down whatever it is you want to remember. Don't be harsh on yourself if you can't concentrate at first. Take your time and allow your body and mind to heal. Most women, in time, get back to their pretreatment levels of concentration.

Sexual difficulties

Sexual relations may not be your top priority during treatment. On the other hand, they've probably been a regular part of your life until now and one of the ways you and your partner achieve intimacy. Losing your sex drive, even if it's only temporary, is difficult.

If you feel exhausted, weak, or nauseous, you'll probably find it difficult to feel sexual. You may have vaginal dryness related to menopause (see section on long-term risks that follows). Talk to your doctor about nonhormonal lubricants. An estrogen ring that delivers a very tiny dose of estrogen to the vagina can also be safely used. Talking with your partner is extremely important, and in Chapter 18, we give you some suggestions for handling this sensitive subject.

Tingling, numbness, and other goodies

Some chemotherapeutic medications, such as Taxol (paclitaxel), may cause *peripheral neuropathy*, nerve damage to the peripheral parts of your body (hands, fingers, toes), which can cause tingling and numbness.

Although peripheral neuropathy gets worse with each dose, it eventually goes away when you're finished with treatment. Paclitaxel may also cause a rash on the palms of your hands and feet. Don't scratch, but rather speak to your doctor about suggesting or prescribing an antiallergenic medication.

Looking at scarier stuff: Long-term side effects

Chemotherapy can have several long-term effects, including menopause and heart problems.

Menopause

Menopause, together with its own accompanying side effects, usually begins around age 50. Some of the chemotherapeutic drugs may precipitate menopause, regardless of your age. Knowing whether that will happen to you is difficult to determine, but the closer you are to age 50, the more likely it is to occur. In younger women, it may be reversible, but there's no guarantee. Essentially, you kind of go through menopause during treatment and then come out of it after you've completed your treatment. Remember, however, that not everyone goes through menopause during chemotherapy.

Menopause has many unpleasant symptoms, including hot flashes, mood swings, weight gain, and symptoms common to aging like losing elasticity in the skin and muscle tone in your body. Dealing with menopause isn't easy when it arrives gradually, but it's even more difficult to cope with when it occurs rapidly. The good news is that women get through this period, and with help and support, you can, too. In Chapter 16, we offer you great suggestions. You may also want to check out _Menopause For Dummies_ by Marcia Jones, PhD, and Theresa Eichenwald, MD, (Wiley Publishing, Inc.), if you want or need more information.

When having intercourse, make sure that you use some form of contraception such as a barrier, IUD, or any other form of nonhormonal contraceptive during the time you're on treatment. If you experience temporary menopause, you can become pregnant, and chemotherapeutic drugs can have terrible effects on the developing fetus.

Infertility

Infertility isn't an issue when you've already had the children, but it's a tough blow if you still were planning to have them. If your menopause is temporary, you may get another opportunity to have children, but if it isn't, this door sadly will close for you.

Talk to your partner, your family, and close friends, and, by all means, allow yourself to mourn the loss. It is a tremendous loss. You can, of course, adopt, if that's something you want to do, but mourning the loss of the children you dreamt of is a process that you'll probably go through. Please look at the chapters in Parts IV and V, where we discuss some of the ways to help you take care of yourself.

Heart damage

Several of the chemotherapeutic drugs, including doxorubicin (Adriamycin) and epirubicin, can cause damage to heart muscles, which can lead to heart failure. Doxorubicin, however, is one of the most effective drugs in terms of killing cancer cells. The risk seems particularly high in patients who receive higher cumulative or total doses of the drug, the elderly, and patients with previous heart disease. Generally you get four or six cycles, and the risk of heart problems usually is only seen when you receive eight or more cycles.

Because heart damage is such a serious risk, you'll probably have a heart scan, which tells you how well your heart is functioning, before starting your treatment. Likewise, your doctor monitors your heart very carefully during treatment.

Leukemia

Leukemia is cancer of the white blood cells that can be caused by some forms of chemotherapy. However, most of the chemotherapeutic drugs that doctors currently use don't have this risk.

Lower quality of life

Survivors, in general, report excellent physical and emotional health five to 10 years after treatment (in one study), but women who had chemotherapy and/or hormonal therapy scored significantly lower on many of the measures of quality of life.

In particular, women who'd gone through chemotherapy reported a worsening of their health and an ongoing difficulty with sexual comfort. Take this into consideration when you're making your decision about whether to have chemotherapy.

Chapter 13

Knowing What to Expect from Hormone Therapy

*O*h those hormones: You love 'em; you hate 'em. When they're circulating through your body and making you the woman you are, developing your breasts and femininity as you mature, helping you ovulate and have babies, and strengthening your bones and muscles, you're naturally grateful.

But when they rage premenstrually, making you grouchy and miserable, you curse them. And when they go away forever, leaving you sweaty and shaky, weakening your bones, and thickening your middle, you naturally mourn their loss. Yes, you guessed it; hormones are an essential part of your life as a woman.

In this chapter, we talk about hormone treatment, but not hormone-replacement therapy (the kind of hormone treatment most people think of), which is for women who are going through menopause and has nothing whatsoever to do with cancer. No, here we describe how hormone therapy, such as prescribing tamoxifen, interferes with cancer cells so they can't grow. Bet you didn't know *that* drug can actually treat cancer *and* prevent it? Tamoxifen can. Tamoxifen is the hormone treatment for premenopausal women, and until last year was the only drug for postmenopausal women. Although more are now available, most women have heard of tamoxifen. Of course, with every treatment come benefits *and* risks, and we describe them to you carefully, so you can determine whether hormone treatment is right for you. Whenever you go on hormone treatment, we describe what to expect during treatment and what questions to ask your doctor.

Throwing a Monkey into the Multiplying Wrench

Ovaries produce two hormones, *estrogen* and *progesterone*. In addition to all that the good hormones do for us, they can actually stimulate the growth of some breast cancers. Traitors!

It turns out that many cancer cells have hormone receptors for estrogen. *Hormone receptors* are the part of the cell to which the estrogen sticks. When estrogen binds with cancer-cell hormone receptors, the cancer cells are stimulated to multiply.

Not all cancer cells have these receptors. The ones that do are called *hormone receptor–positive,* and the ones that don't are *hormone receptor–negative.* If cancer cells that are hormone receptor–positive are treated (in a test tube) with tamoxifen (meaning that as you grow them, you put liquid tamoxifen on them), it halts the cancer cells from multiplying by blocking the effects of estrogen. A similar reaction takes place when you take tamoxifen. If your cancer cells are hormone receptor–positive, and you are treated with tamoxifen (in pill form), then it halts the cancer cells from multiplying by blocking the effects of estrogen.

It's wonderful news that tamoxifen can stop the uncontrolled multiplication of cancer cells. On top of that, it's also a great improvement over what women had to go through during the past to stop hormone production: removing their ovaries surgically (*oopherectomy*) or irradiating them via a procedure known as an *ovarian ablation*. Although these methods still are used in some cases, they're used only in very specific and rare circumstances.

So surgery and radiation have been replaced by . . . a pill. Yes, you read that right. Tamoxifen is administered as a pill, so you won't have any needles poking in your arm, intravenous catheters, or cold medicine dripping poison in your veins. Just a glass of water and a pill and that's that. Like all medications, however, tamoxifen has side effects and even long-term risks, but it is far less toxic than chemotherapy.

HRT for cancer?

Many people understandably become confused about the difference between hormone therapy *for breast cancer* and hormone replacement therapy *for women going through menopause.* Is it any wonder? Both have something to do with hormones (mostly estrogen). *Hormone replacement therapy* provides estrogen when a woman's body no longer makes it; *hormone therapy* for cancer, on the other hand, prevents cancer cells from multiplying.

The next important discovery that was made is that tamoxifen didn't act in only one way; researchers found that it acts differently in different parts of the body. Think of it like this: It's like a one-person band, playing more than one instrument and creating different melodies that apply to different parts of the body.

- ✔ **In the breast cancer cells:** Tamoxifen blocks estrogen receptors in the breast cancer cells by acting as an *antagonist* (or competitor). The estrogen and tamoxifen rush to grab on to the hormone receptor of the breast cancer cell, but tamoxifen ultimately binds with them so they can't multiply.

- ✔ **In the bones and lipids:** Rather than being a competitor in the bones and lipids, tamoxifen acts as a facilitator (or *agonist*). In other words, it helps the estrogen reach the bones and lipids, which, in turn, has tremendous positive effects. It helps preserve the density of women's bones, protecting them against *osteoporosis* (thinning of the bones).

- ✔ **In the uterus:** Tamoxifen acts as a facilitator in the uterus, helping estrogen reach the uterus, which unfortunately results in increases in cancer of the lining of the uterus, or *endometrium*. (You find out more about endometrial cancer in the next section.)

Because it interacts one way with hormone receptors in one part of the body and another way with hormone receptors in other parts of the body, tamoxifen is referred to as a *selective (discerning) hormone-receptor modulator.* Actually, if you really want to impress someone, you call it a *selective estrogen-receptor modulator (SERM).* Tamoxifen was the first of the SERMs ever discovered. Learning from it, other similar drugs have been developed, such as raloxifene or other types of antihormonal breast cancer treatments discussed later in this chapter.

Putting Tamoxifen on the Scale: Weighing Risks and Benefits

The benefits of tamoxifen in treating breast cancer are substantial. The combined results of a study indicate that when tamoxifen is taken for five years

- ✔ It reduces the annual odds of recurrence by 47 percent, a relative risk ratio that means the reduction in risk when compared with a group of similar women who weren't prescribed tamoxifen.

- ✔ It reduces the annual odds of death by 26 percent, which again is a relative risk ratio. See Chapter 8 for an explanation.

So what do these relative risk ratios mean for *your* survival? After taking tamoxifen for five years

- If the cancer had spread to your nodes before it was prescribed (which is an indicator of a poorer prognosis), it increases your likelihood of survival by 11 percent.

- If the cancer had not spread to your nodes before it was prescribed (which already is a very good prognosis), it increases your survival likelihood by 6 percent.

There's more! This benefit was seen equally in women of all ages. Yes, that means pre- and postmenopausal women. And, there's even more! Even after women stop taking tamoxifen after the prescribed five years

- It continues to reduce the risk of recurrent breast cancer by 33 percent, when compared with women who had never taken it.

- It continues to reduce the risk of developing new breast cancers by 47 percent when compared with women to whom tamoxifen never was prescribed.

- The benefits continue for at least ten years after women stop taking it.

But as is true with all good things in life, nothing is perfect. Risks associated with taking tamoxifen are that it

- **Isn't effective in some women.** It's ineffective in cancer cells that don't have hormone receptors. That's why testing to determine hormone-receptor status is so critical. Being hormone receptor–positive tells you that you're a candidate for hormonal therapy.

- **Triples the risk of postmenopausal women developing endometrial cancer.** Endometrial cancer is cancer of the lining of the uterus. Very few women actually develop endometrial cancer. (In other words, the risk is low. Only three in 1,000 women taking tamoxifen develop endometrial cancer, and only one in 1,000 women will die from it.)

Endometrial cancer usually results in vaginal spotting or bleeding, so it can be caught early. Whenever you notice unusual bleeding or spotting, tell your doctor immediately. And don't forget to see your doctor for your pelvic exam at least once a year.

Preventing breast cancer

Tamoxifen is the *only* drug approved by the Food and Drug Administration (FDA) for reducing the risk of breast cancer in women who are at high risk for developing the disease. Although the future may hold more such beneficial drugs, at the moment, tamoxifen stands alone.

So far, three clinical trials have been completed of women who were at high risk for breast cancer and were treated *prophylactically* (as a means of prevention of the onset of breast cancer) with tamoxifen. When the results of these studies were combined, researchers discovered a 42 percent reduction in relative risk of these women developing breast cancer. These findings are exciting, but remember that the figures refer only to *relative risk*, which means for the group as a whole when compared with a similar group of women who didn't take tamoxifen.

What all this means for *you* is that you must know the *absolute risk reduction,* which is the actual reduction in risk for women like *you*. The amount of risk reduction actually depends on *your* individual level of risk. The higher your level of risk, the more tamoxifen can reduce it.

Scoping out Other Hormone Treatments

Inspired by the success of tamoxifen, researchers continue their pursuit of other types of medication that will be equally or more effective than tamoxifen in treating women with either early or metastatic breast cancers with fewer side effects. They also are searching for drugs that likewise are effective in treating cancers that are resistant to tamoxifen.

Other types of hormonal treatments currently are under investigation, and new results become available all the time, so check the Web sites of the American Cancer Society, the Susan G. Komen Foundation, or the National Cancer Institute. Their addresses are listed in Chapter 24. Some of these new treatments are described in the sections that follow.

Aromatase inhibitors

Aromatase inhibitors (AIs) inhibit an enzyme that converts *androgen* (male hormone present in woman) to estrogen. They are important because most of the circulating estrogen in postmenopausal women comes from the conversion of androgens to estrogens. Inhibiting these conversions, therefore, lowers the levels of estrogen that are available to the cancer cell.

Combining chemo and HRT

Hormonal treatment, at times, may be combined with chemotherapy. In women whose tumors are hormone receptor–positive, this combined treatment appears to be more effective than either treatment alone. Check out Chapter 12 to find out which combination of treatments is recommended for you.

Interestingly, aromatase inhibitors don't work in premenopausal women, because most of their circulating estrogen is made in their ovaries.

An entirely new generation of aromatase inhibitors, such as anastrozole (or Arimidex) and letrozole (or Femara) and exemestane (or Aromasin) have been shown to be as effective, and in some cases, more effective than tamoxifen in treating postmenapausal women with metastatic breast cancer, while producing fewer side effects. As a result, aromatase inhibitors have become the treatment of choice for many newly diagnosed hormone receptor—positive metastatic breast cancers.

Ask your doctor whether anastrozole or tamoxifen is the better choice for you.

Although these drugs are effective, they nevertheless can cause *osteoporosis,* so you need to check your bone density on a regular basis whenever you're taking an aromatase inhibitor.

Pure antiestrogens

Testing started only recently on pure antiestrogens, such as fulvestrant (Faslodex). These drugs destroy estrogen receptors (burn, baby, burn!) Although early results indicate that fulvestrant is as good as anastrozole in patients with metastatic breast cancer, no results have been reported about its effect on women with earlier stages of breast cancer. Stay tuned!

Derivatives of tamoxifen

Toremifene (Fareston) is a tamoxifen derivative that is as good as tamoxifen in patients with metastatic breast cancer. Ask your doctor whether this is the right drug for you.

Sticking It Out During Symptoms

Although hormonal therapy is closing in on perfection, it still has side effects and a few long-term risks. But just because you're on hormonal treatment doesn't necessarily mean that you'll experience them.

Sweating through the side effects is a drag

The more common side effects of tamoxifen are hot flashes, vaginal discharge or dryness, and irregular menses in women who are premenopausal. Doesn't sound very exciting, does it? But although these can affect the quality of your life, especially your sex life, we have some great suggestions in this chapter and in Chapter 19 on how to triumph over them.

Hot flashes

Anyone who never has experienced hot flashes doesn't understand what the fuss is all about. After all, it's just a flash of heat, isn't it? Well, not quite. Imagine yourself sitting at your desk when without any warning whatsoever you feel waves of heat rising up your chest, neck, and face. Your face becomes red, and sweat pours down your neck, back, and forehead, all in the span of merely an instant.

Clearing up misleading myths

Many women are reluctant to go on tamoxifen because they're concerned about becoming depressed or getting fat, but these concerns are *not* side effects of tamoxifen.

✔ **Depression or mood swings:** Some early studies reported an increase in depression or mood swings in women taking tamoxifen; however, more recent studies that have tracked women from the start of treatment, throughout it, and after it, found no increases in the risk of depression, anxiety, or psychological distress. Good news, indeed!

That said, you nevertheless may experience depression. Anyone can. If it happens to you, ask your doctor to evaluate you for antidepressants, which have been found to be extremely effective.

✔ **Weight gain — not!:** Here's something that only women can understand. It's about putting on weight. Even though tamoxifen decreases the risk of developing breast cancer, many women (yes, I mean you) won't start taking it because they heard that it makes you put on weight! (I told you only women could relate to this!)

Okay ladies; let's stop that myth right here and now. Placebo-controlled studies have been conducted, which means some women get the medication and others don't and no one knows who's getting it and who isn't, and guess what! Tamoxifen *does not* cause weight gain. Yes, chemotherapy *does*, but not tamoxifen.

I remember seeing a television show in which the leading lady, during a hot flash, began stripping at a restaurant, removing layer after layer of clothing, but the only way she found relief was standing in front of an open freezer in her underwear with a look of utter bliss on her face. That's a hot flash! Unfortunately, they often come in groups, not singly, and waking up in the middle of the night in pajamas and a bed that are soaking wet isn't unusual.

Fortunately, when you undergo hormonal treatment without chemotherapy these symptoms will disappear in time (although it may take several years). Speak to your doctor about medications that help make these symptoms less severe.

Vaginal dryness and discharge

When you're one of the unlucky ones to experience this side effect, and almost a third of the women on tamoxifen do, vaginal dryness or discharge can cause you real discomfort, even outside of sexual relations.

Talk to your doctor about nonhormonal lubricants. An estrogen ring, which delivers very tiny doses of estrogen to the vagina, may be used whenever symptoms are severe. (See also Chapter 19 for some saucy tips on rekindling your sex life.)

Looking at scarier stuff: Serious effects

The other potential serious effects of tamoxifen include cataracts, thrombophlebitis, and endometrial cancer. The last two are potentially life threatening, although fortunately they occur only rarely.

Cataracts

Although rare, an increase in cataracts has been reported among women taking tamoxifen. Three women in 1,000 are at risk of developing it.

Thrombophlebitis and other rare risks

Fewer than 1 percent of women are at risk for *thrombophlebitis,* a clotting in the veins of your legs, and strokes, when taking tamoxifen. Death from thrombophlebitis is extremely rare (one death per 1,000 postmenopausal women treated for five years).

Whenever you have a history of the following conditions, you should not take tamoxifen except in special circumstances where you're closely monitored by your doctor.

Memory and thinking

Here's an interesting twist: In a study of residents in a nursing home, women who were taking tamoxifen experienced less frequent episodes of Alzheimer's disease and were better able to care for themselves than women who weren't taking tamoxifen. However, when women on tamoxifen (others, not the ones in the nursing homes) were asked how they were doing, they reported an increase in memory problems, even though no decreases in thinking and processing thoughts were observed. The answers obviously aren't clear yet on this issue (although I must say that I like the idea of not getting Alzheimer's). More studies are underway in this field.

✔ ***Deep vein thrombosis.*** Blood clots in the veins deep in your legs. (These are not varicose veins or the red, lumpy veins on the surface of your leg.) The risk of blood clots is increased in anyone who's inactive. So if you're taking tamoxifen, your doctor will ask you to temporarily stop the drug to reduce the risk of clots when

- You break a leg.

- You're temporarily laid up from any major surgery, or otherwise immobilized.

  Right after surgery is an especially bad time. Doctors prefer waiting at least until you resume a normal level of activity before prescribing tamoxifen. (Well, you don't have to be playing basketball three times a week, but, on the other hand, you can't be sitting on the couch watching movies all the time either!)

  Don't worry. Whenever something happens and you're temporarily laid up (like if you must have major surgery or you're injured in some other way totally unrelated to the cancer), temporarily stopping tamoxifen *reduces* the risk of blood clots.

  However, even though deep vein thrombosis is a very rare side effect, if you're on tamoxifen, you must let your doctor know immediately whenever you notice any pain or swelling in *one* leg. This doesn't mean swelling of both your ankles when you've been on your feet all day.

✔ ***Stokes.*** A stroke occurs when the brain is deprived of blood. Symptoms depend on the part of the brain affected and may include loss of speech, vision, the ability to move an arm or leg, or in severe cases, even death. Strokes can be caused by blood vessels in the brain clotting or clots in other vessels moving to the brain. Among women older than 50 who are taking tamoxifen for five years, the increase in number of strokes per 1,000 women per year is only one. No excess of strokes is seen in women younger than 50.

> ✔ *Transient ischemic attack.* Symptoms are blurred vision or temporary loss of movement of the arm or leg, which are also warning signs of a stroke. For women older than 50, an increase of only one TIA per year was recorded among 3,000 women taking tamoxifen for five years.

Uterine-lining (endometrial) cancer

Tamoxifen increases the risk of endometrial cancer in postmenopausal women who have a uterus. Obviously, you can't get cancer of the uterus if you don't have one! However, the incidence of this kind of cancer is low, only two to three cases for every 1,000 women who have a uterus and are treated with tamoxifen. Your risk is greater if you've ever been on hormone replacement therapy (HRT) or are overweight.

Whenever you're taking tamoxifen, you must be monitored with a pelvic exam once a year. Likewise, you must let your doctor know immediately whenever you experience any abnormal bleeding.

Future Prospects

Although this chapter provides the basic information, be sure to ask your doctor for the latest news in the exciting and hopeful new area of hormone therapy. Endocrine (hormone) therapy of breast cancer is a very active area of research, and treatment recommendations are changing all the time as new information becomes available. Some areas that are being studied include

> ✔ Drugs that block the chemicals in the brain that cause estrogen and progesterone to be produced (called *LHRH-agonists*) and result in temporary menopause. These drugs are being studied alone and in combination with tamoxifen in premenopausal women.

> ✔ The best order in which to give tamoxifen and aromatase inhibitors and what women specifically will benefit from one treatment or the other.

Chapter 14

Giving Complementary Therapies Kudos

During the last ten years, millions of Americans have turned to complementary and alternative therapies as a way of preventing disease or treating symptoms. In the United States today, estimates point to about half of those affected by cancer as having turned to or considered these methods.

In this chapter, we explain the difference (and there is a very big difference) between complementary and alternative therapies, describe the risks and benefits of some of these treatments, and most important, help you make informed therapy choices by evaluating the risks and benefits.

Defining Terms: It Matters

The first step in being able to evaluate any of these methods is distinguishing between alternative and complementary therapies. Unfortunately, most people still use these terms interchangeably. But important differences exist between the two.

Avoiding alternative therapies

Alternative therapies are the kind of therapies that are used instead of *conventional medical treatment* (scientifically tested and proven to be safe and effective) to prevent or cure disease. Based on the most up-to-date scientific information, doctors strongly urge you not to use any therapy *in place of* the recommended medical treatment for your breast cancer.

Alternative therapies are extremely dangerous because

✔ They cannot cure cancer or cause *remission* (halt the cancer temporarily), despite claims to the contrary.

✔ When you take alternatives instead of a medical treatment that's known to be effective, you delay your receipt of medical treatment that is needed to help you.

Sometimes the makers (and more important, the sellers) of alternative therapies make claims that are totally false. Various sellers of alternative therapies have claimed that their products

✔ **Can cure cancer.** As much as everyone wants to find a cure, not even the best medical treatment that's been carefully studied each step of the way claims to be able to cure cancer. The most that medicine claims are years of remission or years of survival. Anyone who claims to have a cure for cancer is selling you false hope.

✔ **Have no side effects.** This assertion is untrue. At the moment, medical research has developed only a few cancer treatments that have minimal side effects because they target only the cancer. This discovery came about after many, many years of rigorous study. None of the people selling alternative therapies can provide any proof whatsoever of their claim to have a treatment with no side effects.

Considering complementary therapies

Complementary therapies are used *in addition to* conventional medicine. This wide range of methods is broadly grouped into five categories. These kinds of therapies can help you deal with some of cancer's consequences and alleviate some of the treatment side effects. However, not all complementary therapies are beneficial; some may even be *harmful*. We tell you how to distinguish between the two in the following section.

Some complementary therapies may also directly affect your medical treatment. For example, taking antioxidant vitamins may render chemotherapy or radiation treatment less effective. Others can cause severe bleeding during surgery or unusual reactions to anesthesia. We strongly urge you to tell your

doctor whether you're taking any supplements or vitamins. Doing so gives your doctor the information needed to provide you with the best treatment.

Distinguishing the Good from the Bad

So, how do you know whether a complementary treatment is good for you, especially when so much information is available out there that it often clashes in contradiction. More important, how do you know which sources to trust?

So much information coming from so many different sources can seem overwhelming, but it won't be if you:

✔ **Know that natural can be toxic.** Don't assume that just because a product *says* it's "all natural" that that means it's good for you. It may not be. Take, for example

- **Castor beans.** These seeds can be extremely poisonous. A terrorist group recently was caught making a lethal compound from them.

  It's naïve to assume that just because something is natural (like castor beans) it's good for you.

- **Beta carotene.** This natural pigment found in mainly yellow and orange fruits and vegetables (such as carrots, squash and oranges), when taken as a supplement, may increase the risk of lung cancer in smokers (although it may play a role in preventing other forms of cancer such as breast cancer).

- **Garlic, vitamin E, and ginger.** All three of these substances can thin the blood and help prevent normal blood clotting. When you're also taking blood-thinning medications or having surgery, these supplements may cause excessive bleeding.

  Similarly, sometimes vitamins or herbal supplements may be toxic when taken in high doses. So, be careful!

✔ **Consider the source.** Evaluate information critically. Just because you read about it or see it on TV does *not* mean that it's right. For example

- **Anyone can post anything on the Internet.** Whenever you don't know the source of the information, don't naïvely assume that it's a fact.

- **Glossy brochures may or may not be correct, depending on the scientific evidence.** You know the ones; they promise that a supplement will boost your immune system or reduce your risk of recurrence. Remember that the purpose of the brochure is to sell you the product.

> ✔ **Ensure the therapy has been tested.** Does scientific evidence back up the claim? Treatments proven to be effective have been all of the following:
>
>   • **Rigorously and scientifically tested according to proven methods.**
>
>   • **Critically evaluated by scientists other than those who conducted the studies.**
>
>   • **Published in academic journals.** These journals publish only those studies that meet the first two criteria.

Get your information from reliable sources. Up-to-date information on complementary and alternative medicines (CAM) is available from The National Center for Complementary and Alternative Medicine, The American Cancer Society, and The Susan G. Komen Foundation. Additional information about these agencies is available in Chapters 23 and 24.

Giving Complementary Therapies a Compliment

The range of complementary therapies is a wide one, and is broadly grouped into five different categories by type. You have the right to decide on your treatment options (more about them can be found in Chapter 9), but we strongly urge you to select the ones that are proven effective.

Together we can climb mountains

An unspoken battle rages over an issue between the public and the medical establishment. The public, including many cancer survivors, has embraced many nontraditional herbs, supplements, and alternative treatments. The medical establishment originally pooh-poohed these methods, referring to all of them as alternative with no scientific evidence for their claims.

A shift during the last decade resulted in a kind of uneasy truce. Many medical centers now sport complementary and alternative medicine centers to study treatments and provide the ones that are found to be effective. The National Institutes of Health (NIH) contain an institute to study and fund studies on these methods, and many other organizations are funding research on these issues.

Doctors no longer simply dismiss these treatments; however, they want scientific evidence to prove that a method is effective. Most patients, on the other hand, still are reluctant to tell their doctors that they're taking herbs, supplements, or vitamins. And that's dangerous to say the least.

Complementing sugar, spice, & everything nice — or not

A recent study of breast cancer survivors found that close to two-thirds use some form of dietary supplements (which is anything that you add regularly to your diet including vitamins, minerals, and herbs) and half use herbal preparations which are herbs derived from the plant including the stalk, leaves, flowers, or roots. The most common are echinacea, gingko, ginseng, and St. John's Wort. Most scientific evidence for these treatments is unknown, inconclusive, or not presently encouraging. Table 14-1 gives the dish on some of the more popular ones.

Table 14-1	Herbs and Supplements	
Herb or supplement	**The (somewhat) good**	**The just plain bad**
Ginger, a plant.	Effective against nausea for motion sickness or after surgery.	May not be effective against nausea during chemotherapy, because ginger affects the stomach, not the central nervous system, which is how chemotherapy causes nausea. Although the taste and smell of ginger has a calming effect, taking large doses in pill form has been shown to cause depression and irregular heartbeats.
Black Cohosh, a plant.	Root that has been found to be effective in treating menstrual symptoms such as menstrual cramps and menopausal symptoms such as hot flashes. Although it's chemicals resemble the effects of estrogen, it doesn't contain the hormone. Some herbalists believe it may be dangerous for people with cancer, while others state that because it doesn't contain estrogen, it's safe for cancer patients.	Scientists caution that it should not be used for more than six consecutive months.

(continued)

Table 14-1 *(continued)*

Herb or supplement	The (somewhat) good	The just plain bad
Echinacea, a genus of wild-growing herb	Widely believed to help fight colds and flu. However, most recent studies have found it doesn't enhance the immune system, and no evidence exists that it increases resistance to cancer or alleviates the side effects of chemotherapy or radiation therapy.	Some caution that when used for more than eight weeks it can cause liver damage or suppress the immune system.
Gingko, an extract of leaves from the ginkgo tree	Aids memory in patients with dementia and improves blood circulation. Some herbalists claim that gingko contains a substance that may block a chemical that causes tumor growth, although there's no scientific evidence to support this.	No studies have been conducted on ginkgo regarding its effectiveness in preventing or treating cancer.
Ginseng, a plant	Although several studies have been conducted to investigate whether it can prevent cancer, the results to date are inconclusive.	Is available in various forms, although because of its expense, it is often diluted or mislabeled.
St. John's Wort, a shrub flower	Has been shown to be effective in treating depression that isn't severe. Some women with breast cancer take it to deal with feelings of depression that may have arisen following their diagnosis. A large study is currently underway to examine its effectiveness with severe depression.	The FDA has issued a public health alert that it may interfere with several other prescriptions you're on, such as oral contraception, digoxin (heart medication), antiretroviral medication (treats HIV). If you're on any other medication, please consult with your doctor before taking St. John's Wort. Also, if you use it in combination with other antidepressants you can have a severe psychiatric disturbance that can even result in death.

Eating to remission

A study recently evaluated the relative benefit and harm to cancer survivors of several dietary factors. Those proven to be beneficial included food safety, which refers to organic and safe food preparation, and losing weight (if you're overweight) *after* recovery. Losing weight during treatment has been proven to be harmful, so if you want to diet, do it only after you've completed your treatment. A seminal study recently published results that demonstrated the huge role obesity plays in cancer risk, (see more about that in Chapter 3.) What's so exciting (and hopeful) about these results is that if you're overweight, you can decrease your risk by losing weight.

Increasing the amount of fruit and vegetables in your diet, decreasing alcohol, eating a vegetarian diet and juice therapies are considered beneficial even though these courses of action haven't been scientifically proven but are strongly recommended by the American Cancer Society.

It's worth mentioning that despite the enthusiasm of the public and the scientific community for the use of soy foods (such as tofu, soybean milk, or soy powder) in preventing recurrence of breast cancer, the findings have been inconsistent. In some studies, soy-based products were found to inhibit the growth of breast cancer cells, while in others, it was found to stimulate them to grow. Some studies currently are underway, but until they are completed, soy can't be recommended, because it may be beneficial for some women but harmful to others.

Reading the buzz on beasties

Some substances are synthesized and produced from chemicals, plants, or other living things, such as blood, urine, or cartilage from humans or animals. Sounds creepy, doesn't it? But many such substances exist, and some are currently being scientifically evaluated while others simply make completely unsubstantiated claims.

Apitherapy or bee-venom therapy

A few laboratory studies have looked at the anticancer effects of some of the active ingredients in the venom of bees, the pollen they collect, and the *propolis* or waxy stuff they use to build their hives. Some claims have been made that cancer cells in a test tube were killed. However, these results have been neither published nor tested in humans.

Cow or Shark Cartilage

Cartilage is an elastic tissue found in many animals. Cartilage from cows and sharks is sold as food supplements, claiming to slow the growth of cancer. No scientific evidence supports this assertion yet, but the National Cancer Institute currently is funding a large trial of liquid shark cartilage extract, together with conventional treatments, in the fight against lung cancer.

Fatty acid from Perna canaliculus

This fatty acid is extracted from a mussel called Perna canaliculus, native to New Zealand and is sold in capsule form in supermarkets in New Zealand and over the Internet. A few years ago, when a local researcher claimed that he found this substance was able to stop cancer, $2 million worth of the capsules were sold the next week. At the same time, another laboratory researcher in New Zealand warned that this substance may promote tumor growth. Public outrage stopped the manufacturer from distributing it, but other companies continue to sell it.

Getting touchy-feely

This group of treatments involves touching, manipulation, or body movement, and is based on the premise that problems in one part of your body often affect other parts of your body. These treatments include a wide range of activities.

Bodywork

Bodywork claims to relieve pain, reduce stress, and promote relaxation by a range of physically oriented techniques that include

- ✔ **Rolfing.** Using fingers, hands, elbows, and knees to apply deep pressure and realign bones.

  Manipulating a bone where cancer has metastasized can result in a bone fracture.

- ✔ **Movement therapy.** Using movement, rhythmic motion, and dance to improve mental well-being. Clinical reports have shown that it helps reduce stress, provides exercise, improves self-awareness and confidence, and improves circulation. Over and above all this, it can help you get fit and enjoy your life. Try it sometime.

- ✔ **Shiatsu massage.** *Shiatsu* (which means finger-pressure in Japanese) consists of pressing fingers on points of the body to open pathways for the body's flow of energy or life force (also known as *chi*).

Many people who have used these methods report feeling more relaxed and therefore more able to deal with whatever challenges they have to face during treatment.

Acupuncture

Tiny needles are inserted into the skin and manipulated. Another version of acupuncture is electroacupuncture, in which electrical stimulation is applied to the acupoints.

Several studies have found acupuncture effective against nausea caused by chemotherapy and anesthesia for surgery. Some studies have found that it may also reduce the need for conventional pain medication.

To find an acupuncturist, ask the proprietors of the herbal store nearest you to recommend someone, or simply look in the Yellow Pages.

Cancer salves

Pastes, salves, or poultices also have been applied to the skin on top of a tumor that is inside the body or directly onto external tumors with a completely unsubstantiated belief that it can cure the cancer. Variations of these ointments may contain a mixture of up to ten different ingredients including Indian tobacco, comfrey, myrrh, and chaparral in a base of olive oil, beeswax, and tar.

No evidence exists that these topical applications can treat any cancers or tumors, and in fact, many severe burns have been reported as a result of using these salves.

Therapeutic touch and polarity therapy

Therapeutic touch and polarity therapy are based on the belief that the smooth flow of energy within the patient's body promotes health, and blockages of that energy field prevent it. A *polarity therapist* applies varieties of hands-on techniques, including twisting the torso, curling the toes, rocking motions, and moving crystals along the person's body. In *therapeutic touch* no actual touching of the patient occurs. Instead, the therapist holds his or her hands above the patient's body, which is believed to release harmful energy from the patient. Although no scientific evidence supports that either of these techniques promotes healing, patients often report feeling relaxed after these sessions. Doctors may refer you for one or both of these therapies as a relaxation tool.

Finding the connection between mind, body, and spirit

Many different types of therapies focus on the interrelationship between the mind, the body, and the spirit. Most have a very positive impact on the quality of your life, by improving your overall sense of well-being. Wiley publishes *Mind-Body Fitness For Dummies* if you want to learn more.

Support groups

Many studies have revealed that support groups are extremely helpful for people going through treatment. By receiving information and offering support to one another, survivors are better able to deal with the extraordinary challenges that cancer poses. We talk about support groups in Chapters 18 and 23.

Support groups vary in

- ✔ **What they offer:** Information to emotional support
- ✔ **Structure:** A closed group or one in which people come and go

> ✔ **Focus:** Listening to working through issues
>
> ✔ **Place:** Face to face or online
>
> ✔ **How they're led:** By a professional or by members

Try out a group and see which one fits you best. Some women prefer one that's face to face in someone's home, whereas others prefer a group run by a professional. Your decision often depends on whether you click with other members. If you don't fit in with the first support group you attend, don't give up. Try another one or go online. So much can be gained from belonging to one.

Imagery

You can also use mental exercises in which you visualize images such as walking along a peaceful beach with blue-green water lapping at your feet, a cool breeze gently blowing your hair and the person you love the most in the world at your side. Mmmm, just thinking about such things makes my shoulders drop from their customary tense position and a calm feeling descends throughout my body. Try it (using an image that appeals to you) and see what response you have.

In *image therapy,* either trained therapists assist you during 30-minute sessions, or you can try it on your own, learning from books or tapes. Image therapy techniques include:

> ✔ Guided imagery, in which you visualize a specific image or goal that you want to achieve (for example, walking cancer-free on the beach)
>
> ✔ Palming, which includes placing the palms of your hand over your eyes and imagining a color you associate with stress (perhaps black) and then a color you associate with calm (perhaps blue)

Yoga

The many different forms and types of yoga use different focuses or methods, with the underlying thread being the use of movement, breathing, and meditation to achieve a connection between the mind, body, and spirit. The sense of calm and relaxation and added confidence can help you cope much better with all that you're going through.

Meditation

Meditation is a mind-body method that combines breathing with concentration or reflection aimed at relaxing the body and calming the mind, which results in a sense of well-being. Many different forms of meditation are achieved through sitting quietly, with closed eyes, and trying to achieve a sense of peace. Other forms of meditation actually are achieved through movement. Tai chi is one example. You can meditate on your own or be guided by a professional. You can explore this ancient art in Wiley's *Tai Chi For Dummies.*

Chapter 15

Regarding Reconstruction

. . . .

In This Chapter

▶ Examining all your options

▶ Considering reconstruction — when and why

▶ Discovering what type of reconstructive surgery is right for you

. . . .

Reconstructing your breasts isn't a part of your treatment. It's an option that you may or may not want to consider. Reconstruction is surgery (actually several different types of surgery that we tell you about in this chapter) to build you a breast to replace the one that was removed because it had cancer cells in it. The option of reconstructing your breast is available if you want it, and its sole purpose is to make you feel good about yourself, your body image, and your sexuality. What a relief! Something that's just for you. Reconstructive surgery is neither a part of all the instructions you seem to be getting at every turn nor a medical necessity. Surprisingly, and quite wonderfully, it's a consideration of your femininity.

Furthermore, you don't need to feel forced into one decision or another, because whether you have reconstructive surgery is a matter of preference, and you get to make the decision.

So, how are you supposed to know what's the right decision for you? And how can you make such a choice when you're already in the throes of dealing with so many other decisions? We wrote this chapter to help you answer those questions. We break down reconstruction (there's an oxymoron for ya!) step by step, so you can review your options carefully through your new-found understanding of the pros and cons and benefits and risks of each of your choices. Take your time when making your decision. After all, it's yours to make and yours to live with. After you read this chapter, you'll know when the time is right for *you* to make *your* decision.

Karen D.

"I had a mastectomy with bilateral reconstruction. Here I woke up with two mounds. It was wonderful. I felt like a woman again. I figured, 'go for the gusto' and now I'm a good sized C/D."

Looking Over Some Options

The first step in guiding your decision is making you aware of the choices you have. When you've had a mastectomy, the three options you have are

- ✔ **Doing nothing further.** Au naturel is just fine for you. You don't want to do anything else after treatment.

- ✔ **Using a prosthesis.** This breast form can be worn in your bra. With your clothes on, it looks completely natural. When and where you wear it is your choice. No surgery's required with this choice, either.

- ✔ **Having reconstructive surgery.** Reconstruction involves building up a breast to replace the one that's no longer there. Sometimes, the surgeon needs to operate on the other breast, too, so that they match up. Several types of reconstructive surgery are discussed later in this chapter.

Basking au naturel

Many women don't want a reconstructed breast. They're just fine with things the way they are. Some of these women simply don't want any more surgery, and others believe that no matter how good the reconstruction is, nothing replaces the real thing. And some of these women simply don't care; with or without a breast, they're just fine. Studies have shown that regardless of their reasons, most women who choose not to have reconstruction feel just as good about their decision as women who choose to have the surgery. Besides, you can always change your mind if you want to. Hey, it's a woman's prerogative!

Ruth R.

"If I had to do it over again, I'd have a double mastectomy. I'm not a feminine woman (no heels or makeup), and I'm small-chested to begin with. It was an easy decision not to have any reconstruction done; I didn't care. But with one breast now, it's just a hassle."

Barb L.

"I have my wedding dress all picked out. I don't wear my prostheses, and no one expects me to for the wedding, either. The dress is form-fitting.

C'est la vie. I walk around like this every day of my life, at work and everywhere. I wouldn't be me otherwise."

Popping in a prosthesis

Breast forms (sometimes called a *breast prosthesis*) are very realistic in the way they look and feel. Most are worn in your bra, but some are attached directly onto your body with adhesive tape. *Breast enhancers* are available if you've had a lumpectomy and don't need a full prosthesis. They're smaller than a full breast form and available in all shapes and sizes.

Prostheses come in all shapes, sizes, colors, and prices. They're made from silicone or foam, and some are covered with latex or a particularly gentle combination of cotton and spandex fibers. They're also available with removable covers that you can take off and wash. You'd be surprised how natural they look in your bra. Most forms are weighted. (Did you think that you'd just be wearing a stuffed sock? No way!) The weight helps them sit correctly and match your other breast. Matching is more than cosmetic; it also helps prevent backache, which can occur when one breast is large and the other isn't there.

Your skin may be sensitive immediately after surgery, so you may initially need a breast form that's particularly soft on your skin and not too heavy. After your scar loses that sensitivity, you may decide that you want another kind. (See the "Breast forms are the mother of invention" sidebar in this chapter for the trick to keeping an unweighted breast form in place.)

Toni G.

"I was continually pressured to reconstruct. I think women also need to be given the alternative of being 'breastless.' It hasn't bothered me at all. Most people don't even notice that I had

a modified radical mastectomy. My boyfriend loves me just the way I am, and we have a great sex life. Entirely too much emphasis is placed on breasts."

Wearing a breast form won't limit your activities. You can do almost everything with these prostheses, including exercising and swimming.

You can buy a breast form that's ready-made, or you can have one made just for you. They're available at specialty stores. The Reach to Recovery volunteer who visits you in the hospital after surgery will give you a list of places where you can find breast forms. See Chapter 10 for more about what to expect before, during, and after surgery. Chapter 24 describes the Tender Loving Care (tlc) program of the American Cancer Society, a nonprofit organization that sells breast forms.

You need to buy a prosthesis that's comfortable and fits. Following these tips can go a long way toward making sure that happens:

- **Shop on a day when you're not rushed.** Make sure that you have some energy that day, too. Prosthesis shopping, like bra shopping for many women, can be rather exhausting and stressful.

- **Ask a good friend or trusted family member to go with you.** Just like buying the perfect evening gown, you want someone to give you an honest (but hopefully flattering) opinion. You'll also need someone to keep your spirits and your energy up. You may be in for a long day.

- **Wear a comfortable bra and a tight-fitting top for this particular shopping expedition.** Doing so helps you determine what looks good and what doesn't.

- **Go to more than one store.** Prostheses are available in many types and styles, but most stores usually carry only one or two varieties. To get a good selection, you may have to make several stops.

Breast forms are the mother of invention

After your mastectomy, you may be given a breast form to wear as a *take-home prosthesis.* This temporary breast form isn't weighted, so it's less likely to hurt your incision. You can also buy lightweight prostheses that won't press on your sensitive scar. However, temporary or unweighted breast forms may not be substantial enough to hold your bra in place. In fact, you may find your bra creeping up around your ears if you had a double mastectomy. Fortunately, women find solutions for most problems, and this one is no exception. Try this trick:

1. Cut a single length of elastic.

2. Shape it into a V form, attaching the point (or bottom) of the V to the front of your underwear.

3. Sew each top of the V onto the bottom of each bra cup.

Voilà! That should keep your bra in place. And remember: Many women who haven't had surgery walk around with elastic and tape and goodness knows what else under their clothes. As long as it doesn't show, who cares?

The breast form you choose needs to fit well. Otherwise, it's just going to drift into the recesses of your drawer or the back of your closet where it takes up precious space, gathers dust, or the kids will find it and use it for dress-up. Take your time finding the one that you feel really comfortable in and that looks good from all sides. The following steps help you find that perfect form:

1. **Check your insurance coverage carefully.**

   If you submit claims for a bra and a breast form, some insurance companies won't cover reconstructive surgery if you opt for it later on. Other insurance companies may restrict you to certain manufacturers' products.

2. **Get a doctor's prescription for the breast form and any special bras you need.**

   A prescription helps you get coverage from your insurance company. In fact, many insurance companies pay for a new prosthesis every few years; however, they probably won't pay for the top-of-the-line forms.

3. **Make an appointment at a specialty store.**

   That way, the professional fitter will be expecting you. Most women's boutiques that specialize in such items have a really wonderful atmosphere that's warm, relaxing, and respectful.

4. **Get fitted.**

   When you arrive at the specialty store, the fitter

   1. **Escorts you to a private room and asks you some questions.**

      She asks you how long ago your surgery was, whether it was a mastectomy or a lumpectomy, and how sensitive your skin is. That helps her determine what type of breast form will be best for you at this point in time.

   2. **Measures you for a breast form and a bra.**

      The fitter measures you for a bra size and for a cup size (comparing your other breast if you only had one removed.) Of course, if you had both breasts removed, you can choose whatever size you want, larger, smaller, or just the same.

5. **Choose a breast form.**

   The fitter brings you a selection of different forms that are right for you. Try them out; put them to the test. Shapes and colors vary (just like women's breasts!). They include teardrop, asymmetrical or triangular, round, and so on. Figure 15-1 shows three of the most common shapes. You can also compare different textures of silicone or foam and weighted and unweighted varieties. The fitter will suggest the ones that are likely to fit you best.

6. Choose a bra.

Actually your choice of der Buestenhalters is more extensive than you may think. In addition to special mastectomy bras that feature built-in pockets for the breast form, you can choose to add a pocket to a favorite bra of your own or to a new one. The specialty stores sell the pockets, and either you, the store, or a dressmaker near your home can sew them into your bra.

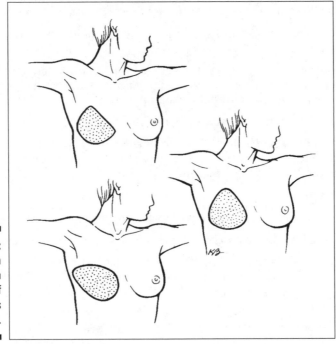

Figure 15-1:
You can choose from a variety of prosthesis shapes.

Yes, the choices are many, and that's why these specialty stores exist . . . so they can turn what can be a difficult process into one where you walk out having found something that you're happy with.

SURVIVORS' SECRETS

Marie C.

"My prosthetic breast is my secret weapon. I'm a DD cup size, and it weighs 7 pounds! I could take it out, hit someone with it, and slip it back in without anyone knowing about it."

Questions to Ask When Considering Reconstruction of Your Breast

Now that you're aware of your options (au naturel, prosthesis, or reconstructive surgery), the next step is exploring reconstructive surgery in a little more depth.

Discuss reconstruction with your doctor, and keep in mind that discussing reconstruction does *not* mean that you have to choose to do it. The first three questions you may want to tackle are discussed in the sections that follow.

Am I risking recurrence?

Studies have shown that you risk no increase in recurrence of breast cancer with any of the breast reconstruction surgeries. However, if the unlikely happens, and you do have a recurrence in the area of your surgery, it's usually in the area of the skin or the scar, not deep inside. In that case, a reconstructed breast *won't* hide the cancer.

As for monitoring your newly constructed breast, continue in the same way you'd monitor the breasts you had before reconstruction: Do breast self-exams (explained in Chapter 2). Sure, the new breast will feel different and may take some time getting used to, but you will. Your doctor will monitor you on a regular basis and will check both breasts, reconstructed or not.

Reconstructed breasts are not routinely mammogrammed, because there's no breast tissue to develop new cancer. Nevertheless, if you had a lumpectomy, you still need to have a mammogram of the breast that was operated on every six months. If you had a mastectomy, you'll have a mammogram of your remaining breast once a year.

Am I eligible for reconstruction?

Almost every woman who's having a mastectomy can have reconstructive surgery at the same time. Only a few women aren't eligible, including women with other serious medical conditions that make having lengthy surgery dangerous, such as severe heart or lung disease.

Making it an option

A very low percentage of women actually have reconstructive surgery. The reason for such a low percentage isn't known, but it's probably because many doctors don't offer all women this option. Doctors may overlook reconstruction if:

✔ The woman is older. Although research shows that reconstruction is safe in older women, many doctors may have the attitude that reconstructing an older woman's breast is not as important.

✔ The woman has more advanced cancer. Studies have found that reconstructive surgery is as suitable in women with later-stage disease as it is for women with early-stage cancer. Chapter 7 talks about stages.

Some women who are offered reconstruction simply choose not to have it, because they don't want to have extra surgery.

So, regardless of whether your doctor offers you this option, be sure that you ask whether you're a candidate for reconstruction.

Similarly, women who need radiation treatment to the chest area may find that the treatment changes their reconstructed breasts. Shrinkage can occur when tissue flaps are used, and that can make the cosmetic appearance less natural. On the other hand, reconstruction with implants or expanders (discussed later in this chapter) may form a hard scar capsule. These are issues you need to discuss with your surgeon. Women who've had radiation prior to reconstruction usually need to have their new breast built by using their own tissue (discussed later in the "Mulling over muscle flaps" section) rather than implants or expanders.

When should I have the surgery?

You can have reconstructive surgery immediately after the mastectomy (*immediate reconstruction*), or you can have it any time from months to years after the mastectomy (*delayed reconstruction*.) See what we mean about women having the prerogative to change their minds? As with everything else in life, each option has its pros and cons.

✔ **The major advantage of immediate reconstruction** is that it saves you the stress and recovery time of a second major operation.

✔ **The major advantage of delayed reconstruction** is that it gives you some time to decide if you really want the extra surgery.

Regardless of whether you choose immediate or delayed reconstruction, you have to have some small additional procedures to adjust the shape of your breast and create a nipple.

Julia W.

"Then we had to decide whether I wanted to have reconstruction, and if so, I had to decide whether to have it at the same time as the breast surgery or go back later and have it. I said there was no way I'd go back later. If I didn't get it all done at one time, they could forget it, because I wasn't crazy about being there in the first place."

Table 15-1 lists additional pros and cons of immediate reconstruction, and Table 15-2 lists additional pros and cons of delayed reconstruction.

Table 15-1	Going At It Right Away
Advantages	*Disadvantages*
You won't have to experience the psychological trauma of waking up to a flat chest where your breast once was. Your surgeon removes your breast and builds up your new breast in one surgery.	If you have medical difficulties (for example, you're extremely obese or are a heavy smoker), you may not be able to withstand the lengthy surgery.
You have one big surgery, and, it is hoped, that will be that. Having one surgery also means you decrease anesthetic risk and need less recovery time. Recovery time also is much quicker than with two surgeries. Small additional operations are likely either way.	Slightly higher wound healing problems.
Surgeons can achieve the best esthetic (beauty) results with this type of surgery by saving the skin of your breast at the time of mastectomy. Using your own skin makes achieving a symmetrical breast easier and limits scarring.	Radiation treatment (which you may need) can make the breast shrink if flaps are used, or cause a hard scar to form around implants with expanders.

Table 15-2	Putting It Off Awhile
Advantages	**Disadvantages**
Gives you additional time to consider how you feel about reconstruction.	Extra skin is needed to cover the new breast, and means either spending a longer time than with immediate reconstruction stretching skin in the mastectomy area or bringing it with a tissue flap from another part of the body (which makes the scars bigger).
Your next surgery will be shorter than a joint mastectomy/ reconstructive surgery, which includes a shorter anesthetic time and a lower risk of wound complications.	You must go through a second complete recovery from major surgery. Total time for recovering from two separate operations is greater than having both procedures done at the same time.
Your cancer treatment will be completed, and you can think of your reconstruction as a celebratory gift to yourself.	You may have to wait for more than a year to finish your cancer treatment before you're able to have this surgery.
	If you want the surgery, but keep putting it off, making time for it may become more difficult.

Begin considering whether you want reconstructive surgery right after your doctor tells you that you're a candidate. If you decide that you want reconstructive surgery, you then need to decide whether you want it done at the same time as the mastectomy. You and your doctor need to be able to plan for the two factors that follow when you decide to have reconstructive surgery along with your mastectomy:

✔ Having reconstructive surgery may affect the type of procedure that's done. For example, if you're having reconstructive surgery at the time of mastectomy, the surgeon can leave the skin that covers your breasts. *Skin-sparing* means that the skin of the breast is kept at the time of mastectomy for use in the reconstruction (see Chapter 10).

✔ Your oncology surgeon needs to line up a plastic surgeon (see Chapter 9 for a full description of your various doctors) so the two of them can coordinate their plans. This is done long before the surgery. You'll have to meet with the plastic surgeon before you decide for sure that you're going to have reconstructive surgery.

Studies have found that most women are unsure at the time of their mastectomy whether they want breast reconstruction. Even though the immediate reconstruction is an option that you have to consider as soon as you know you're having a mastectomy, please don't feel pressured to make a decision. Speak with your partner and close family, and don't feel like you have to make your decision right away. If you're unsure about reconstructive surgery when you schedule your mastectomy, don't feel pressured to do it. You can always have it later.

So Many Options, but Just One Chest

So you're taking the plunge and having reconstructive surgery, but now you're wondering what kinds are available and what kind you should have.

Think of the options the same way would in choosing a hairdo. Look at all the possibilities; they seem endless, don't they? But when you look more carefully, you find that they really aren't. I mean if your hair looks best when it's short and curly, then long hair styled like Cher's isn't really an option. Women with very thin hair can consider one set of styles, while those with luscious waves can consider another. You get the idea.

The same goes for reconstructive surgery. Here are the two main options:

- **An implant or expander.** An implant is the simplest surgical technique and involves placing a saline (or salt-water) filled sac under the chest muscle during surgery. An expander is like a balloon. Later, the plastic surgeon fills the expander with salt water (gradually, over a period of time) to match the size and shape of the other breast. It's used because, even with skin-sparing surgery, there is never enough skin to match the size of the other breast (that's because of the removal of the nipple and the scar).
- **Muscle flap procedures.** This surgery involves using your own tissue to recreate a breast.

Both of these procedures give you a breast mound, but no nipple. After you have one or other breast built, you can chose whether you want a nipple reconstructed and discuss with your doctor the best way to do it. Nipple reconstruction usually is done in a procedure that's separate from the breast reconstruction surgery. See the "Opting for nipple reconstruction" section later in this chapter.

The type of reconstructive surgery you can have depends on

- **Your body type and breast size.** Some reconstructions (for example, using expanders or implants) are more suitable for women with small breasts; others (for example, muscle flaps) are better suited for women with larger ones.

✔ **Which option you prefer.** The amount of surgery and recovery time varies considerably. Your preference will, of course, become clear to you after you talk with your surgeon.

✔ **Whether you're going to have radiation treatments on your chest.** When radiation treatments are called for, breast reconstruction is an area of controversy. If you need radiation after surgery as part of your treatment (see Chapter 9) then implants may not be advisable because radiation can cause a scar to form around the implant (called *capsular contracture*, since the capsule contracts), and thus change the shape of your breast. Instead, some surgeons recommend reconstruction with flaps when your likelihood of needing radiation is high. Others, however, prefer starting with an expander to see how things look and saving the more extensive flap reconstruction as a later alternative if you're unhappy with the outcome of the implant.

Make sure you discuss *your* particular options with your surgeon who will be able to advise you and make recommendations based on your particular needs and on his or her medical and surgical expertise.

At this point, talking to the surgeon who will perform your reconstruction is crucial, unless for some unlikely or unusual reason, your oncology surgeon will be doing the reconstruction. When you meet with the surgeon, ask these questions and more to get the answers you need to make the best decision:

✔ **What are your qualifications, expertise, and experience?** Try to find a plastic surgeon who specializes in breast reconstruction. Find one who can perform the entire spectrum of reconstructive techniques rather than someone who tells you they only do implants.

✔ **For which types of reconstructive surgeries am I eligible?** Can I choose between all the options (listed in this chapter) or am I restricted to only a few because of my particular circumstances (for example, because of my very large breasts)?

✔ **Which kind of reconstruction do you recommend and why?** If I have a choice between several types of surgeries, what are the reasons you'd choose one over the other in my case?

✔ **When do you recommend that I have the surgery? Why?** If I have a choice about when I should have the surgery, what are the reasons you'd recommend one time over the other in my case?

✔ **What kind of realistic results can I expect? Can I see some reconstruction photographs?** Looking through the photographs is very important because most of us imagine we'll have another breast exactly like the one that's no longer there. However, this often takes more than one surgery to achieve, so it's very helpful to know what you can expect, so you know what you're facing and what you can achieve.

If your surgeon listens to your questions and takes time to answer them, and you see in the photographs what can be achieved, you've struck gold — stick with that surgeon. If, on the other hand, the surgeon blows you off, telling you what you should do without listening to you, quite frankly, I'd go elsewhere.

Slipping your chest an implant

The most common form of implants in use today are filled with saline (salt water.) A *permanent implant* generally is full when it's inserted. Permanent implants are inserted when the skin has stretched enough to accommodate the full implant after your mastectomy. When the skin needs to be stretched to accommodate the implant, your surgeon first inserts an *expander*, which is like a deflated balloon that the plastic surgeon later (gradually) fills with salt water to match the size and shape of the other breast. The type of implant that's used often is a decision made during surgery, when surgeons find out exactly what they have to work with. Both types of implants are put in the same way in the same place.

If your surgeon inserts an expander, you can count on visiting the surgeon repeatedly during a period of about 4 weeks so that additional saltwater solution can be injected into a valve opening under your skin. Adding a little more fluid each week enables the skin to stretch slowly. Of course how much water is added over what period of time is dependent upon how big the breast needs to be, how much skin is present, and how much pain pulling the skin causes.

After the expander and skin reach the size of the other breast, you may have another small surgery in which the expander is replaced with a permanent implant. Some expanders, however, are designed to stay in your chest permanently, so, if that's the case, you won't need the next surgery. Ask whether your doctor recommends that you have a permanent expander placed or one that has to be replaced. This will be determined by your particular circumstances (for example, if you have small breasts, this is a great option). As with every procedure, pros and cons are associated with permanent and with temporary expanders, so be sure to discuss these with your surgeon before deciding on whether you'll have the permanent expander or the one that needs to be replaced.

Mulling over muscle flap procedures

Muscle flap procedures use flaps of your own skin, fat, and muscle to reconstruct your new breast. This tissue is taken from other parts of your body, including your back, abdomen, or buttocks. Because this tissue is taken from your own body, it's often referred to as using *autologous* (your own) tissue flaps. With a muscle flap procedure, the tissue can be shaped to match your own breast, and you end up with a much more natural-looking breast than is possible with implants.

Two general types of muscle flap procedures can be used to build your breast.

✔ *Pedicle* **(attached) flap:** In this procedure, the surgeon begins removing muscle, skin, and fat from either your back or your tummy (areas of your body that have muscle and fat and are in close proximity to your chest), but leaves the blood vessels attached. The surgeon then pulls the piece that's been dislodged (remember it's still attached by the blood vessels to your back or tummy) under the skin, into the breast area and sews it on there. The opening that was made on your back or your tummy is then sewn up. So the new piece that's now a part of your breast remains attached to the blood vessels (which give it nutrition and keep it alive) from your back or tummy. You can joke that you now have a "back boob," but then not many people would get it, would they?

✔ **Free-flap:** In this procedure, the surgeon cuts out a piece of skin, fat, muscle from any part of your body that has a lot of fat and muscle (usually the abdomen) and then sews it onto the breast area. This procedure obviously differs from the (pedicle) attached flap. Because body parts need a blood supply to live, and in this case they've been completely detached, the surgeon must patiently and carefully reattach (or sew) the cut blood vessels in the tissue to the blood vessels under the armpit or in the chest wall. This method must be done under a special surgical microscope because the blood vessels are so tiny. That is why this particular surgery is time-consuming and requires special expertise called microvascular (blood vessel) surgery. Imagine sewing two parts of a tiny blood vessel together!

Each of the muscle-flap surgeries has its own pros and cons, shown in Table 15-3 below. Talk to your doctor for recommendations.

Table 15-3   Comparison of Attached and Free-Flap Procedures

Attached-Flap	Free-Flap
The still attached tissue must be pulled through the body, (in other words, from back to chest) which may cause temporary damage to the areas through which the tissue is pulled, in addition to the breast area and the area from which tissue was taken.	Doesn't have to affect any parts other than the breast area and the area from which the piece was taken.

Attached-Flap	Free-Flap
The surgeon doesn't have to have the specialized vascular (blood vessel) expertise.	Requires specialized expertise to sew up blood vessels under a microscope.
Shorter surgery.	Surgery takes longer because of miniscule, detailed, and precise surgery.
Lower risk of flap dying.	Higher risk of flap dying (although rarely occurs).
Higher risk of flap hardening and patches of fat dying.	Lower incidence of flap hardening.
Excellent cosmetic results.	Excellent cosmetic results.

The most commonly performed reconstructive surgery is an attached flap, because it has excellent results, and few surgeons have the expertise to do the free-flap microsurgery, which also is much more time-consuming. If you decide to have an attached-flap surgery, you'll have either a transverse rectus abdominis muscle (TRAM) flap surgery (tummy) or a latissimus dorsi muscle flap surgery (back), depending on where the tissue is taken from.

Transverse rectus abdominis muscle (TRAM) flap

The most common surgery is called a *transverse rectus abdominis muscle flap* (TRAM flap to its close friends). Your surgeon takes skin, fat, and muscle from the lower abdominal (tummy) wall, together with their own blood supply, and tunnels them under your skin to your chest to create a breast as shown in Figure 15-2. The result of this kind of surgery can be seen in Figure 15-3.

Guess what? As an added benefit, you also get a tummy tuck out of the procedure, because pulling the muscle upward tightens the muscles on your abdomen. (Hey, if you'd known this, you'd have had this surgery done and forget the breast cancer, huh?)

Latissimus dorsi muscle flap

When tissue is taken from your back and used in an attached procedure, it's called a *lattisimus dorsi muscle flap,* because that's the name of the muscle across your back that the tissue is taken from. Because the latissimus dorsi muscle isn't big enough to build a breast in most women, it usually is accompanied by an implant under it. Figure 15-4 illustrates the procedure and Figure 15-5 shows how it looks after reconstruction.

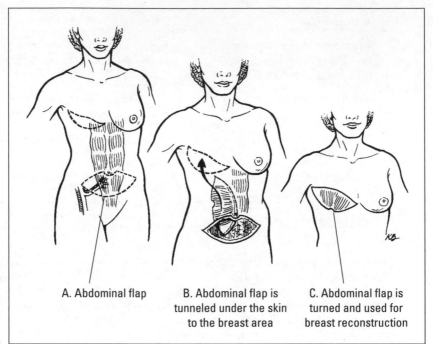

Figure 15-2:
TRAM Flap
Procedure.

A. Abdominal flap

B. Abdominal flap is
tunneled under the skin
to the breast area

C. Abdominal flap is
turned and used for
breast reconstruction

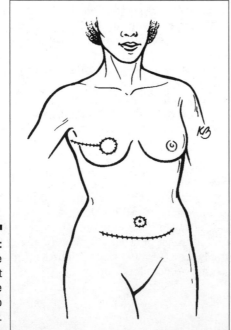

Figure 15-3:
Appearance
of breast
after the
TRAM flap
surgery.

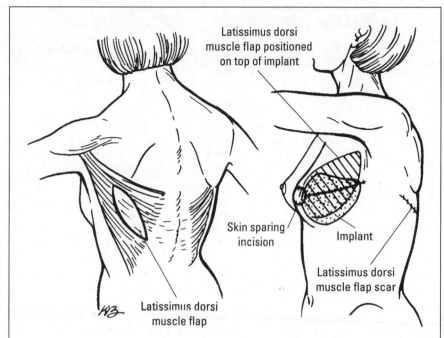

Latissimus dorsi
muscle flap positioned
on top of implant

Skin sparing
incision

Implant

Latissimus dorsi
muscle flap scar

Latissimus dorsi
muscle flap

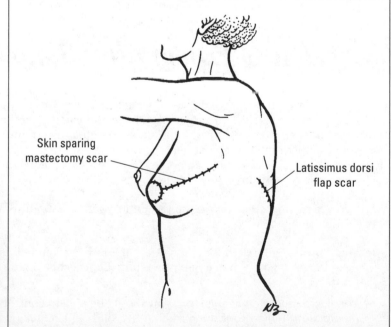

Skin sparing
mastectomy scar

Latissimus dorsi
flap scar

Opting for nipple reconstruction

So your breast was rebuilt, and you're getting used to it (see Chapter 19 for more about the feeling and sexual aspects), it's healed well, and it's settled into its final shape and size. And now you want a nipple. Well, we can get you a nipple!

The surgeon can construct your nipple several ways, using an artificial implant or skin flaps or skin grafts — using your own tissue. Skin may be taken from your inner thigh or your ear to create the part of your nipple that sticks out, or extra skin on the breast mound may be used. Tissue from your own nipple or from the other nipple can't be used because of the risk of microscopic cancer in the nipple.

The *areola* (the colored part on which the nipple sits) is made by tattooing the skin around the nipple with flesh-colored dye to match your other areola. This technique gives it a very realistic look. (Pretty cool, huh? Now you can compete with those young dudes whose bodies are covered with tattoos! Of course, you don't need to show them yours if you don't want to.)

The two disadvantages to a reconstructed nipple: The nipple won't have the sensation that your old one did, which is why most women don't opt to have nipple reconstruction surgery, and it may stick out a little all the time (but not as much as an erect nipple). If you think you may be interested in nipple reconstruction, see Chapter 19 on intimacy for more suggestions on stimulation.

Knowing What to Expect after Surgery

We cover what to expect before, during, and after surgery in great detail in Chapter 10, but we thought we'd give you a little info here, too. Regardless of what type of reconstructive surgery you have and whether you do it at the same time as a mastectomy or later on, you're going to go through a period of recuperation and adjustment. If you don't experience any complications, you'll probably be able to go home after a few days, depending, of course, on the type of surgery you've had.

While you're recuperating but before you enter your next marathon, keep these things in mind:

- ✔ You'll probably be tired for a few weeks if you've had an implant and even longer if you've had a flap procedure. Expect this fatigue and plan for it.

- ✔ You'll experience some pain, but you should be able to control it with medication. Talk to your doctor about the kind of pain meds you can use.

✔ You need to avoid strenuous physical activities or lifting immediately after surgery. Your doctor tells you when you can do certain exercises.

✔ The scars take several years to fade and never completely disappear. After the wound has healed completely, ask your doctor if you can use a scar-removing cream or Vitamin E, although there's nothing that really eradicates scars.

✔ Take your time in healing and talk to other women who've gone through the same surgery whenever you can. They can tell you about the procedures they've had and provide great after-surgery mending advice, like how to walk proudly with what you have. They'll understand better than anyone else, and they'll welcome you to the club with warmth that'll bowl you over.

Chapter 16

Duking It Out with Recurrence

*Y*ou've had your breast cancer treatment, and you've lived through it. You've had surgery, endured a chemotherapy regime that you wouldn't wish on your worst enemy, tolerated radiation that left you with sensitive skin, or undergone hormone treatment that leaves you dripping-with-sweat hot at the most inopportune times. You went through all that just so you can live. After treatment, you're eating healthier food, exercising regularly, and seeing your doctor for follow-ups as scheduled. And now they're telling you that the cancer is back!

Take special note that not all recurrences are the same and that a world of difference lies between a local recurrence and distant recurrence. Your prognosis and treatment options vary considerably depending on the type of recurrence you encounter, the location, the characteristics, and, of course, the choices that you make.

Reckoning with Recurrence

A *recurrence* is defined as cancer that comes back after you've completed treatment. Bring the following symptoms to the attention of your doctors. Although they probably mean nothing in particular, they *can* indicate possible symptoms of *metastasis,* which means that the cancer has spread from the breast to other parts of your body via the lymphatic or blood systems:

✔ Ongoing, chronic pain that doesn't relent, is not arthritis, and is not related to anything specific you're doing (such as exercise).

✔ Chronic cough and/or shortness of breath that's not related to a cold, and that persists despite attempts at treatment.

✔ A persistent headache that lasts for weeks and can leave you sleepy and nauseous.

✔ Unexplained weight loss.

X-rays (mammograms, chest X-rays, or bone scans) or blood tests may be prescribed by your doctor to determine if the cancer has returned.

How and why does the cancer come back? Recurrences usually happen because your treatment didn't destroy all the original cancer cells. One or more of the following reasons can cause this kind of recurrence:

✔ You received systemic treatment (chemotherapy) designed to kill all the cancer cells, but a few survived undetected. Some cancer cells are born resistant to drug therapy, and some develop resistance during treatment.

✔ You received radiation therapy to the breast to kill any remaining cancer cells, but some were resistant to radiation, so the cancer returned.

✔ You had breast-conserving surgery when, in your particular circum-stances, what you really needed was a *mastectomy,* which removes the entire breast (see Chapter 10). Rest assured that this rarely occurs.

The three different types of recurrence are local, regional, and distant. Each is different in terms of what you can expect your prognosis and treatment to be. Ask your doctor what kind of recurrence you have. In general

✔ *Local recurrence* occurs in the same general area where your original cancer was and can mean that your treatment consisted of either of the following:

 • A breast-conserving surgery (lumpectomy and radiation), and the cancer either returned to the same or very close to the original site or a new primary tumor developed in a part of your breast other than where the original tumor was located. Although the latter actu-ally is a new cancer, it nevertheless is referred to as a recurrence.

 • A mastectomy, and the cancer returned in or under the skin of the chest wall, near the mastectomy scar.

✔ *Regional recurrence* indicates that cancer has returned to the lymph nodes under your arm (often referred to as an *axillary recurrence*). Recurrences in lymph glands that are farther away (for example, in your neck or above your collarbone) from your original cancer site also are considered regional.

✔ *Distant recurrence* means that the cancer has spread to more distant parts of the body, usually the lungs, bones, or the liver.

A quandary in which women with breast cancer are placed: On one hand, if you worry too much about recurrence, feeling your bones, nodes, and poking at your abdomen, and are terrified that every pain and twinge and lump and bump is a recurrence, you don't really have a life anymore. On the other hand, if you put it all out of your mind after treatment, ignore the obvious, and disregard doctor appointments, you refuse to let it spoil your life, but you also risk ignoring a life-threatening problem. Neither of these extremes is helpful, and yet both are understandable.

The key is finding the balance that's right for you. Here are a couple of helpful guidelines:

✔ Never neglect a follow-up appointment with your doctor or clinic. If you have to miss an appointment, make sure that you reschedule.

✔ Always share with others, regardless of whether with family, friends, or support groups. Many studies have revealed the emotional benefits and helpfulness that support groups can provide. See Chapter 23 for options.

Predicting the Future, Part II

You already received plenty of statistics during your first go-round with breast cancer, but what about now? How likely are you to have a recurrence? And, if you have one, you'll probably want to know

✔ What kind will it be

✔ What treatment can be expected

✔ What prognosis can be expected

The variety of factors that go into providing answers to these questions is described in the following sections.

Predicting the likelihood of a recurrence

So how likely are you to have a recurrence? Is it 100 percent (no way, not even close!)? So what is it then? Cancer isn't one disease; it's a whole bunch of them, and so much variation exists that you can't just throw out a number and hope that it applies to most women. Predicting the recurrence of cancer just doesn't work like that. The answer (again) is: "It depends." However, before we discuss the likelihood of your cancer recurring, remember that a prediction is just that, a prediction, not a hard and fast rule.

Although predicting how likely you are to have a recurrence is possible, such predictions are statistical projections and, therefore, give you only partial information. Table 16-1 provides some of those projections.

Barbara B.

"I was so freaked out when my doctor called to tell me I had cancer again. I thought after 15 years I'd be fine forever. I called my sister, boyfriend, and my best friend. They all came over to take me to the doctor to talk. The doctor was upset, too, because I was doing so well. After the surgery, I was feeling sorry for myself, but I realized that what's important is doing whatever you have to do to fight this rotten disease. And here I am now."

After breast-conserving surgery

Following breast-conserving surgery, the incidence of local recurrence is less than 10 percent during the first ten years after surgery, and in cancer centers that do considerable amounts of this kind of treatment, the incidence of recurrence is only 5 percent to 6 percent during that same ten-year stretch.

The good news is that the risk of local recurrence has steadily been decreasing ever since breast-conserving surgery first was performed more routinely in the late 1970s. The decrease occurred mainly because of

- Improvements in mammography
- More detailed evaluation of the breast tissue that's removed
- The use of chemotherapy and/or endocrine therapy for most women

Axillary recurrence occurs in the lymph nodes under your arm. It occurs only rarely in fewer than 2 percent of women who have had an *axillary dissection,* or removal of the lymph nodes (see Chapter 10).

Supraclavical recurrence occurs in the lymph nodes located above the collarbone. The chance of supraclavical recurrence is dependent upon the number of nodes under your arms that are involved when your cancer was originally diagnosed and how you were treated at the time.

Paula M.

"I was in remission for four years, during which I had reconstructive surgery. Following my reconstruction, I was told my chest X-rays showed that my breast cancer had spread to my lungs. This time the cancer was inoperable, and I began aggressive chemotherapy treatment, which lasted 30 months. I've been in remission since 1985, and I'm living my life as a healthy, spiritual woman. My experiences have made me a better person, more giving, more compassionate, and certainly happier to be living what I consider to be a charmed life."

Distant recurrence (also called *distant metastases*), which spreads to more distant parts of the body, is the same regardless of whether you had breast-conserving surgery or a mastectomy and is dependent upon many different factors, including

- The number of nodes involved when you were originally diagnosed
- The original size of the cancer in the breast
- The treatment you received

Table 16-1	Likelihood of Recurrence Following Surgery	
Type of Recurrence	*Following Breast-conserving Surgery*	*Following Mastectomy*
Local	• Less than 10 percent in first ten years after surgery. • 5%–6% in first ten years if treated at a cancer center that does a lot of this treatment. Local recurrence is unlikely in first two years. Between years 2–6, the chance is 0.5%–1% per year. After six years, most cancers that appear in the same breast are new cancers, not recurrences.	Depends on: • Number of nodes that were involved originally. • The size of the original tumor. • Whether radiation therapy was part of the original treament. If tumor was small and nodes were negative, likelihood is less than 5%. If four or more nodes are involved, the likelihood is much higher (approx. 30%).
In axillary nodes	Less than 2% if axillary nodes have been removed.	Less than 2% if axillary lymph nodes have been removed.
Supra-clavicular	Depends on number of nodes under your arm with original cancer and how you were treated at the time.	Depends on the number of nodes under your arm with original cancer and how you were treated at the time.
Metastatic	Depends on: • Number of nodes with cancer when originally diagnosed. • The size of the cancer in the breast. • The treatment you received.	Depends on: • Number of nodes with cancer when originally diagnosed. • The size of the cancer in the breast. • The treatment you received.

(continued)

Table 16-1 *(continued)*

Type of Recurrence	Following Breast-conserving Surgery	Following Mastectomy
Metastatic *(continued)*	For example, if your tumor was less than a centimeter in diameter and none of the nodes were affected, the likelihood of a distant metastatic recurrence of cancer is less than 10 percent. On the other hand, it if had spread to four or more nodes, it's approximately 60 percent. That's why chemo or hormone therapy is given.	For example, if your tumor was less than a centimeter in diameter and none of the nodes were affected, the likelihood of a distant metastatic recurrence of cancer is less than 10 percent On the other hand, it if had spread to four or more nodes, it's approximately 60 percent. That's why chemo or hormone therapy is given.

After a mastectomy

The risk of local recurrence after a mastectomy depends on the number of nodes to which the cancer had spread, the size of the tumor, and whether radiation therapy was part of your treatment.

If you had a small tumor and the cancer hasn't spread to your nodes, the risk of local recurrence is less than 5 percent. On the other hand, if the cancer had spread to four or more nodes, the risk of local recurrence is approximately 30 percent. This greater risk is why radiation therapy is recommended for women whose cancer has spread to four or more nodes.

Of even greater concern, however, is that half of the women who develop a local recurrence of the cancer are also likely to develop a *metastatic recurrence* (meaning a recurrence of the cancer in a more distant part of the body, such as the lungs or bone) at the same time or within a few years. More than one-third of women who have a local recurrence after a mastectomy unfortunately develop *metastatic disease* (a metastatic recurrence) either at the same time as the local recurrence or a few years later.

Predicting treatment and outcome

The first step in treatment is an evaluation to determine whether the recurrence is confined to a local or regional area or whether it has spread to another part of the body and, if so, to what parts. Your treatment and predicted outcome may vary greatly depending on these factors. In the following section, we discuss treatments and predicted outcomes for only local and regional recurrences. Treatment for distant metastases is discussed later in the chapter.

For local recurrence when you've had breast-conserving surgery

Here's some really great news: Most local recurrences after breast-conserving surgery can be surgically removed and do not increase your risk of dying of cancer.

Treatments for local recurrence include the following:

- **Mastectomy:** This course of treatment may be disappointing because you've managed to keep your breast for all this time. We discuss mastectomy in great detail in Chapter 10. You can have an immediate reconstruction (discussed in Chapter 15); however, radiation treatment that you received as part of your original treatment may influence the type of reconstruction.

- **Chemotherapy:** Whether this form of treatment is used to treat you after a local recurrence is dependent upon whether you received chemotherapy your first time around.

  - If you didn't receive chemotherapy in your original treatment, doctors determine whether chemotherapy is the right treatment option now based on several of the same characteristics that are used to assess women who are prescribed chemotherapy originally. We discuss chemotherapy in full in Chapter 12.

  - If your original treatment included chemotherapy, you and your doctor will determine whether you receive it again based on how long it has been since you completed chemotherapy, what type of chemotherapy you received, and the size of the recurrence.

- **Hormone treatment:** Hormone treatment is considered an option whenever your recurrent cancer cells contain the *estrogen receptor,* which is explained in Chapter 13.

For local recurrence when you've had a mastectomy

It doesn't seem fair that you can have a recurrence after a mastectomy, does it? Fortunately, treatments do exist for a local recurrence after a mastectomy. These include

- **Surgery:** If the recurrence is small and localized, it will be removed surgically. When the recurrence is scattered about the skin of the mastectomy site, surgery usually isn't done.

- **Radiation therapy (RT):** RT should always be given after a local recurrence if it wasn't given at the time of the mastectomy. It will be administered to your chest wall and even the area above your collarbone since it's very likely that the lymph glands have scatterings of cancer cells in them, even if the cancer found is small and localized.

- **Chemotherapy:** Unfortunately, after a mastectomy many local recurrences are followed soon after by distant metastases. Chemotherapy often is considered, depending on whether you received chemotherapy before and how much time has elapsed since you completed that regimen. The doctor also considers what particular regimen you received and the size of the recurrence.

- **Hormonal therapy:** If your tumor is hormone receptor–positive, you'll be placed on hormonal therapy in addition to receiving RT.

Your predicted outcome after a chest-wall recurrence varies a great deal and depends on many factors, such as how long after surgery it occurs and whether it has spread to other parts of the body. Discuss this information with your doctor, because each woman's situation is different.

For regional recurrence after you've had either type of surgery

If you had no axillary surgery or a sentinel-node biopsy, a regional recurrence in the axillary nodes will be treated by surgery to remove the effected nodes. You may also have radiation therapy.

If you have an axillary recurrence after you've already had an axillary dissection (which is rare, in fewer than 2 percent of cases), it may be treated surgically or with radiation therapy, depending on the specifics of the recurrence.

In deciding whether you receive chemotherapy or endocrine (hormonal) therapy, the same factors are considered that were addressed in your original treatment (see Chapter 9), as well as what treatment you received before recurrence developed (in other words, at your first treatment).

Providing you with any specific information about your predicted outcome is impossible because it varies so much from person to person and depends on so many factors.

Getting Nasty with Metastasis

A *distant recurrence* is also known as *metastasis,* which means that the cancer has spilled out of the breast and spread via the lymphatic or blood systems to other parts of the body. Breast cancer most commonly spreads to bones, lungs, or liver. On rare occasions, it can spread to the spinal cord and brain.

As mentioned previously in this chapter, if you have any of the following symptoms, make sure that you bring them to the attention of your doctors because they can point to metastasis:

- A new, ongoing, persistent pain that doesn't relent, isn't arthritis, and isn't related to anything specific you're doing (such as exercising)

✔ Chronic cough and/or shortness of breath that isn't related to a cold and persists despite attempts at treatment

✔ A persistent headache that lasts for weeks and can leave you sleepy and nauseated

✔ Unexplained weight loss

Many women die of metastatic breast cancer. But equally important is the fact that many women with metastatic breast cancer live with the disease for many years. The average number of years is between two and three; however, between a quarter and a third of women with metastatic breast cancer live five years, and about 10 percent live more than ten years.

Predicting metastasis prognosis

What determines how long you live? You know the answer: It isn't one factor but rather a combination of many. We discuss these factors in detail in Chapter 9, but in general, they are

✔ **The length of time between your initial diagnosis and the recurrence.** The longer it's been, the better your prognosis is likely to be.

✔ **How aggressive the cancer is.** The less fast it grows, the better your prognosis is likely to be.

✔ **Whether the cancer has spread to one spot only or to several parts of the body, to which part or parts of the body the cancer has spread, and to what extent it has spread.** The cancer may have spread to the bones and remained there, or it may have spread to other organs, most commonly, the liver or lungs.

Targeting metastasis treatment

The two primary goals in treating women with metastatic breast cancer are

✔ **Maintaining or improving the quality of life.** This primary goal includes making sure that any cancer symptoms are controlled. If that isn't happening for your loved one, insist on it. Why should a woman suffer?

✔ **Prolonging life.** Treatment with this purpose in mind depends on the qualities of the cancer, such as how aggressive it is and where the metastasis is, and may include the entire range of possible treatment options (all of which are described in detail in Chapter 9). Recent clinical trials have shown that more effective treatments have extended the lives of women with breast cancer.

From Plan A to Plan B and so on

Although doctors and researchers still don't understand why, all tumors eventually stop responding to hormonal therapy. That's when chemotherapy is given. If the chemotherapy stops working, another type of chemotherapy is tried. Different chemotherapy regimens can be tried one after the other. During the last ten years, researchers have found many more kinds of chemotherapy that can be used in women with metastatic cancer. In fact, many of the newer chemotherapy or hormonal treatments now have far fewer side effects than when they first came out.

You and your loved ones being closely involved with all the decisions is important when reviewing your choice of treatments with the doctors, determining whether to be on treatment, ensuring that side effects are minimal, and maybe even making difficult decisions such as knowing when to stop treatment. (For more information about how family and friends can be effectively involved, be sure to check out Chapter 20.)

Accepting the inevitable

The inevitable arrives. That's when no more treatments are available or when you decide to stop treatment.

If you want to ensure that *your* wishes are respected, make sure that you have a living will (see Chapter 17) and that you appoint a guardian. Most people find it incredibly difficult to talk about such issues, often hushing you up with, "Don't talk like that, you're going to live forever." They don't react that way because they don't want to help but rather because their own fears are making your demise so difficult for them. However, making your wishes known clearly and legally while you're still well enough to do so is very important. If your family can't help you with this, then be sure to ask for the social worker at the hospital.

Asking Your Doctor

If you're diagnosed with a recurrence, you need to ask your doctor these questions:

SURVIVORS' SECRETS

Carol M.

"Fear will live in your head, right next to that positive attitude that you must keep. Fear that the breast cancer will come back, that it will strike the other breast, or that cancer will show up somewhere else always is present. Personally, I don't think there's any way to eliminate the fear, only ways to control it. As the famous saying goes, 'There's nothing to fear but fear itself.' You will have it, but fear doesn't have to rule your life with every little bump, ache, and pain."

✔ What type of recurrence do I have?

✔ What is my prognosis? The answer to this question may not be easy news to hear. If you choose to know, make sure that you have someone with you to provide support.

✔ What treatment options do you recommend? What are the pros and cons of each of these options?

✔ Will you describe my available treatment choices and help me decide what best meets my needs?

✔ What happens if I decide I don't want any more treatment? Will you work with me on that?

Chapter 17

Boxing Back at the Double Whammy: Health Insurance and Money Woes

*I*t doesn't seem right. You're facing so much already, and now, to top it all off, you have to deal with financial and insurance problems. Unfortunately, that's the reality of a breast cancer diagnosis, even more so with the rise of health maintenance organizations (HMOs) and limitations on insurance coverage. As frustrating as these woes may be, facing them head-on can help you prevent substantial problems in the future. Dealing with these problems one step at a time makes them more manageable.

Uncovering Your Insurance Coverage

The first step in dealing with medical insurance is finding out exactly what your insurance covers. That means reading the policy and all that awful fine print. It's a pain in the neck — literally — but it can make an enormous difference financially. Wiley Publishing's *Insurance For Dummies* by Jack Hungelmann can tell you more.

Asking the right questions

The important things to know about your insurance are what procedures it covers (or doesn't) and how much your maximum coverage is. Here are some helpful questions to ask your insurance agent and some of the language (Insurancespeak) he or she may respond with

- ✔ How much of *my own money* do I have to spend before my health plan kicks in? How much do I have to pay for *each doctor's visit*? (Insurancespeak: *yearly deductible and copay,* respectively.)

- ✔ Are all breast cancer treatments *covered?* (Insurancespeak: *Specific illnesses/treatments excluded.*) What if I need several rounds of chemotherapy or radiation? If not all are covered, which are not? How can I appeal this decision?

- ✔ Are all my hospitalization costs covered, or do I have to pay for some myself? (Insurancespeak: *Days of hospitalization in a year; hospital costs covered.*)

- ✔ Can I choose a doctor out of network, and if I can, how much will I have to pay? (Insurancespeak: *Choice of medical provider.*)

- ✔ Does the policy cover a clinical trial? Are there special circumstances under which it can?

- ✔ If I have a recurrence, what does the plan cover and what do I have to pay for myself?

- ✔ Is reconstructive surgery covered in this plan? Does it cover *all* the costs involved including anesthesia and hospital charges? Do I have to have reconstructive surgery immediately or if I choose to have it later, will the insurance pay for it? (The Women's Health and Cancer Rights Act of 1998 states that all insurance companies that cover mastectomy must also cover reconstructive surgery and surgery on the other breast to make both breasts even.)

Popping pills

Medication coverage can become another headache. Ask your insurance company

- ✔ How much of my prescription medication costs do you cover?
- ✔ Do you cover experimental drugs?

There may be some medications (to help control pain, for example) that the insurance company won't cover. In that case

- ✔ Try to appeal to the insurance company. First, call the toll-free patient number and ask to speak to the customer service representative (it helps if you're not angry with her). Speaking to a human being helps make the situation a reality. She'll usually advise you about the additional paperwork the doctor may need to send to the insurance company for the appeal to go through. Let your doctor's office know exactly what's needed and ask them if they can fax that information to the insurance company. This process can involve many phone calls and paperwork, so this may be a perfect job to allocate to a friend or family member who wants to help.

✔ Ask the social worker at the hospital for a Drug Assistance Program (a program run by a large group of pharmaceutical companies that may offer free medications to people whom they consider eligible). Or you can find out about whether you're eligible for this assistance yourself by going to www.helpingpatients.org/. There are many participating drug programs, each with its own guidelines, so it's best to inquire at this site directly.

✔ Ask your doctor or pharmacist whether less expensive or generic drugs are available.

Filing the paperwork

Filing insurance paperwork is seldom flawless and often confusing. Bills and payments cross in the mail. The same bill is sent more than once. The insurance company denies claims that it should approve. Claims are disapproved because of missing paperwork or a missing signature or because of a misclassification of the item by the hospital. These are but a few of the things that can and do go wrong.

Here are a few suggestions to help minimize your understandable frustration:

✔ Set up a filing system to organize all your bills. Wanting to throw them all in a pile to deal with later is the easy way out and can result in disastrous financial consequences. If neither you nor your partner has the energy to do this tedious work, ask a friend to help.

✔ Make a copy of each of the bills for your records.

✔ File each bill with the insurance company as soon as you receive it, even if you don't remember whether it covers that particular item. (If it doesn't, the insurance company will let you know!)

✔ Keep a paper copy of each transaction.

✔ Record the names of the insurance company representatives with whom you speak, the date, and any decisions they make. Doing so saves you many headaches in the long run.

✔ When the insurance company refuses to pay

• Appeal the decision in writing. Ask your insurance agent to whom the appeal should be addressed.

- Ask the doctor's office or hospital for help in filing the appeal. They've done it many times before.

- Ask the insurance company to reply in writing.

✔ Contact your state insurance office. That office may assist you with the appeal process and definitely offers plenty of other good advice. Check in the phone book under State Government or go to www.naic.org. From there you can ask for information by state.

Lodging a complaint

When you've done everything that you can, and you still believe you suffered an injustice, you can file a complaint against the insurance company through the organizations listed in Table 17-1.

As you begin this process, ask the hospital's social worker to assist you. The social worker has the necessary expertise and will be glad to help. The *National Coalition for Cancer Survivorship* (NCCS) offers a very helpful booklet (at minimal cost) and even a training course that can assist you with all your questions about health insurance.

Table 17-1	Filing an Insurance Complaint		
To File a Complaint Against	**Contact**	**Web Site**	**Phone Number**
Private insurance company	State Insurance Commissioners	www.naic.org.	Click Information by states. Look in the phone book for State Government or click on your state on the Web site shown at left.
HMO (Health Maintenance Organization)	State Insurance Commissioners	www.naic.org.	Click Information by states. Look in the phone book for State Government or click on your state on the Web site shown at left.
Federally qualified HMO	The Centers for Medicare and Medicaid	cms.hhs.gov.	Look for information by state. Look in the phone book for State Government or click on your state on the Web site shown at left.

To File a Complaint Against	Contact	Web Site	Phone Number
Private employer insurance, union self-insurance, self-financed plans	U.S. Department of Labor, Employee Benefits Security Administration	`www.dol.gov/ebsa/.`	Look by topic for health-care plans by type. Depends on the state. Look in the phone book for State Government or click on your state on the Web site shown at left.
Veteran's benefits	U.S. Department of Veteran Affairs	`www.va.gov`	1-877-222-8387.
Medicare	U.S. Social Security Administration	`www.medicare.gov`	1-800-633-4227
Medicaid	State Department of Social Services	`cms.hhs.gov/medicaid/stateplans`	Find all the phone numbers on the Web site by state.

Finding yourself sans insurance

You'd be surprised how many people find themselves without medical insurance at some time during their lives. Maybe you just left your job or your ex-husband's insurance no longer covers you, or you decided to start your own business and you're thinking who has money for insurance? Besides, you were in perfect health, so you thought you'd get it later and now. . . . So what happens when you find yourself without insurance? Although they aren't cheap, you do have some options. Table 17-2 lays them out. Ask the case-worker at the hospital or clinic for assistance in locating them.

Table 17-2	Insurance Options	
Who It Is	**What They Do**	**Where to Find Them**
Independent brokers	A broker may be able to find you a health insurance plan that's affordable. It will usually be group rather than an individual insurance policy.	Look in the yellow pages under Insurance.

(continued)

Table 17-2 *(continued)*

Who It Is	What They Do	Where to Find Them
HMOs	A broker may be able to find you a health insurance plan that's affordable. It will usually be a group rather than an individual insurance policy.	Contact the HMO in your area. They usually have one period during the year when they offer open enrollment to anyone, regardless of their health.
Employment benefits	Getting a job with a company that offers benefits is a shoo-in for receiving insurance. Of course when you're ill isn't exactly the time to be looking for a job, but at some point in the future, or when you feel well, you may want to consider this option. If you're employed and have insurance benefits, don't leave your job until you've found out whether you can continue with the same insurance benefits. Sometimes conversions aren't possible, and even if they are, they can be extremely expensive.	Ask the human resources department or check your employer's Web site.
Disability Insurance	You may have disability insurance as part of your employment benefits.	Ask your human resources department or check your benefits information.
COBRA (Consolidated Omnibus Budget Reconciliation Act)	Nope, not a snake. A law that ensures that if you leave your job, you can continue receiving your health insurance for a set period of time (usually a year and a half). You must pay for the coverage.	www.dol.gov. Click on the search function, and type in COBRA.
HIPAA Insurance (Health Insurance Portability and Account-ability Act)	A law that ensures no discrimination based on preexisting conditions. This way you won't lose your insurance if you have to move to another job or city.	www.dol.gov. Click on the search function and type in HIPAA.
Health Insurance Risk Pools	Risk pools are based on the HIPAA law. Some states sell health insurance to people who otherwise aren't able to get it because of a preexisting medical condition. This insurance is expensive but often is the only option.	Look in the phone book under State Government.

Who It Is	What They Do	Where to Find Them
Insurance from Professional Organizations	Many professional or alumni organizations offer insurance coverage. Make sure that it's a *guaranteed plan,* which means you can be insured regardless of your medical history.	Call or check the Web site of any professional organization to which you belong or were a member of and can rejoin.

Getting Money from the Feds (for a Change)

The United States government provides several other insurance options or health-care resources for which you may be eligible.

Medi-what?

Medicare? Medicaid? After figuring out the difference between these two, you're likely to need a medivac. Take out the "medi" in both words, and you're left with "care" and "aid," which refer to the respective services that each provides.

Medicare

Medicare provides health insurance for retired people who meet one of these qualifications:

- Are at least 65 years old, a citizen, and either worked for (or had a spouse who worked for) at least ten years in a job that was Medicare-covered
- Are permanently disabled
- Have been receiving Social Security Disability payments for at least two years

This insurance plan is divided into two separate parts, each providing different benefits.

- **Part A:** Covers care in a hospital, certain approved institutions, or at home.
- **Part B:** Covers medical tests, doctor's fees, and a few other similar services. Part B is not automatically provided. You must pay for this part of the coverage.

Medicare does *not* cover all medical expenses or all medications. It provides for

- ✔ **Basic health coverage.** Most doctors and hospitals accept Medicare payments and services covered under the HMO plan. But — and here's the catch — you have to use HMO's health-care providers.

- ✔ **Drugs prescribed only while you're in the hospital.** Because Medicare covers only medications that you're given while you're in the hospital, you need to consider purchasing (yes, you have to pay for it) additional Medicare insurance policies to cover medications you'll need when you're not in the hospital. You can do this through a Medicare- and state-administered plan called *Medigap*. (They fill in the gap.) Basic Medigap insurance plans exist, but the amount and types of coverage vary by state. Some states have supplemental plans called Medicare Select plans.

Medicaid

This program provides medical assistance for people with low income. Generally (although this varies by state — see next paragraph) this includes

- ✔ Families with low income who have children
- ✔ People who receive Supplemental Security Income (SSI) because of a permanent disability
- ✔ Children younger than 6 and pregnant women whose family income is very low
- ✔ Others who may be eligible to receive Medicaid for a limited time only

Medicaid is operated jointly by federal and state governments, and although the federal government intended it to provide medical care for the nation's poor, each state decides on its own criteria about

- ✔ Who's eligible to receive Medicaid
- ✔ What services are and are not covered
- ✔ How much it will pay the provider of your treatment

Because these factors vary so much between states, be sure to ask a hospital social worker to assist you in finding out whether you're eligible, or go to the Medicaid Web site (cms.hhs.gov/medicaid/stateplans) where it's easy to go through your state's plans to find who you need to contact to get the right information.

Because Medicaid is jointly sponsored by federal *and* state governments, beware that

- ✔ Because each state sets different policies regarding what its Medicaid program provides, you may or may not be eligible in your state.
- ✔ Medicaid isn't accepted by many doctors or hospitals.

Speak to your hospital about a discount on your medical bill if you're on Medicaid. You must show evidence of your financial situation, and getting this discount won't be easy, but you don't lose anything by trying. Ask your hospital social worker to advise and assist you in this process.

Dishing up more assistance

In addition to government-backed assistance, you may also be eligible for several other programs, including the ones discussed in Table 17-3. To find out, ask the hospital social worker or caseworker to let you know

✔ Whether and for which programs you're eligible

✔ How and where to apply

✔ What documentation you need to apply

Table 17-3	Getting Help from Government Agencies	
Who It Is	*What They Do*	*Where to Find Them*
Medical assistance	Assistance provided for people with a low income and dependents to pay for items such as medical expenses or medication. Varies from state to state.	cms.hhs.gov/med icaid/stateplans/) www.medicare.gov
Hill-Burton Program	Some hospitals and clinics receive Federal support so that they can provide free or low-cost services for people who can't afford care (but not for people with Medicare or Medicaid.) Each hospital makes its own decision what programs to pay for.	www.hrsa.gov/ osp/dfcr 1-800-879-4422
Veterans' benefits	If you're a veteran or the dependent of a veteran, you're eligible for health benefits from the federal government.	www.va.gov 1-877-222-8387
Social Security Disability Income	Benefits to people whom the Social Security defines as disabled. You must meet Social Security Administration criteria to qualify. Once you do, receiving the benefits takes many months. (Getting assistance in filing this claim is better than doing it on your own.)	www.social-security- disability- claims.org/

(continued)

Table 17-3 *(continued)*

Who It Is	What They Do	Where to Find Them
Supplemental Security Income (SSI)	Federal support if you're disabled and haven't worked much, or when you did work, you received a very low income. (Getting assistance in filing this claim is better than doing it on your own.)	www.social-security-disability-claims.org/
Aid to Families with Dependent Children (AFDC)	Assistance provided by the federal government and the state to low-income families with children younger than 18. You may be able to receive Medicaid through this program.	www.acf.dhhs.gov/programs/afdc/

Paying Out of Pocket

You'll have out-of-pocket expenses even under the best financial circumstances. Don't panic! Hospitals and doctors have come to expect patients to ask for payment plans or extensions. You can do it, if you take just one step at a time.

Taking stock of your finances

A different perspective on your life often accompanies a diagnosis of cancer, and money is one aspect that is of lesser importance. But for practical purposes, money matters must be dealt with, especially when you're a single parent or someone who's been surviving from paycheck to paycheck.

✔ Don't wait until you're drowning in a sea of bill collectors and unopened mail piled as deep as the ocean on the kitchen table. Get a handle on the situation. Now! Doing so gives you back a sense of control over your life.

✔ If your bills are too confusing or overwhelming to manage on your own, never hesitate to ask a friend or relative who's got accounting or other financial experience, and if not, someone who can help you get them organized. You'll be ever so glad that you did.

Where do you start? Well, sit down with a pen and paper and follow these four steps:

1. **What are my assets?**

   - List estimated income and benefits.

   - List all stocks and bonds or other investments.

   - List all your assets, including your house, car, and household furniture. (Don't worry, we're not selling anything; compiling these lists of your assets just gives you an idea of what amount of money you can raise if you had to in an emergency.)

2. **What are my expenses?**

   You can estimate your regular expenses, but add up all the medical expenses that your insurance won't cover. Ask your doctor's office, the hospital social worker, or other survivors for an estimate. This amount is variable, but you have to start somewhere.

3. **Subtract your assets from your expenses.**

   Depending on whether you're facing emergency circumstances, decide whether you want to include your grandmother's pearls and your prized antique barrister's bookcase.

4. **Calculate how much extra money you need to cover your costs.**

After you've taken these steps, you can decide in which direction you want to head.

Getting help

Whenever money woes find you biting your fingernails into nubs, don't panic. Get help instead. Numerous organizations can help you take stock and provide support.

Ask the hospital social worker for referrals to

- **Organizations** that provide transportation and lodging during treatment, such as the American Cancer Society.

- **Federal and state programs** that provide assistance for people without any or meager sources of income.

You can also consider

- **Asking your church or synagogue for help.** For example, your church can play host to a fundraiser for your hospital bills.

- **Asking your friends or family whether you can take out a loan from them.** Get the friend's discount: low interest.

- ✔ **Getting a home-equity conversion.** You can convert part of the equity you have in your house into cash if you're at least 62 and own (or are close to owning) your house.

- ✔ **Pulling from your retirement fund.** Speak to your financial advisor about this avenue, because you may be eligible for a hardship loan.

- ✔ **Selling your assets.** That's right. Off to the auction house they go.

- ✔ **Consolidating your credit-card debt into one card.** Be sure to use the one with the lowest interest rate and make regular payments even if they're only small ones.

If your finances become unmanageable

- ✔ Make an appointment with the nearest office of the Consumer Credit Counseling Service, a nonprofit organization that can help you consolidate and pay off your debts. A CCCS representative can speak to the creditors for you. The number is in the phone book.

- ✔ Attend the "Taking Charge of Money Matters" workshop, geared especially to cancer survivors and their families. It's free! To find out whether it's offered in your community, call 800-227-2345 or go to www.cancer.org.

Considering last resorts

The time may come when you're at your wit's end and you're down to your last resort. This differs from person to person. Maybe you can't pay most of your bills and you don't see a way that you'll be able to pay them anytime in the future. You may even be at risk of losing your house, with the electricity only one check away from being cut off and the kids going off to live with their dad because you just can't afford to keep them. This is a tough place to be in, but it can be a reality. When you do reach this point financially, consider

- ✔ **Filing bankruptcy.** This is a last-ditch resort, but it's always available. Speak to a lawyer or legal aid office about it.

- ✔ **Borrowing against or selling your life insurance living benefits.** In some circumstances, you can borrow from or sell your life insurance policy for cash (called *viatical loan or viatical settlement*); however, doing so is a consideration best left only for when you're terminally ill. Companies buy your policy from you at around 60 percent to 80 percent of its value. Before you consider this last-ditch option, please be sure to carefully explore the advantages and disadvantages.

Looking to the Law

Some laws are designed to look after your rights, and knowing about them when you're sick is extremely important. In addition to the laws discussed in the "Asking the right questions" and "Lodging a complaint" sections earlier in the chapter, others have been passed to protect you.

Keeping your desk warm: Your job

Meeting with your supervisors and filling them in about your illness is a good idea, so they understand why you have to take time off. Patients with cancer are entitled to exactly the same rights and benefits as other employees, even with regard to hiring and promotion.

When you're in the process of being physically assessed, whether you tell your boss about what's happening is up to you. After your cancer has been diagnosed and the doctor has described the extent of your illness (see Chapter 7) and your treatment plan (see Chapter 9), it's definitely time to talk to your boss.

You may not know precisely how long you'll be out of the office, but your doctor will give you an estimated timeline. Other than the surgery, most of your treatments are outpatient. You may be pleasantly surprised to realize that you feel well enough to go to the office more often than you thought you would.

Some specific laws that are in place to help protect you are the

- ✔ **Americans With Disabilities Act (ADA).** This law protects the rights of people with disabilities. Although in most cases, breast cancer won't leave you disabled, in case it does, you're protected under this act. Discrimination against people with disabilities is prohibited, and your employer must make reasonable accommodations to enable you to continue doing your job.

- ✔ **Family and Medical Leave Act (FMLA).** This law requires employers of more than 50 people to allow up to 12 weeks of unpaid leave, which you can use to take care of yourself or to take care of a family member who is ill.

Whenever you have reason to suspect that you're being discriminated against because of your illness, keep a log of to whom you told what, when you told them, and what their responses were. This information will be helpful in the event you need to take legal action in a situation of unfair treatment.

Protection in the hospital

The Patient's Bill of Rights was adopted by the American Hospital Association to ensure that patients received the best care, while protecting their rights. (All hospitals should have one. Usually it's displayed prominently, but if not, ask to see it!)

As a patient you have the right to

- ✔ Considerate and respectful care
- ✔ Information (that's understandable) about your condition, treatment, and your projected outcome
- ✔ Discuss treatment options with the doctors (except in emergency situations)
- ✔ Confidentiality about your condition
- ✔ See your charts
- ✔ Provide the hospital with information in advance (Hospitalspeak: *advance directives*) about how you want to be taken care of in case of dire situations

Protecting your advance wishes

If you want to, you can make your own decisions (with the help of your family) about how you want to be taken care of in case you become terminally ill and too sick to provide directions. Decisions like these are known as *advance directives.* Preparing advance directives ensures that the instructions you give are followed.

The Patient Self-Determination Act (PSDA)

- ✔ Encourages you to make your own choice about the type of care you want to accept or refuse if you become too ill to make your own decisions. For example, if you are terminally ill, what do you want the hospital to do if your heart stops? Resuscitate you or not?
- ✔ Requires all treatment facilities that accept Medicare or Medicaid to abide by your advance directives.

If you're considering advanced directives (sounds a little like a preemptive strike, doesn't it?), decide whether you want to provide

- ✔ **A living will.** You write and sign this document and give it to the hospital (with a copy going to a loved one to keep). It tells the medical team whether you want them to withhold or provide you with certain treatments, such as life support.
- ✔ **Power of attorney for healthcare.** This designation also is called the *durable power of attorney,* and in it, you appoint someone to make health-care decisions for you when you're no longer in a position to do so. Talk to your partner before deciding whether he or she is the one for this responsibility.

Keep a copy of your living will and your power of attorney with you and tell your close family and friends where you keep it in case you can't get to it when it's needed. Don't forget to provide your lawyer with a copy.

Part IV:
Living Life After Diagnosis

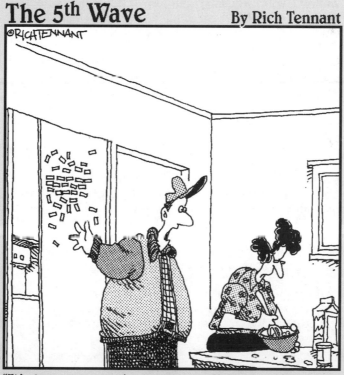

The 5th Wave   By Rich Tennant

"It's been two months since your diagnosis, and I know you're reluctant to talk about it. But we've got to start discussing it in some way other than messages left on the refrigerator with these tiny word magnets."

In this part . . .

Looking after yourself is crucial. Chapter 18 shows how every woman, regardless of treatment option or demands on her time, can find ways of making some chicken soup and dealing with the many emotions that flow in the wake of being diagnosed with and treated for breast cancer. Chapter 19 talks about reacquainting you and your partner with the sexual intimacy (and some saucy suggestions for enhancing your love life) you may not have experienced for a while, overcoming inhibitions of how someone new may feel about your new body, and simply finding ways to love your new body. Chapter 21 addresses the best ways of telling the children about your illness and how knowing how to tackle this issue calms everyone's fears. In this part you also find out how to face the extraordinarily strenuous challenges of surviving this difficult journey as a primary caretaker and how to rely on the help that your family and friends want to provide (Chapter 20).

Chapter 18

Putting on Some Chicken Soup: Looking After Yourself

*W*hen you're diagnosed with breast cancer, your life changes forever. Regardless of your predicted outcome (and chances are high that it's good, if your cancer was caught early), fear has been introduced into your life. Maybe the fact that you might get breast cancer never even crossed your mind, or maybe it's always been a nagging fear in the back of your mind. Either way, it's here now and you must deal with it. And you will. In this chapter, we give you some tools to help you do just that.

Dreading the Diagnosis

The time right after you're diagnosed is the most difficult part of the journey. Ask any breast cancer survivor, read any book, review any study — the time just after you receive the diagnosis is tougher to deal with than any other part of the treatment you go through.

Shattering your world

The devastation that you feel about the news you've just received is totally understandable and for good reason:

✔ **Your life's been altered dramatically.** There you were, taking care of the family, your home, and your life, working, playing sports, having fun, and meeting the challenges and demands of daily living. That's all different now. In an instant, your life simply isn't the same any more. You may feel as if your old life's been abruptly taken away from you.

✔ **Most people think that being diagnosed with cancer means they're going to die from it.** That isn't always the case any longer. You may feel like you've been handed a death sentence, even though the doctor told you that, with treatment, you have a very good chance of a great outcome. Chance? What's he talking about chances? You'd never even thought about death and now the doctor can't even give you a guarantee.

✔ **The fear of the unknown rears its ugly head.** What's going to happen to you? Who's going to take care of the kids while you're in treatment? And your job: What about that big deadline that's approaching — not to mention money?

Riding the wave of emotions

Each woman reacts in her own unique way to the news of being diagnosed with breast cancer, but any way that you feel is perfectly fine. You may feel

✔ Frightened of not knowing what's going to happen

✔ Terrified at the possibility of facing death

✔ Angry at the injustice of life

✔ Intense sadness at the possibility of losing your breast

✔ Dread at facing the treatment ahead

✔ Depression so deep that it feels as though you're grieving

The fact is you're experiencing all these emotions either one at a time, one after the other, or all jumbled up at once. The emotion may come in waves, or it may come in spurts. You can't predict it, and you can't control it.

Here are a few important things to remember about feelings:

✔ Feeling awful is completely understandable and perfectly normal. In fact, if you weren't, that in itself would be a cause for concern.

✔ Allowing yourself to go through, or experience, those feelings is important. Don't block them out or run away from them. Doing so only makes it worse in the long run. Go ahead and cry and let someone you love hold you and rock you. Now is the time to express your feelings.

✔ Getting angry is tricky. When you feel anger (and you will), try to express it. Talk to people you trust and tell them how angry you feel, hit the pillow, shout up at the sky. Yelling at your loved one (which is what we often do, isn't it?) isn't helpful since it may result in him or her pulling away. (Which is the last thing you need!)

✔ Knowing that you won't feel this way forever, that it'll get better, and you'll get through this dilemma is perhaps most important.

Nevertheless, you may still require a referral to a psychologist. Call your doctor whenever you experience one or several of the following emotional situations *continuously* for more than three to four weeks:

✔ Crying spells that you can't stop

✔ Depression or hopelessness

✔ No interest in yourself and what you used to be involved with before treatment

✔ Inability to take care of your responsibilities

✔ Insomnia or sleeping too much

✔ Lack of appetite or energy

When depression is treated, you'll notice such an improvement in your life — you'll feel joy and pleasure again, be able to sleep and have more energy.

Stepping Through This

One of the best strategies for dealing with such an overwhelming situation is to tackle it one step at a time. You may think that you have to act immediately, but in most cases, you have time. You can help prepare yourself in many ways for the next phase, beginning with treatment. You can

✔ Take a week or two to enable you to think, feel, process, and plan.

✔ Get a journal and a pen and write down your questions, concerns, and all the stuff that you have to take care of.

✔ Use the following steps as a guide.

Recognizing the survivors at your side

You are not alone. More than 2 million women in America today are breast cancer survivors. You may be surprised by how many of them want to (*and*

Jen H.

"What a relief it was to come across a cancer survivor's Web site. The first few weeks after my diagnosis, I slept little, if at all. I spent numerous hours on the Internet, just searching for stories of people my age in similar situations, and all the information I could find about breast cancer. I would not wish my situation upon anyone, yet it is a comfort to know that I am not alone."

will) support you throughout the months ahead. Countless support groups and programs across the country exist and survivors staff most of them.

The bottom line: Get some support. You can do it online, by phone, or in person, and someone is available who's glad to offer you help. (See Chapter 23, where we list many helpful resources.) She's been in your shoes and can understand better than anyone how you're feeling. What's more, she faced the same terrors and made it to the other side. Call her; she's waiting for you.

Acquiring information

Find out as much information about breast cancer as you can. Reading this book is a perfect start. For example, did you know that every woman diagnosed with breast cancer faces a very different journey? Each woman's particular form and stage of cancer (see Chapter 7), her prognosis (see Chapter 8), and her treatment options (see Chapter 9) are very different.

Part of what causes the uncontrollable fear and anxiety is not knowing what to expect, or for that matter, what you can do about it. So understanding your *particular* diagnosis and treatment options can help you feel more empowered and in control of your life. You *don't* need to get a degree in medicine or in cancer research; in fact, sometimes knowing too much can make you feel confused. So get the knowledge about your individual circumstances and watch how you get your power back. Or if you're more comfortable not knowing all the options, your doctor can help you make the right choice.

Iris K.

"Educating myself on choices, striving to understand this new vocabulary of breast cancer and chemospeak, and being my own advocate helped me. Having the support of my husband, family members, and more friends than I ever knew I had helped me become a survivor."

Becoming a part of your team

Reclaim yourself by playing an active part in your treatment. You may be feeling as though everything's out of your hands and that you have no say in what happens. Get involved in choosing your hospital and your treatment. Ask questions and explore your options. We explain this fully in Chapter 9.

Building your own cheerleading squad

It's unanimous. The number-one predictor of how well you'll do psychologically is having a support system. The secret isn't so much that your loved ones take away your emotional pain (I sometimes wish that they could, don't you?), but rather it's that having their support can prevent you from becoming severely depressed or remaining terrified. Think of it as the people version of antidepressant drugs.

If one prescription were to be filled for getting through this period, it would include

- Building family members, friends, relatives, and colleagues into a team rallying to support you. Don't kid yourself; no one can do it alone. (Well, maybe one person in a million, but imagine how hard it must be for her!) Your cheerleading squad can do whatever needs doing. See Chapter 20 where we give them the suggestions.

- Relying on breast cancer survivors to provide you with the comfort, support, and understanding that you need. Check out Reach to Recovery or other similar programs that we describe in Chapter 23.

- Joining a support group that works for *you*. Many are out there. (See Chapters 23 and 24 to find the right one.)

Taking care of business

The final step before you begin your treatment is getting your life in order so that you can focus only on getting better. Make sure that you

- Talk to your children (see Chapter 21)

- Talk to your boss and human resources office at work about time off and the benefits to which you're entitled (see Chapter 17)

- Organize your insurance and finances (see Chapter 17)

Karen D.

"Don't be intimidated by your doctors. If you're not used to the medical world, dealing with breast cancer can be very scary. But if you're well informed, you can stand on your own."

Preparing yourself mentally

You can mentally prepare yourself for the start of treatment in many different ways. Much of it depends on how you view life. Check out the following suggestions:

- ✔ If you have a spiritual or religious belief, now's the time to draw strength from it.

- ✔ Many other relaxation techniques can help you through treatment, including meditation, yoga, and breathing exercises (which we describe in Chapter 14).

- ✔ Many women find that keeping a journal of what they're going through and their feelings is helpful, both at the time of treatment and later on.

- ✔ Having a heart-to-heart talk with your partner, in which you tell him or her how you feel and ask for what you need, is extremely important.

Of course, you may have your own way of coping with stress that you've successfully used in the past. Just remember that you need to take the time to take care of *you*. Now's the time to put on that batch of chicken soup.

Regardless of what your treatment is, it isn't going to be easy. Suffering from nausea, weight gain, and hair loss takes its toll. In Chapters 10, 11, and 12, we provide you with many helpful suggestions for dealing with these, so that you can feel good again, physically and mentally.

Birdie H.

"The most important thing you have to do when you join the sisterhood of breast cancer survivors is finding a good support group. It doesn't necessarily have to be a cancer support group, just so you have a group of people who can help you cope with what is so rapidly changing in your life."

Toeing the Line after Treatment

The moment you waited for, lived for, longed for is here at last. Your treatment is over; it's done! You can't believe it: no more hospital visits, no more of that dreaded chemotherapy (maybe now that hair will start growing back in and you can throw away that stupid cap already), and best of all, you get your life back.

So what's wrong with you? How come you're feeling so confused and sad? When you should be feeling grateful, here you are down in the dumps. Don't be hard on yourself; it's normal. Many women are more scared after treatment than they are when they were getting treatment. That's why many institutions have support groups for patients after treatment as well as for those undergoing treatment.

Feeling up and feeling down

Experiencing a feeling of void is normal for several reasons. You've been through such an intense period in which everything has been prescribed for you: "Be here at this time." "Get that treatment at that time." "You need to bring a spare set of clothing, and don't forget your treatment card." By the time it's over, you don't even know whether you can think for yourself again.

And don't forget that during treatment you had to focus on getting through it, without much time or energy left for philosophical thoughts about the meaning of life. Now you're overwhelmed with feelings. How *are* you going to get your life back? And how do you want to spend the rest of it?

All your support team members are happy to be able to have their lives back again. Don't take their reactions the wrong way, they were happy to be there for you, but now they must get back to their own responsibilities. Suddenly, you're no longer surrounded by this fine group of loving friends. You're alone with all those thoughts and feelings they helped you get through. So, feeling a void is normal.

Learning to accept your body is an essential part of accepting yourself. In Chapter 19, we discuss ways of exploring and embracing your new body and talk frankly about ways to rekindle intimacy. Oh yes, it certainly *can* be done!

And just about the time you've accepted this greater solitude, all those other issues well up and you have to deal with looming questions, such as "Is it going to come back?" and "Will I ever be able to have sex again?" Please read Chapter 19 to see that life can really go back to normal.

Wrestling with the fear of recurrence

Learning to live with the nagging fear of recurrence is something that all breast cancer survivors struggle with. It's more difficult in the beginning as you wonder, "What's that ache?" or think, "I've never felt *that* pain before."

How can you get through this fear? Try

- ✔ Setting up your regular follow-up appointments with your doctor and asking many questions.
- ✔ Speaking and sharing your thoughts with other survivors.

Some days are more difficult than others, like the anniversaries of the date you were first diagnosed or when a close friend finds out she's had a recurrence. However, a day will arrive when you realize that you haven't thought about the cancer at all. Not for an entire day! Then a week, then...

Wanting to go back to your life, to live again and not think about cancer or treatment or hospitals is perfectly normal. But never skip a follow-up visit! Denial is a very potent defense, and it's understandable if, at times, you just want to pretend that the cancer never happened. Just don't pretend when it's time for that all-important follow-up visit. It's your life that's at stake.

Managing menopause

One of the most psychologically (and physically) difficult side effects of chemotherapy is developing early *menopause*, the stopping of your menstrual cycle. Chemotherapy, radiation therapy, and tamoxifen can cause your menstrual cycle to become irregular. Your cycle may also stop completely, either permanently or temporarily.

The older you are when you're diagnosed with breast cancer, the more likely you are to go through menopause (if you have chemotherapy); however, being young unfortunately doesn't mean that you're immune.

Carol M.

"Fear will live in your head, right next to that positive attitude you must keep. There's always the fear that the breast cancer will come back, that it will strike the other breast or that cancer will show up somewhere else. Personally, I think there is no way to eliminate the fear, but only to find ways to control it. As the famous saying goes, 'there is nothing to fear but fear itself'. You will have it, but fear doesn't have to rule your life with every little bump, bruise, ache and pain."

Despite these irregularities, you *can* become pregnant during these treatments. Chemotherapy can be very toxic and may cause birth defects, so you must take precautions and use birth control while undergoing treatment.

Your doctor will advise you on appropriate birth control options and on the issue of when it's safe to become pregnant after being diagnosed with breast cancer. In general, most doctors advise against pregnancy for the first two years after you're diagnosed with breast cancer. New data suggest that after the two years following a diagnosis of breast cancer, pregnancy doesn't increase the risk of your breast cancer coming back.

Women who undergo menopause normally (in other words, not because of chemotherapy) often experience many physical and emotional changes. Because the process usually is gradual, menopause gives the woman the opportunity and the time to adapt to these changes. Unfortunately, the process isn't so gradual when it happens in conjunction with chemotherapy. These changes take place rapidly, and it's therefore more difficult to adjust to them.

Symptoms

Some of the symptoms that accompany menopause include

- **Hot flashes:** A heat wave, unrelated to the temperature or any activity you're engaged in, rises suddenly and rapidly from your chest and up to your forehead, leaving you bright red and dripping with sweat as if you'd just ran up a very long flight of stairs. This often occurs at night, resulting in soaked bedclothes, disturbing your sleep, and leaving you exhausted and irritable. Hot flashes during the day also are common and can be very uncomfortable, not to mention potentially embarrassing.

- **Vaginal dryness during intercourse:** This potential side effect can have a tremendous impact on your sex life. We offer solutions in Chapter 19.

- **Light spotting after intercourse:** The lining of the vagina thins after menopause, so you may experience light spotting after sexual activity. This is normal, nothing to worry about.

- **Mood swings:** Women often experience mood swings during menopause as a result of changes in hormonal levels. You may experience crying, irritability, or feelings of helplessness unrelated to actual events.

- **Weight gain:** This may occur even when you don't eat any more than you always have. So as soon as you can, begin following a healthy diet and exercising at least a few times a week. You'll be so glad that you did. (For more about the importance of diet and exercise, see Chapter 3.)

Unfortunately, menopause varies from woman to woman, and your doctor won't be able to predict how long your menopausal symptoms will last.

Menopause does not mean madness: Dealing with symptoms

So what can you do about these really unpleasant symptoms? Here's the bad news: Hormone replacement therapy (HRT) is not an option. Some women who go through menopause are placed on HRT, which helps abate menopausal symptoms. However, because this therapy is hormone-based, it's not an option that you can consider since estrogen may cause cancer cells to grow more rapidly and increase your risk of developing a new cancer.

Don't worry, you are not doomed to suffer the madness of the incessant hot flashes and menopausal mood swings. Fortunately, there are several effective nonhormonal drugs that have been shown to decrease hot flashes and other menopausal symptoms. Ask your doc. Also, herbal remedies, such as Black Cohosh (described in Chapter 14), can be effective in some women.

Accepting the pain of infertility

For most women, having children brings meaning to their lives, making them feel complete and providing hope for the future. Although most women who get breast cancer are older and already have children, this scenario is by no means always the case.

Annually, thousands of women are undergoing treatment for breast cancer but have not yet begun their families, either because they're still young or because they've chosen to postpone having children until later. Unfortunately, infertility is a possible consequence of breast cancer treatment. Chemotherapy sometimes leaves you infertile (although radiation and tamoxifen never do).

The realization that you may not be able to have children can be especially painful and difficult to deal with. After all that you've been through, the impact of this realization hits with twice the intensity, and you may experience a tremendous feeling of loss. You may also experience feelings of anger at the injustice you've experienced or jealousy and resentment toward women who have children. All of these feelings are normal and understandable. Sharing your feelings with others who've gone through similar losses can be helpful in keeping you from feeling alone in your loss.

Addressing the issue head-on

If you want to consider having children after your treatment, speak with your doctor first. When considering this life-altering decision, you have to think about your prognosis. Doing so is a very tough issue to face, because it means taking into account what chances you have of raising your baby. This issue is a painful one to face; however, by knowing as much of the reality as can be predicted, you can consider your options knowing exactly what challenges you may have to face and what your chances are for success.

Considering other options

If you're still hoping to have children, several other options that you can consider include

- **Trying to get pregnant after treatment is complete.** The most recent research shows that pregnancy after treatment is not harmful to your outcome. After your treatment is officially declared complete, if you're not sure whether you're infertile, discuss the possibility of a pregnancy with your doctor. Remember, however, that your attempts may not result in a pregnancy.

- **Cryonic preservation of embryos or embryo donation.** Freezing your embryos is an option. However, it may prove to be a costly and time-consuming project that requires the assistance of a gynecologist who specializes in such methods. The problem is that the process requires large doses of hormones to stimulate ovulation before your cancer treatment. The good news is that tamoxifen can safely stimulate ovulation!

- **Adoption.** Although this option is obviously not a decision that you have to make right away, it's one that you can keep in the back of your mind for consideration at the right time.

Preparing for the Rest of Your Life

Here's the best news. Yes, cancer can adversely affect your life, but many breast cancer survivors report that their lives have been altered for the better. Going through such a traumatic experience and coming out on the other side revealed so much about themselves that they hadn't known or realized before.

Roberta H.

"Throughout the awful, horrible year that I spent undergoing breast cancer treatment, I learned so much. Some things that I experienced, I could have done without; others have been true blessings. I discovered that others really care about my family and me. Strangers who saw my bald head told me they'd pray for me, and they meant it. Food appeared daily at our doorstep for weeks on end, lovingly prepared by friends from many walks of life. People organized to make certain I had transportation to treatments when my husband had to work. Others called regularly just to chat and let me know I wasn't forgotten. My husband learned what I do all day, how to pay the bills, and where the insurance policies are kept. We both learned that we haven't spent nearly enough years together yet, that we're still deeply in love, and that looks aren't all that important."

Carol M.

"After the depression, after the acceptance, after the healing, I hope you're ready to give back. Being able to help someone else is very rewarding. I think you'll find that it took breast cancer to teach you how to really live."

They discovered that

- ✔ Their priorities in life had changed.

- ✔ Their current lives held so much more meaning.

- ✔ They wanted to focus on the more important aspects of their lives and pay less attention to the more mundane aspects.

- ✔ Their sense of self-worth increased significantly after they realized they'd weathered a life-altering storm.

- ✔ Their relationships with close family and friends were more meaningful.

- ✔ They were able to be much more compassionate toward others.

If you think this is the case with only a few women, you're wrong. A recent study — the largest ever conducted of breast cancer survivors — found that most survivors were doing extremely well physically and psychologically five to ten years down the road. The chances are great that you'll soon be one of them.

In time, many breast cancer survivors give back to the community, and they do so in many different ways. They become volunteers who greet newly diagnosed patients, run support groups, answer crisis calls, raise funds for research, or advocate for better laws so that others don't have to suffer. Their contributions are priceless.

When you're first diagnosed is not the best time for you to begin taking care of others. It's the time to take care of you. When you do, in no time at all, you'll be the one doing the giving, and someone else will be receiving.

Chapter 19

Rekindling Intimacy After Treatment

*W*hen you were diagnosed with breast cancer, you had other things to focus on, such as whether you were going to live or die. Then came treatment, and frankly, sex probably wasn't at the top of your agenda at that time either. But now that you've been through those things, it's different. You've nearly or completely finished your treatment, and you're facing your life.

For most of us, making love is an essential part of an intimate relationship, a way of experiencing closeness with a loved one and an integral part of what makes us feel alive. Most people don't talk about overcoming barriers to intimacy after treatment, because after you get cancer, it seems as if you're no longer supposed to be a sexual human being. Nothing could be farther from the truth. In this chapter, we open the doors to rekindling your intimacy.

First Cancer, Now This?

Will treatment affect your sex life? More than likely. (But just because that's true doesn't mean that the effects last forever.) Which symptoms you develop and what changes you undergo depend on your age and the form of your treatment. For example, chemotherapy and tamoxifen can sometimes reduce your sexual desire, but radiation rarely has that effect. The dose and the amount of time you're treated also are factors. The length of time that these symptoms persist varies from woman to woman.

Carol M.

"What could be more intimate when you undress for the first time and your mate sees that awful incision and the drainage tubes hanging out of your body? Or when he cries right along with you as he feels your pain as he helps change your bandages and applies ointment to the cut? Or when he helps you into the shower for the first time or washes your hair in the kitchen sink? Or when we lie in bed and discuss our fears and hopes for the future? To me this is the real intimacy in a marriage. This was the good part of breast cancer, because I never felt more loved and more connected to anyone in my whole life and never will again."

Here are some symptoms you may develop after breast cancer treatment:

- ✔ Decreased sex drive
- ✔ Vaginal dryness (which may result in pain during intercourse)
- ✔ Hot flashes
- ✔ Weight gain
- ✔ Depression

Unfortunately, doctors often don't discuss with their patients how breast cancer treatments affect their sexuality and sex lives. The reason: Doctors often are so focused on saving your life that they may not recognize or realize how important your sex life is to you. That's why you may have to initiate discussions about this issue with your doctor.

Despite menstrual irregularities that treatment causes, you can become pregnant while undergoing treatments. Chemotherapy and tamoxifen can cause birth defects, so doctors strongly advise that you to take appropriate precautions and use birth control during treatment.

Sexy study

A recent study of breast cancer survivors who are five to ten years postdiagnosis revealed that survivors who experienced the most symptoms that got in the way of their sex lives (such as hot flashes, vaginal dryness, or lowered sexual desire) had received chemotherapy. The good news is that many of the survivors reported that even when they experienced these symptoms, their negative sexual side effects lessened with time. Here's the best part: Most survivors reported no decline in their sexual interest or sexual pleasure. That's plenty to look forward to.

SURVIVORS' SECRETS

Kim G.

"When my husband initiates sex by fondling my breast, and he switches to my left breast, which is the one that was operated on, I can move his hand back over to my right breast. At that point I can become very interested in what my husband is doing. After surgery, my left breast lost major feeling and became a dead area for arousal purposes. Unfortunately, my husband doesn't spend the required time to keep my interest going; he moves on to other areas that may arouse him but not me. That said, our sex life is terrible for me and good for him.

Having sex right now is too painful for me. This has been going on for a year now. My husband says that he still loves me and acknowledges there are other ways. However, we have not explored these options. At this point, I equate sex with pain, and I'm not interested in it in any way, shape, or form. Sex after cancer has its drawbacks. The conditions you suddenly get after your body has undergone an invasive medical and surgical attack are not always discussed at length by the medical community."

If the Bed's A-Rockin' . . .

You can overcome each sexual side effect. Sex therapists offer tried-and-true strategies, and many cancer survivors have successfully used them. (The strategies, not the therapists.)

Feeling randy

Your desire for sex may be reduced. If you do feel a lessening in your sexual desire, don't despair. It hasn't left you forever. Consider keeping a desire diary. Here's how:

1. **Buy a pen and a blank book and keep them with you at all times.**

2. **Whenever you have a sexual thought or feeling, jot it down.**

   Record the time of day, where you were, what you were doing, and who else was there.

3. **Record what you did about your desire.**

4. **Keep this journal for a month.**

5. **After a month has passed, look at your diary.**

   Do you see any desire patterns? Do you feel more desire:

- At certain times of the day?

- Around certain people?

- In certain settings?

6. **Create situations in which you can feel such desire.**

You can do this on your own at first to make you feel more comfortable. After you feel comfortable, grab your partner, and get him or her involved.

If you find that you never feel any sexual interest for months, consider seeking professional help from a gynecologist or therapist.

Being sensitive to your breasts

Various breast cancer treatments may impact your sexual life.

Radiation can cause your breasts to be red and sore, similar to the way a sunburn feels, and they may either be very sensitive when touched or lack sensitivity at the site of the scar. If you've had a mastectomy, you no longer will have a nipple that may have been a source of sexual pleasure. Touching the scar may feel uncomfortable or even hypersensitive. The skin of your chest (from the collarbone to your ribs) usually is numb during the first year or two after surgery. As feeling begins to come back to your skin, the sensation often feels strange (not the same as before surgery). Sometimes, it even feels painful.

If you've had a breast reconstruction, you may feel *more* sexy and attractive. After all, you now have the breasts you always wanted. However, because the nerves that supply feeling to the skin of your breast area were cut during surgery, the area around your reconstruction also is numb during the first year or two after surgery. You may not have any sensation to the nipple, or the sensation may return but not at the same intensity and in a different way than it felt before.

Joanne B.

"There was no change in our level of intimacy after the mastectomies. However, in my narrow experience, the breasts are part of the sexual act, and I worried a bit about my husband's response. It made no difference to him, although he had previously enjoyed my breasts. However, now I do not remove my nightgown, and make sure it covers my upper chest throughout."

Roberta H.

"I took a direct approach and asked him how he felt about the way I looked and what effect it had on his desire to be intimate with me. I talked to him about my fears, my self-image, and my love for him. He told me of the fears he'd had — first that he'd lose me, later that he might hurt me, and then about his physical and emotional fatigue from caring for me and our family. Most important, he told me that what mattered and what inspired his desire for me wasn't my appearance but rather my self and the love and trust we'd developed over the years. Although I still need to hear that every now and again as I adjust to my new appearance, the need is less often now. We talk privately more than we did precancer and enjoy each intimate moment much more intensely, perhaps because we realize how close we came to "until death do us part." We've both had to rediscover (to some extent) the mechanics of sex to accommodate the changes in my body, but it has been with excitement that we're still together rather than with regret for what is gone."

Getting back on the horse

Chemotherapy and tamoxifen may reduce vaginal moisture, which can result in painful intercourse. Even though these symptoms can be extremely upsetting and can adversely affect your sex life, most women find that talking about them with their doctors is very difficult. Don't let it be so difficult — especially when proven ways of overcoming these problems are available. Talk to your doctor. He or she can give you advice to help with the dryness and soreness.

Carol M.

"I think sex and intimacy can be two entirely different things. And, I can tell you that having a mastectomy (oh, what a 'kind way' to say something so horrible) . . . having a breast cut off does dramatically change one's sex life. With a breast gone, some of the physical things I used to do with my husband could no longer be done. There were no longer two breasts and that wonderful gully in between that he loved. I think this frustration, coupled with feeling very ugly and deformed, caused me to cry in his arms the first several times we made love. I was one of the lucky ones, though, since he kept reassuring me that he loved me no matter what. So in time, our sex life was as great as it always had been."

Peg I.

"My husband told me that I was not my breast. It was a part of me, but not my self worth. I was a sexual person on my own without it. I didn't feel like the disfigured person that I could have felt like."

Intimacy isn't just about intercourse. In fact, it doesn't have to be about intercourse at all. Whatever you and your partner feel comfortable with is what's important. The key to intimacy is understanding, feeling love for, and enjoying each other.

Talking as preforeplay

Most couples don't talk much about their sex lives. However, talking to your partner about it after your cancer treatment is important. Yes, doing so may be difficult for you, and it may feel very embarrassing, but things have changed. Although most people want sex to be spontaneous and unplanned, those expectations may not be realistic, especially right after your treatment. Let your partner know when you're ready to talk about it or even to begin touching again.

If you're to resume a sexual relationship, your partner needs to know

✔ Whether you're ready to have sexual intercourse. Don't do it until you're *both* ready. We talk more about resuming intercourse later in the chapter.

✔ When and how you want to show your breasts.

✔ What works and what doesn't. Use words or guide with your hands.

✔ What makes you comfortable with your breasts. Experiment with what and how you feel most comfortable. Buck naked or wearing these things and any combination thereof:

- Pajamas
- Bra
- Prosthesis

One single session of talking won't likely have you raring to go. Take your time, talk it over during the course of days, weeks, or months. Ah ha! Ready to get down to the nitty-gritty?

Keep in mind that the nitty and the gritty are relative. Sex therapists recommend that during the first few times you engage in intimate contact, you do not engage in actual intercourse but instead try gentle touching or massaging. Avoid touching the breasts and genitals, not because such actions are not pleasurable, but rather because the goal is to help you both feel relaxed and comfortable with each other's bodies again and to feel sensual pleasure. Here are some steps you can take to get there:

1. **Plan a time when you'll have quiet without interruption.**

2. **Create a soothing, relaxed atmosphere.**

   You know the drill: candles, soft music, a bearskin rug, new batteries . . .

3. **Agree ahead of time that if you feel any discomfort or pain, you'll let your partner know.**

   Here's the key: Be honest but not rude. You don't want to convey rejection. If something your partner does hurts or doesn't feel right, avoid shouting, "Don't touch there, fool!" Gently move his or her hand to another part of your body or tenderly say, "That still feels sensitive, but this feels good."

4. **Massage away.**

   Employ all your senses: Touch, taste, smell, sight, and hearing. You can even giggle and cry if you want.

   Did things go well? Great. Nitty-gritty continues. If not, stop for now and get back to it when the time is right again.

5. **Okay, *now* add breast and genital touching.**

   Make sure that you're comfortable with saying what feels good and what hurts. Be sure to use strategies described in the "Lubing you up," "Thanks, Dr. Kegel," and "Feeling the flex" sections that follow whenever you need to.

   Maybe you've tried all these suggestions and still feel uncomfortable during intercourse. But you really want to have sex. Try a position — anything other than the missionary position — where you can control the movement, so that if deep penetration is painful, you can make the thrusts less deep. Use pillows and blankets (building blocks, big pieces of furniture, whatever it takes that is secure) to support any part of your body. With patience, love, and good communication between you, you'll find a way.

Lubing you up

Dry as a bone has taken on a whole new meaning for you. Between treatment side effects and trouble getting aroused, you're battling vaginal dryness, and that's no fun for anyone. Luckily, you have plenty of help. You can try using

   ✔ **An estrogen ring.** Your doctor inserts this device (available by prescription only) into your vagina during an office visit. The ring releases very tiny doses of estrogen (too low to be a risk), which lets the vagina lubricate itself.

✔ **Vaginal hormone cream.** Your doctor can prescribe vaginal hormone cream. If used daily for a month, it rebuilds your vagina's lining. After that, you use it once a week or every other week. You can't continue using it daily because the dose of estrogen is too high.

✔ **Lubricant.** A lubricant helps keep your vagina moisturized during sexual activity, which is really helpful. Make sure that you get one that's uncolored and unscented because colorings or perfumes can irritate your vaginal lining. Astroglide and Replens are popular, easy-to-find lubricants.

✔ **Vaginal moisturizer.** You can use a vaginal moisturizer several times a week, regardless of whether you're engaging in sexual activity. Because this moisturizer keeps the acidity at a normal level, it also can prevent yeast infections.

Thanks, Dr. Kegel

If you feel pain during intercourse, you're more likely to tighten the vaginal muscles in the future — often without even being aware of it. Gaining control of your vaginal muscles helps you relax during penetration.

Kegel exercises help you control your vaginal muscles, which, in turn, helps you relax them when you want to. They're really easy:

1. **Next time you urinate, stop the flow midstream and hold it for a few seconds.**

2. **Relax those same muscles.**

   Your urine should flow again. Taking these first two steps simply helps you pinpoint the muscles you need to exercise. Don't stop your flow every time you urinate.

3. **Practice flexing those same muscles when you're not urinating.**

4. **Flex, count to 3, and release.**

   Do these tensing-and-relaxing movements several times in a row two or three times every day.

Feeling the flex

Sometimes, even though you do these exercises, intercourse still may be painful or difficult for you. When that's the case, you or your partner can stretch your vagina before there's any penetration.

1. **Make sure that everybody's in the mood.**

   Marvin Gaye can help.

2. **Lubricate your finger or your partner's finger.**

   Use a personal lubricant; avoid combining culinary arts and coitus.

3. **Very slowly slip the finger into your vagina.**

The O is good to go

Fortunately, your ability to have orgasms is not affected by treatment. (Phew!) Having orgasms depends on your ability to feel aroused and relaxed, so please don't get upset if it takes time for you to achieve this state. Go easy on yourself, and make sure that your partner does, too.

You've just finished a rigorous treatment, so let this part of your sex life take its course. If you find that achieving an orgasm becomes an obstacle, consider seeking professional help from a gynecologist or sex therapist.

4. **Use Kegel movements to relax your muscles and slowly move the finger in deeper.**

   Once that feels comfortable, try using two, and then three fingers. This may take several attempts. Use plenty of lubrication, plenty of time, and plenty of patience.

If you've tried all of these ideas but you're still experiencing pain, please consider getting help from a gynecologist or a sex therapist.

Going beyond the Physical

Physical pleasure isn't the only kind of pleasure that's involved in sexuality. You also need to consider psychological pleasures. When a change has occurred in your body, you may feel less attractive or less appealing, and you may have to get used to being just plain different. Don't give up. We have suggestions.

Focusing on your positive attributes is a very important aspect of going through treatment. Here's one practical suggestion:

1. **Find a time when you have uninterrupted quiet.**

2. **Stand in front of a mirror.**

3. **Really look at yourself and ask the following questions:**

   • What parts of my body do I look at most?

   • What negative thoughts do I have about the way I look?

   • Has cancer changed the way I look? How?

4. **Put on your most beautiful clothes.**

   Get all dolled up with your wig, makeup, and jewelry. Dress the way you like to look.

5. **Stand in front of the mirror again.**

6. **Ask yourself what three positive things you can say about yourself?**

Revisiting your image

You have several ways of dealing with some of the changes you've experienced in the way you look. Feeling anxious or uncomfortable is completely natural when you haven't been physically intimate for a while, so talk about it. Share your feelings with each other if you can. Taking things one small step at a time is a great start.

The good news: In the same study of breast cancer survivors we describe in the "Sexy study" sidebar earlier in this chapter, most of the women reported that many years after diagnosis, they still had the same body image that they originally started with. What that means is that even if you feel as yucky as they come after your treatment, things do get better.

7. **Say them out loud.**

   When you can't find at least three positive things to say, try again another day. Do this until you've given yourself at least several (more than just one!) compliments.

8. **After you achieve this goal, congratulate yourself.**

9. **Get naked and stand in front of the mirror.**

   Remember that the goal is finding the good things about you. If you can't do that at first, take a few deep breaths and try again. You can find good things about you. Look, they're right in front of you. Now that you've practiced standing in front of the mirror naked and beautiful, you'll feel much more relaxed when your partner looks at you.

If after you've tried this exercise several times, you've ended up in tears or without any positive things to say, consider getting help from a professional therapist. In fact, if you can't do anything without crying, get help right away. If you're not sure whether you're depressed, check out the warning signs in Chapter 18.

Roberta H.

"We knew intimacy after my treatment would be an issue that we'd have to deal with sooner or later, so before it began, we decided as a couple to deal with it through better communication. We reaffirmed our love and commitment to each other early on and relied heavily on that commitment. I promised to fight to live and stay with him, and he promised to love and support me in sickness and in health. The same promises we made 23 years ago, but with a new insight into what those vows really meant. . . .

"I won't lie. I wish I could be young, slim, and symmetrical again. It's a real shock when I catch my image in a mirror. I keep expecting to see the 20-year-old who's my inner self-image. She may not be visible to the casual observer, but my husband knows where to find her, and that's all that matters."

Chapter 20

Helping the One You Love: A Chapter for Family and Friends

In This Chapter

▶ Dealing with the diagnosis

▶ Traveling through treatment

▶ Considering the consequences

▶ Finding solutions

▶ Being friends forever

*W*hen someone you love is diagnosed with cancer, it affects the entire family and circle of friends. It's like a mobile; anything that happens to one part affects the others. When one piece of the mobile is damaged or broken, the rest of the mobile becomes off balance. It keeps moving, however, until it achieves a new balance. The same can be said about your family and friends.

It may be your wife, daughter, niece, or cousin who's just been diagnosed with breast cancer. She might be your best friend, irreplaceable neighbor, close colleague, or your workout buddy. Regardless of the nature of your relationship, you love her and want to be there for her throughout her journey.

What do you say? What do you not say? Taking care of your loved one and worrying about other pressures can seem overwhelming. How can you help? And most important, how can you help when you're feeling devastated and scared yourself? Being there for her and taking care of yourself at the same time isn't always easy, but remembering that it can be done is important.

TIP

Working in some boss time

You may consider taking time off from work to be with your loved one during her treatments. Finding out whether (and how) you can modify your job responsibilities can buy you much relief. You may want to sit down with your boss and discuss how long you think you'll be out from work (your loved one's doctor can help by giving you an estimation). You may need to get a letter or form from the doctor. Some of the things you can do to accomplish these ends include

✔ Educating yourself about the Family and Medical Leave Act, which requires employers with at least 50 employees to provide up to 12 weeks of unpaid, job-protected leave to eligible employees for certain family and medical reasons.

✔ Speaking to your boss about the possibility of taking extra time off. Doing so may not be easy, but frequently a compromise can be reached.

✔ Finding out from the Human Resources Department whether your employer recognizes any special circumstances (such as a catastrophic illness) for which you can take time off without sacrificing your salary or your job.

✔ Finding other ways to keep in touch with your office even when you must be at the hospital. (What would we do without cell phones, laptops, and e-mail?)

Hearing the Verdict

After hearing about your loved one's diagnosis, you face many challenges in the months ahead, especially when you're the primary caretaker. Yet hearing that someone you deeply love has cancer is probably one of the worst moments you'll ever experience.

The word *cancer* sounds ominous, but did you know that *most* women survive breast cancer? Additionally, breast cancer isn't one single diagnosis; moreover, many different forms and stages of breast cancer exist. Some require minimal treatment and have a 98 percent survival rate, while others are more extensive and require a heavier treatment load. What's more, a woman's prognosis varies considerably depending on an entire host of factors.

Knowing what to expect and what you're facing enables you to begin planning and to be able to tackle what needs to be done. So the first step is finding out *exactly*

✔ What type of breast cancer your loved one has (see Chapter 4). Is it infiltrating ductal cancer (the most common type) or one of the rarer types?

✔ How far it has spread, if it all. (Chapter 7 tackles this topic.) Has it spread to the lymph nodes under the arm?

✔ What her prognosis is. Chapter 8 can help you understand what a prognosis is and give you an idea of what your loved one's is.

✔ What treatments she will require. Choices abound; what type she receives depends on her cancer and her decisions. Chapter 9 reveals more.

Finding out all this information may take time and quite a few medical tests, so try not to become too frustrated when you don't have all the answers right away.

Set realistic expectations and manageable goals. Adjusting your goals to the realities of the current situation can help your entire family. A diagnosis of cancer doesn't mean that all your dreams and aspirations are dead, but rather it just means that now may not be the time for pursuing them.

Tuning In

Remember all those times when you tuned her out? Well, now's the time to actively listen. Regardless of what she says or how she says it, hearing her now is a gift. Any ways that you can show her you're paying attention to what she's saying are added bonuses. Look into her eyes when she talks, stroke her hair, hold her hand; whatever you're both comfortable with. If your partner feels uncomfortable with these actions, think about what she would have liked before her diagnosis and go with that. If you've never reacted to your partner in these ways before, now's the time to start.

Your reaction to the diagnosis may differ from that of your loved one. She may be terrified, kind of like a deer in headlights, feeling powerless to do anything, or you may be the one feeling this way while she moves full steam ahead (see Chapter 18 for more about how she might be feeling). Whatever the case, you need to make yourself available in myriad ways. For example, what you say to the kids is so important that we devote all of Chapter 21 to that purpose.

To each other

A woman who's just been diagnosed needs to know that you're there for her, regardless of how bad it gets or how long it takes. She's probably terrified and in need of plenty of reassurance and comfort.

The best thing you can do is make sure that she knows that you love her and you'll be there for her, no matter what the circumstances may be. Tell her that as many times as she needs to hear it in as many different ways as you can say it: words, actions, notes, songs, or any other way you come up with.

From a partner's perspective, your loved one is going through treatment that takes a physical and emotional toll on her. The kids are scared, angry, or clingy, and require plenty of reassurance, all of which takes time and effort that quite simply isn't easy to come by. You're exhausted, scared, and sometimes feel angry and frustrated (which usually is followed by guilt for having those feelings), and on plenty of occasions, you're bound to feel overwhelmed.

Studies reveal that couples who are honest with each other, sharing their thoughts and feelings and working together to find solutions, keep their marriages alive and strong through these difficult times. Many even report growing closer and more intimate than before cancer, because of their intimate and honest sharing. If you've never treated each other this way before, now's the time to start. If you need help, plenty of information is available (see Chapter 23).

At the hospital

No, you don't have to get a degree in medicine, but being in the know and an active member of the treatment team sure helps. Understanding the medical challenges that your partner faces, what her treatments entail, and how she can best get through this dilemma gives *you* the tools you need to become her coach and confidante. That way you can cheer, guide, and support her all the way. You'll welcome the sense of control and achievement this insight provides you, and she'll relish and appreciate your active support. You can

- ✓ **Get information from the many available sources.** Chapters 23 and 24 give you lists of resources from which to start. Having your hands on this book, after all, is a great advantage, too.

- ✓ **Develop alliances between you and members of the medical team.** Treatment team members are great allies, and Chapter 9 tells you more about them.

- ✓ **Ask her doctors for *specific* information about what to expect.**

- ✓ **Be upfront about asking questions.** Don't be shy or afraid to pursue answers.

- ✓ **Attend appointments and make sure you're at the hospital when the doctor plans to be there.** Take notes when you speak with the doctor.

- ✓ **Support your partner in all the decisions that must be made.**

Carol M.

"You'll find that friends and family aren't quite sure what to say or how to react. I found the best way to handle these episodes was to forgive them whenever they say something totally inappropriate and use humor to break the ice. My friends felt helpless and wanted to really do something to ease the pain. My advice is to let them. It makes them feel better and you, too. Helping allows them to take an active part in your recovery and creates a bond that transcends traditional friendships and even some family relationships."

Calling in the reserves

No single person can handle the job of helping your loved one through this breast cancer alone, regardless of how competent you may be. It's time to call in the reserves. Gather a team of workers. Wait! You already have this team. It's made up of family, friends, and colleagues, and don't forget that members of your church or social organizations usually want to help, but often don't know how. Now isn't the time to be shy about asking team members to enroll. (You can always pay them back later when they need your assistance.)

Call the group together and try this:

1. **Make weekly assistance charts.**

   Include

   - Tasks that need to be accomplished. Include job descriptions.

   - Expertise required for each task. Can you drive?

   - When the tasks need to be done . . . 9 to 5? The night shift?

   Table 20-1 shows an example assistance schedule. Use the table to create your own list that meets your needs.

2. **Ask members of your team to sign up for the times and duties they prefer.**

   Sign up backups in case of emergencies.

3. **Assign tasks to team members who are unsure about what to do.**

   Maybe a team member doesn't know what job he or she is best suited for or doesn't mind which responsibility he or she is assigned.

SURVIVORS' SECRETS

Karen D.

"Let people do things for you, and accept help, no matter how independent you may think you are. People truly want to help you out; sometimes, they don't know what to do for you. Ask them to do something according to their skills to make them and you feel better. A friend's friend was a massage therapist, but I couldn't afford her $60 an hour. She insisted on coming to my house for a special cancer rate of only $30. So I got regular massages. It was wonderful. I normally wouldn't be so extravagant on myself."

4. **Set up a conference when a change in therapy or follow-up visit is planned or if you anticipate your support team (family and friends) may be away.**

   Devise new plans or strategies to meet each of these new situations. You'll be so glad you did.

Table 20-1	Example assistance schedule		
Task	*Description*	*Time Needed*	*Who's Doing it*
Driving to and from the hospital			
Taking the kids to school			
Taking the kids to soccer practice			
Taking the kids to doctor appointments			
Grocery shopping (See attached list)			
Cooking			
Laundry			
House cleaning			

Brushing Up on Your Bedside Manner

Many unknown, unscheduled, and unexpected demands are made on the family during your loved one's treatment. Recognizing these challenges enables you to prepare and places you in a position to find the best ways of dealing with them. What is it that you're being asked to do?

Hands-on healing

Seeing a sick loved one is not something with which most people are familiar. You're going to get your hands dirty in the most literal of senses, and that may be covering new ground for you. You can do it. Sickness is an intimate, less-than-beautiful thing, but you can dive in headfirst. Help her heal by

- ✔ **Giving her medication.** How difficult can it be to hand out a few pills? What if a few different medications must be taken at various times of the day, with or without food, with or without water, on an empty or full stomach, or some combination of the above? Maintaining a chart can help you take care of the "I forgots!"

- ✔ **Dressing and taking care of the wound.** The nurse will show you how to change the dressing on your partner's wound if necessary before she's discharged from the hospital, but most women go home without any bandages. Chapter 10 describes the procedure, too. Whenever you're uncomfortable with this assignment, ask a family member or friend to assist.

- ✔ **Disinfecting the indwelling catheter.** The *indwelling catheter* (a device under the skin that is connected to a vein in the chest or neck — no more needles in your arm!) requires regular disinfecting to prevent the risk of infection. Many hospitals train family members to do it and provide the tools that are needed for administering such care at home. If you're queasy about doing this job, a relative or friend can (or may already) be trained, or you can take your partner to the hospital every four weeks or so to have the nurses do it. (You'll probably have to wait in line!)

- ✔ **Bathing and dressing her.** She'll usually be able to do these things herself, but during treatment, she may be too ill or too weak to do much of anything. Consider bathing her as your loving and giving act for her.

- ✔ **Watching her.** As the person closest to your partner, you're the one who becomes her observer, monitoring progress and watching out for possible side effects. You're probably the one who determines when it's time to take her to the emergency room and when she can be taken care of at home, and that's an awesome responsibility. You're the one who has to make certain that your loved one does what she's supposed to do (and make sure that she follows doctors' orders!).

Sponging the soap

Having someone give you a bath is a luxury few people ever experience. Now is the perfect time for you to do this for a loved one with breast cancer. The kind of bath she needs depends on what can and cannot get wet. For example, if she has an indwelling catheter, it must be kept away from water, so cover it with a clear (and clean) plastic bag taped down on all sides. The plastic bag covering may not look professional, but it works wonders! Cover all the other parts that need to be covered in a similar way. Run a few inches of warm water in the bathtub (check it with your elbow to make sure it's just right — neither scalding nor freezing.) Place a nonskid mat at the bottom of the bathtub. This step is very important because she shouldn't make any sudden lurching movements. If she can sit in the bath, help her carefully into it. If she can't (or you can't bend too deeply), you can get a special bath stool from a medical-supply store that she can sit on in the water. Use a clean, soft sponge or cloth and a nonallergenic soap and wash her back, legs, feet, and the arm on the side that hasn't had surgery. If she wants to wash her vagina herself, allow her that dignity. Don't wash her hair in the bathtub until the doctor gives her the okay to use running water. (It's amazing how handy a kitchen sink is for washing hair!) Don't bend into the bathtub from a standing position, but rather sit or kneel on a pillow on the floor. You won't get as tired or risk hurting your back. Have a large, soft, clean towel ready close by, and when she's ready, gently wrap her in it. By finding out how to properly give someone a sponge bath, you've just given that person a most loving gift.

Being her advocate

Sadly, you can't assume that she's receiving the best medical care just because she's at the best hospital. In today's medical climate, on many occasions, you must become your partner's *advocate* (speaking and acting on her behalf). Here are some situations in which doing so may become necessary:

✔ When it takes a while for your partner to get pain medication (because of hospital staff shift changes and the likes), check to make sure the doctor has ordered the meds (no doctor's orders, no medication). If the doctor has to be called in, check to see that the nurse has been able to do this. If you get no response and your partner is still in pain 45 minutes to an hour later, don't hesitate to ask again.

✔ During a trip to the ER, especially when you have to wait and your partner becomes distraught, go to the desk and ask for help.

✔ When your partner doesn't understand part of her treatment or feels overwhelmed, call her doctor for her.

✔ If the doctor uses language that she and you don't really understand, ask your doctor for clarification.

✔ If your partner needs letters of verification for work, get them from the doctor or nurse for her.

✔ When your partner needs prescriptions filled, go to the pharmacy and pick them up.

Being a kick-butt personal assistant

Your partner may not be able or may not want to be responsible for all the aspects of her treatment. For example, she may be too worn out to call for prescription refills. She may be too nauseated to go to work. She will need your help at these times. You're going to be expected to assume other responsibilities, such as

✔ **Scheduling appointments.** Your partner may have to go to the clinic for any number of reasons: to consult with the doctor, to be monitored by the nurse, or to have a test. Unless she's being treated in a small hospital, several people are involved in her care, and all want to make appointments at times that are the most convenient for them. Coordinating these appointments to make the best use of her time (and yours) is up to you. When you don't, you stand a good chance of making multiple trips to the hospital every week.

✔ **Playing chauffeur.** Regardless of how well you schedule your appointments, many visits and extensive waiting times are required, and delays and unscheduled tests and procedures are the norm. You can expect plenty of waiting for long periods of time. Such a taxing schedule soon begins interfering with your work schedule.

✔ **Picking up prescriptions.** Picking up medicines can be difficult, especially when

- Your partner requires medications that most pharmacies don't carry.
- It's the middle of the night and she needs them urgently. (Actually, helping her plan for such an event in advance will usually prevent this.)
- The insurance company won't cover them.

✔ **Organizing and paying medical bills.** Dealing with insurance (see Chapter 17) and sorting out medical bills can be overwhelming. Paying for items that insurance doesn't cover (and there are many) can seriously strain your finances.

Balking at the Consequences

You're kidding yourself if you think that you can breeze through your partner's breast cancer infirmity. Being aware of the challenges enables you to prepare more effectively and more efficiently, even though you may not be able to solve all the problems. You may want to *do* something — talk to the doctor, organize, plan, get on with it, especially when you're a take-charge sort of person. Reality is different.

What you as the primary caretaker are expected to do sometimes seems impossible to achieve. Knowing this means that you must do the best with what you have, ask for lots of help from family and friends, and move on from there.

The situation is not one that you can easily control, because you often can't predict what lies around the corner, and as such, all the work you put into anticipating and planning doesn't always help. When you've always been someone who's in charge of your life and able to take care of your family, this realization can come as a real blow to your ego.

Taking care of your partner physically and emotionally, making sure that the kids are adjusted and happy, keeping up with your job's demands and earning a living, and managing the household (you forgot to take the trash out last week, and the dog's chewing the rug) is enough to make an adult cry (and seek out a really good therapist).

The pressures of having to put your own dreams and aspirations on hold can often cause feelings of anger and resentment. Add to that your fears of losing her or wondering how the family will manage without her, and you're probably feeling like a powder keg ready to explode. For you, free time becomes a distant memory, and when combined with the many sleepless nights you've endured, little is left to wonder about your road to feeling more tension, frustration, or depression.

Roberta H.

"I appreciate how so much more difficult it is for men being in a relationship with a breast cancer survivor. Men already are predisposed and socialized into keeping their feelings to themselves, and a good many of them will be at that mid-life crisis age anyway and have family and employment responsibilities, so we need to applaud the men in our lives. They are victims, too, but they're also such a huge part of our healing. For many of us, our marriages and families are the primary reasons we *have* to live."

You're so wrapped up in helping that you haven't thought about yourself for a while. Or you've realized just how long it's been since you've done something for yourself, by yourself, and it's tugging at your last nerve. So, what can you do?

- **Acknowledge your feelings.** Ignoring them won't make them go away; they'll just build up and cause you more frustration until you feel like you can't control it anymore.

- **Join a support group.** Go in person or go online.

- **Consider getting help from a counselor or religious leader.** Sometimes, a fresh perspective is just what you need.

- **Know when to seek professional help.** Being able to do so is key for your entire family. Forget soldiering on; make an appointment when

  - You and your partner end up arguing about how you expect each other to act.

  - The kids are crying or clingy, and you don't know how to help them.

  - Resentment and anger are two of your main feelings. Do you feel resentful when you see other families being happy? Do you find yourself feeling angry that you have this burden and others don't?

  - You're not sure how the financial pressure will be resolved.

  - You don't know how to ask for help, and even if you did, you wouldn't know whom you should ask.

    If ever you entertain *any* thoughts about hurting yourself or another person, please stop, take a deep breath, and call one of these numbers below (all are available 24-7):

    911 and ask for the Suicide Hotline

    1-800-227-2345 American Cancer Society

    1-800-221-2141 Y-Me Breast Cancer Organization

Chapter 18 describes more warning signs. Remember that you're grieving, too, and chances are you may be experiencing depression and not even know it. Call a hotline, ask your doctor for a referral to a therapist, or chat with the nurses at the hospital. They can tell you who to see. Taking care of yourself means you're better equipped to take better care of your partner.

Being the Kind of Friend You Want to Be

When you have a friend or acquaintance with cancer, although you may want to help, you probably don't know how, and more important, you don't know what to say. The good news is that you need to concern yourself with only a few "don't dos." Otherwise, there's a whole bunch of things that you can do. You're not responsible for fixing everything and making sure everyone is happy. So what are you responsible for?

Know what you're good at and do it. Don't wait to be asked to do something, because you can do any of the following:

✔ Ask for the job list and sign up for the things you can and will do.

✔ When a list doesn't exist, suggest two or three things that you're good at, explain when you're available to do them, and then just do the work.

✔ Try to assist on a regular basis. Don't take on more than you know you can carry out because you'll burn out and drop out.

✔ Remember that even a small task like taking a child to the park every Wednesday afternoon is a gift.

Many people are comfortable *doing* something; it's the person-to-person inter-action they find tough. What to do (or not do)? Table 20-2 gives you the goods.

Table 20-2	Do's and don'ts for the friendly friend
Do	**Don't**
Listen. You don't have to find a solution; you just have to be attentive and hear what she's telling you.	Say, "Everything will be alright." By saying that, you're stopping her from sharing her worries or fears.
Respect her wishes. If she wants to be alone for a while, let her have the time alone.	Say, "If you need anything at all, let me know." Offer, instead, whatever it is that you *are* prepared to do. And then do it.
Let her have her feelings: If she wants to cry, pass the tissue. If she needs to wail, let her do it. She doesn't always need cheering up. Mourning is part of the process.	Say, "Oh, don't say that," if she does share her fears or worries with you. What she needs is someone to listen and hear her, and if you falsely reassure her, you're cutting her off.
Something to help.	Promise anything that you can't guarantee or take on something you can't carry out. If you know you can only send a card and can't provide any practical help, then send the card and don't say you'll do anything else.

Chapter 21

No Kidding Around: Talking to Your Children

*W*hat should you do about the kids? Tell them? Not tell them? If you do talk to them, what should you say? What if you make things worse? In this chapter, we answer all these questions and provide guidelines and tips developed by experts in child psychology. After reading this chapter, you'll know what to do and what not to, and you'll feel much more comfortable about talking to your children about your breast cancer. Being comfortable doesn't make it easy, of course, but you'll find that it helps the kids adjust much better to your illness.

Giving Myths the Boot

For many parents, talking to the children is one of the most difficult things they have to deal with on their breast cancer journey. Regrettably, many myths and misperceptions cloud the issue of how to deal with children whose mothers are diagnosed with breast cancer, and these misconceptions often end up causing more problems in the long run.

Here are some of the myths and misconceptions, combined with the truths that kick them out the window. Turns out that the cold, hard truth is much better for the kids.

▸ **Myth:** Children can be sheltered and protected from reality.

Truth: You would like to protect your children from pain and suffering, but, in reality, that isn't possible. Trying to shelter them from the reality won't protect them in the long run. Instead, it can cause much more pain and insecurity later on.

✔ **Myth:** If I don't say anything, they won't know.

Truth: Children learn by not only listening to what you say but also by watching the way you act. No matter how old they are, children notice when something's wrong. If you don't tell them what it is, they'll think it's something so terrible that it can't be talked about. What's more, their own imaginations combined with their fears will conjure up all kinds of terrifying possibilities, usually much worse than reality.

✔ **Myth:** If they know the truth, they'll be emotionally damaged.

Truth: Children are resilient, and in the long run, adapt better knowing truthful information. The energy you expend keeping a secret safe places an added strain on you, and that's energy that otherwise can be put to good use helping you (and them) get through your upcoming journey.

So if the things that are usually right — helping your children stay children as long as possible and keeping them safe — aren't the right thing to do in this situation, what are you supposed to do? Read on.

Helping Kids Adjust

Following certain proven guiding principles contributes greatly to the healthy adjustment of a child whose mother has been diagnosed with breast cancer.

Don't go pulling a Pinocchio

The best thing you can do to help your children is tell the truth, so your children aren't left guessing and creating their own truths. Let the following principles be your guide.

✔ **Make sure that _you_ talk to your children.** That way they won't over-hear it from others, which only increases their terror and distrust.

✔ **Never ever lie.** Lying only causes harm in the long run.

✔ **Begin by asking what your children know about cancer.** Don't assume that you know what they know; you may be very surprised. For example, they may have heard from friends that people with cancer die, and now whenever they hear the word cancer, they associate it with death.

✔ **Tailor what you say to the ages of your children.** Children process information differently at different ages (as we discuss in the next section). Explain the illness and the expected side effects so that they can know what to expect.

✔ **Talk about how their mother's illness will affect them.** Reassure your children that they'll be cared for (tell them who will do it) and explain how they'll have someone taking care of them.

✔ **Never deny the feelings of your children.** You can reassure them that things will get better, but let them know that whatever they feel is valid at that moment.

✔ **Address magical thinking.** Young children have *magical thinking* and may feel that something they did caused the illness. For example, a child may be thinking, "I didn't tidy my room like she asked me and now she's sick because of me." Children rarely speak of these things, so you need to bring it up. Emphasize that your condition is not their fault, and that they weren't responsible for the illness in any way.

✔ **At the end of your conversation, ask if your children are afraid of anything.** They probably will be. Ask what it is, and address their fears openly and honestly.

✔ **Realize that you may have to explain more than once.** Repeating information and providing answers to new questions can be par for the course when dealing with your children. (Remember how many times you have to ask them to pick up those dratted building blocks?)

✔ **Recognize that telling your children about your breast cancer will take a toll on you, too.** Make sure you have someone to support *you*.

Making what you say age appropriate

Children of various ages can hear information very differently. They differ greatly in terms of the amount of information they can process, the type of information they understand, their reasoning, and their needs.

Talking with toddlers

Children ages 2 to 7 process information in a very concrete way and can digest only a little information at a time. Gear what you say into bite-sized bits of simple information. For example, "Helen told you that when someone's sick, they have to go to the hospital for ever and ever and never come back. Well, that's true sometimes, but *not* all the time."

Let your children know in advance that certain side effects may occur, so that they're not taken off guard when it happens. For example, "The medicine mommy's taking will make my hair fall out, so I'm going to look a little bit funny, but I'm still going to be *your* mommy. Then when mommy's hair grows back again, you can brush it nicely for me. Want to?"

Reassure your children that they're going to be looked after: "When mommy goes to the hospital, Nana's going to come stay with you. Won't that be nice?" If they get upset, don't deny their feelings. "I know you want your mommy to take you to the park, but I can't when I'm in the hospital. So why don't we ask Nana if she'll take you?"

Amanda C.

"I was afraid breast cancer might run in the family or that I might get it from being around her. I found out that it can run in the family, and that I'd have checkups for it later . . . but it isn't like a cold or the flu; you can't get cancer from someone else. Now, I'm not afraid of people with cancer."

Finally, ask about your children's fears: "Is your Teddy scared? What's he scared about? Let's talk to Teddy and see if we can make him all better, okay?"

Preparing preteens

Children ages 7 to 11 or 12 can process information, may already have some knowledge about cancer, and are able to start finding solutions to problems. Therefore, you can be more detailed in explaining to them what's happening to you. Tell them that you have cancer, but reassure them that you're going to be okay. Warn them about side effects of the treatment — tell them that you're going to be bald like their grandpa, for instance, or that you have an upset stomach when you feel nauseated from chemotherapy.

Ask what your preteens know about cancer: "So Johnny told you that people with cancer die, right? Well, that only happens *sometimes*. But you know what? Most people with cancer usually get better, and they don't die. Did you know that? It's the truth." Explain about cancer. You can make a drawing if you find that it helps, or even use toys as props. For example, "Remember when you found out about cells in school? Well, you know how in our bodies there are a million, billion cells that grow nice and slow. Well, cancer is a cell in your body that grows too fast and makes a lump, and the lump is cancer, and that's what made me sick."

Describe as much as your children can hear and understand about your treatment and the side effects, so they know what to expect: "Mom's going to the hospital for surgery, and she'll be home in two days. But you know what? Then she's going to have treatment that's going to make her a little bit sick. Weird huh? Medicine that makes you sick? It makes you sick because it's so strong, but it also makes you better afterward; it kills the cancer cells and when they're gone, Mom'll be getting stronger and stronger."

Involve your children in the process as much as possible. Your partner might say, "Mom's going to be too tired the first day, but I'll come get you and take you to visit her after that, okay? And your Uncle Tom's going to come stay with us for a week while Mom's resting, and he's going to take you to your soccer games, so you won't miss your tournaments. How does that sound?"

Debbie D.

"My son was 7 when I was diagnosed with breast cancer. Being somewhat precocious and curious, we answered all his questions directly. He asked if I would die, and we explained that everyone dies, in God's own time. A few days later he told me I'd be healed. He explained, 'God heals in two ways. He'll either cure the body you have or take you to heaven for a new one.'"

Dispelling blame is a way that addresses possible magical thinking: "The doctors told us that no one can cause someone else to get cancer. Cancer isn't a punishment, and it isn't because of anything *you* or anyone else did. Do you understand that? Remember that time you got mad at Mom and you yelled at her? I knew you were thinking about that. Well, it had absolutely nothing to do with Mom's cancer." Finally, ask about your child's fears: "Do you want to ask me anything else? I don't know everything, but I'll be glad to let you know what I do know."

Dishing to teenagers

Because of their ages and stages of life, adolescents and teenagers face unique difficulties. Teenagers often are confused about their own feelings and can be particularly sensitive to being different. All these factors make them even more vulnerable when their mother is diagnosed with cancer.

The teen years are the ages when young people begin defining their own identities and developing a separation from their parents. However, the mother's illness pulls them back into the family, often away from their friends and other activities.

The combination of these factors can become overwhelming for teenagers. Feelings of inability to help the parent coupled with the additional responsibilities they shoulder and difficulties with expressing their feelings can result in teenagers acting aloof or becoming angry, acting out, or becoming overly involved in their parent's care. Kids who were fighting or angry with their mothers prior to diagnosis have a particularly difficult time adjusting.

Several strategies can help in this difficult situation. You can

- ✔ Enable your young adult to continue with his or her normal activities as much as possible.

- ✔ Make sure your teens have time to hang out with their friends or by themselves.

- ✔ Even if teenagers must take on additional responsibilities, do everything in your power to prevent *parentification* of the child (where the child becomes the parent of the parent).

✔ Talk with your teenagers about their feelings. Acknowledge them, and if necessary, refer them for professional help.

Talking about death

Talking about death is one of the most difficult things for adults to do, and some go to extraordinary lengths to avoid it. On the other hand, a parent's death is the fear that's uppermost for children. They're terrified not only of losing the parent who's sick, but also the other parent.

Don't think that if you *don't* talk about death, no one will think about it. Don't think that if you *do* talk about death, you'll be putting ideas into your children's heads — you won't. Death was probably the first thing on your child's mind when she heard about your illness. Fortunately, in most instances of breast cancer, death isn't a risk, and telling your children that will come as an enormous relief to them. However, if death is a possibility, you'll have to talk to the kids about it.

Tell your children the truth:

✔ If there's a high chance of you surviving, say so: "The doctors told me I would live a long time, so please don't worry about me dying. I promise that if it *ever* becomes a possibility, I'll let you know, okay?" Giving your children that reassurance helps them let go of the terror in their hearts.

✔ If there's a high chance of you not surviving, find a way of telling your children. Ask your family's religious leader or the hospital's social worker for assistance. Many support groups and professionals can help you with this difficult message.

One of your children's biggest fears is not having a loving adult to care for them. Letting them know who will take care of them provides a sense of security and relieves the terror of potential abandonment, even if there's no risk of you dying. As a parent you want to help your children deal with the world, and if you can talk about these things with them, you'll be giving them an encouraging message: They don't have to struggle alone.

Keeping kids, kids

Adults are often tempted to share their difficulties with teenagers, turning them into young adults with additional responsibilities or confidantes. A recent study found that many women with breast cancer considered their teenage children their confidantes and anchors. Although turning young teenagers into "mature responsible adults" may appear to be a positive step, it actually contributes to an unhealthy process of turning teenagers into parental substitutes, thus robbing them of the ability to form their own identities, and can have long-term negative consequences.

Keeping Life on Track

A change in a child's life can be extremely frightening and provoke feelings of insecurity. Several strategies help provide your children with a sense of safety and confidence.

Keep on going to soccer

As much as possible, try to keep the children's routines the same as before, even when doing so means soliciting the assistance of friends, relatives, or neighbors. No matter how strong you or your family think you are, you're bound to run into times when it isn't possible for the family to manage alone. We talk more about getting support in Chapter 18, but here are some specific pointers:

✔ **Let the children remain at home instead of sending them off to live with a relative.** Keep them at home whenever doing so is at all possible. Being away from home increases your children's sense of abandonment and builds their fantasies about the unknown terror that's taking place at home.

✔ **Draw up a weekly schedule in which you indicate which child does what when.** For example: "Monday 6:30 a.m.: Johnny eats Cheerios for breakfast. He hates plain milk, so please use chocolate milk. 7:00 a.m.: The bus arrives exactly on time. Please make sure he has his lunchbox and $1.00, which he often forgets." All this attention to detail may seem excessive, but it ensures that your children's routines and preferences are kept.

✔ **Set up a way for the children to communicate with their mother.** C'mon, it's the 21st century, you can do it: The telephone, cell phone, personal digital assistant text messages, handwritten notes, or e-mail are potential avenues of communication when your children aren't able to visit.

Ruth R.

"One thing that helped in explaining my cancer diagnosis to my son was that he was young enough not to know what cancer was, so it wasn't an innately scary word. It was freaky thinking here I am, a single parent, and I've adopted a child who already has lost two parents (he was orphaned at age 2½). I didn't share this with my son, but he expressed to me the normal fear of my dying. He felt better once he knew the identity of the best friend that he would live with if anything happened to me and that he would have the ongoing support and involvement of my parents and brothers. Twice in the last year he's had a dream where I'm driving away, abandoning him. I don't know if the dream is because of the cancer thing, the adoption thing, just a regular kid's fear, or all three."

Continuing discipline

Children may react to stress by acting badly and lashing out at their care-taker or even their ill parent. You may feel that being lenient with children whenever they react that way is the right, loving, and logical approach to take. However, the fact is that doing so can result in many more problems than you'd ever expect. When children are allowed to get away with negative behavior that normally isn't permitted, it can indicate to them that the situation is much more serious than they ever imagined, because no limits are placed on their behavior. Surprisingly, that can add to their terror.

Keeping up with previously established limits often takes more work and effort on behalf of the caretaker, but it helps the children to know their boundaries. Tell children that you love them very much. You can imagine how frightened they must be feeling, so let them know that you're available whenever they want to talk to you. Remember that in spite of their fears, bad and destructive behavior is not allowed.

Talking to teachers

One of the most helpful steps that you can take is talking to the child's teacher. Doing so helps in so many different ways, because it

✔ **Prepares the teacher.** He or she knows to look out for problems that may arise and can be of assistance when and if they do. The teacher can alert you if grades start slipping or your child begins misbehaving in class. Make an appointment to see your child's teacher (or if you can't go in person give him or her a call). Explain what your treatment plan is, how long it will take, what side effects you may experience. Writing down dates of surgery, chemotherapy, and other appointments may also be helpful, so that the teacher can be alert to your child's behavior at these times. Consider asking the teacher to explain what's going on to the other kids, for example: "Tommy's mother is getting treatment that makes her hair fall out."

✔ **Ensures an understanding of the special stresses that your children are facing.** That way the teacher can do whatever is needed, making sure that your children aren't teased but instead are provided with extra attention whenever they may need it. Because children may act out in school, letting their teachers know about your situation helps to ensure that the teacher doesn't simply become angry with the child but instead understands the source of the problem and finds the right way to deal with it.

✔ **Lets the teacher know what warning signs to look for.** Letting the teacher know what's going on in your child's life enables him or her to recognize if and when your child needs to be referred to the school counselor for additional guidance.

Keeping the kids in the loop

Another way to help children cope is keeping them involved as much as possible.

✔ **Tell them about surgery.** Children may have built up extraordinary fantasies of what surgery means. Let them know that mommy had special medicines before the operation, so she was fast asleep and couldn't feel any pain.

✔ **Allow them to see their Mom as soon as she feels comfortable.** That way they can see that she isn't in pain or distress, and most important, that their mother hasn't abandoned them.

During this time, explain to them that mommy may have some pain from time to time, but this will go away in a few days.

✔ **Explain what the tubes, monitors, and beeps are.** If you can, buy younger children a doctor set, so they, too, can be doctors, and the instruments become toys. Don't assume that children are terrified of hospitals; usually, they're extremely curious and fascinated by all the gadgets.

✔ **After doctor visits, try to share some information with the children.** Otherwise, they'll see the adults talking in a huddle or getting quiet whenever doctors walk into the room and assume that a catastrophe has occurred.

✔ **Give each child a duty.** Doing so enables your children to play an important part as their mother recovers. For example, ask them to water the plants, bring in the mail, take out the garbage, or other similar chores.

Amanda C.

"I had a very hard time not worrying about the cancer, and I started getting bad grades on my schoolwork. Going to school every day wasn't very easy. I heard my aunt telling my grandmother, 'The whole family needs counseling.' So I went to our team's guidance counselor. She helped me out a lot. We talked about all the different emotions and what to do when I felt angry. She gave me some bubble-wrap to pop and that helped me get rid of my anger. She also gave me a pass to come to her office if I ever needed to see her, and that made me feel good. I still keep it in my book bag."

Roberta H.

"Kids will surprise you. When my 9-year-old son came home from school and was told I was home after my mastectomy, he came running in to greet me. I was trying to adjust a blocked chest drain at the time without the benefit of my right arm, and so I was unsuccessful in covering my incision in time. I was worried what trauma seeing such a train wreck would cause a sensitive young boy and didn't know what to say to him. He taught me a very important lesson. He stopped still for a moment, and then said, 'Eow. Yuck! Oh well, at least you're still alive.' Then he carefully hugged and kissed me on my uninjured side and ran off to do his homework."

Preparing for Problems

Despite all your efforts to make life seem normal and ensure that your children feel safe, secure, and loved, someone eventually will feel overwhelmed. Children aren't always able to verbalize their feelings in these circumstances, so their behavior is the best indicator of how they're coping.

Don't be surprised if your child begins to regress. Little ones who are recently toilet-trained may require diapers again; toddlers who loved nothing more than playing outside may become clingy; and kids who were running to the school bus may become reluctant to leave the house.

If you notice a change in your child's behavior and it continues for a few weeks, that's a sign that your child is in distress. Try the following:

- **A support group for children whose parents have cancer.** Mixing with other children who are in similar situations normalizes their lives, and through a series of activities (art, playing with doctor's instruments, and so on) they're able to learn about cancer, illness, and separation. Such groups are available through your local hospital.

- **A therapist with expertise in this area.** This step is especially urgent whenever your children show any of the following symptoms of great distress that persist:

  - Violence toward others or destructive behaviors toward themselves

  - Anxiety so high they're unable to engage in normal activities

  - Refusing to get dressed, bathe, or go to school

  - Unable to sleep or experiencing ongoing nightmares

  Your doctor may be able to help you find a child counselor or someone to talk to.

Part V:
The Part of Tens

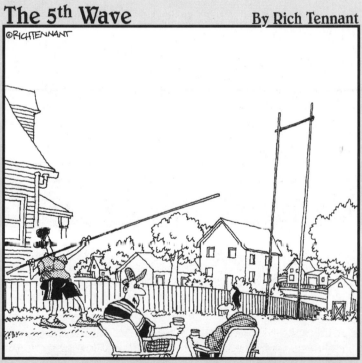

The 5th Wave   By Rich Tennant

©RICHTENNANT

"Don't get me wrong. I think it's great that Barbara decided
she wanted to start exercising more after her surgery."

In this part . . .

This part gives you helpful information in handy groups of ten (or more). Here you'll find such useful lists as ten excellent hospitals around the country, and ten-plus resources you can turn to for additional information, support, and professional guidance.

Chapter 22

Ten Best Hospitals for Breast Cancer Treatment

*I*f you're fortunate enough to have a choice of treatment centers, take this advice: Evaluate, evaluate, evaluate. Studies have found that patients treated by specialists in hospitals that treat many breast cancer patients have a 3 percent to 14 percent better chance of surviving than those who are treated in facilities that don't get as many breast cancer patients.

If your doctors work in a treatment center that conducts research, you can feel pretty confident that they're in the know and up-to-date on the latest advances in the field. But don't be fooled. Not all research is created equal. To receive funding from top-dog funding agencies like the National Cancer Institute, American Cancer Society, and Department of Defense, researchers must go through a rigorous scientific review. Only the very best are funded. And you want the best.

TIP

Any treatment center can call itself a "Comprehensive Cancer Center," but only those centers that have been designated as such by the National Cancer Institute (NCI) are recognized as particularly outstanding for their treatment of cancer. You can find 39 such centers in the United States. You can check at www.cancer.gov and click on Cancer Centers Program to see whether a comprehensive cancer center is located in your area.

We want you to receive the best care that you possibly can get. So in this chapter, we describe ten of the best places to receive cancer treatment. Other centers and hospitals not mentioned here may be equally as good, but we simply chose one from each part of the country, so that you can find one close to you. For a full listing go to www3.cancer.gov/cancercenters/centerslist.html, and click on your state to find the Comprehensive Cancer Center nearest you.

Okay, now for our top ten. Drum roll, please. . .

Abramson Cancer Center at the University of Pennsylvania: Philadelphia, PA

Internet: pennhealth.com/health/hi_files/cancer/

Phone: 800-789-7366

The Rena Rowan Breast Center is part of the larger cancer center. Its 40 doctors and researchers form the backbone of a multidisciplinary team approach to treatment. This cancer center is known nationally for its expertise in mammography, ultrasound, core biopsies, and magnetic resonance imaging (MRI) in diagnosing breast cancer, and for its expertise in radiation therapy in the treatment of the disease. This center also has extensive expertise in genetics and genetic research. You can make an appointment by calling the toll-free number above, or you can log on to the Web site above and click on "Making an Appointment" and then choose the "Electronic Appointment Request," and complete the form. You should be contacted within one business day.

MD Anderson Cancer Center at the University of Texas: Houston, TX

Internet: www.mdanderson.org

Phone: 800-392-1611

MD Anderson Cancer Center is one of the largest cancer centers in the United States, with more than 60,000 patients receiving treatment each year. Although the MD Anderson Cancer Center treats many Texans, almost one-third of its patients come from across the United States and abroad. It's one of the top research institutions nationwide, and it receives more research grant funding from the National Cancer Institute than any other cancer center. Because of its many ongoing clinical trials, 15 percent of patients at the center participate in them. Needless to say, this center has consistently ranked among the top two cancer centers in the country.

To make an appointment online, go to www.mdanderson.org/patients_public/new_patients/.

Memorial-Sloan Kettering Cancer Center: New York, NY

Internet: www.mskcc.org/mskcc/html/44.cfm

Phone: 800-525-2225

One of the most well known cancer hospitals, the Memorial Sloan-Kettering's Cancer Center, has its own breast center, the Evelyn H. Lauder Breast Center. More breast cancer patients are treated there than at any other cancer center in the United States. A special surveillance breast program is available for women at high risk for breast cancer where careful screening and monitoring is performed. The Memorial Sloan-Kettering Cancer Center is well known for its research into sentinel-node biopsy and its aggressive approaches to chemotherapy.

To make an appointment online, go to www.mskcc.org/mskcc/html/8616.cfm.

Lynn Sage Breast Center of the Robert H. Lurie Comprehensive Cancer Center: Chicago, IL

Internet: www.cancer.northwestern.edu/index.html

Phone: 312-926-3021

Northwestern Memorial Hospital is one of the foremost academic medical centers in the country. In conjunction with the Robert H. Lurie Comprehensive Cancer Center of Northwestern University, it conducts many clinical trials.

Its breast cancer center, The Lynn Sage Breast Cancer Center, directed by our own Dr. Monica Morrow, a coauthor of this book, provides a multidisciplinary approach to treatment and research. The program of Northwestern received international acclaim for its groundbreaking research in antihormonal treatments, especially tamoxifen, and for its contribution to clinical research on the effectiveness of breast-conserving therapy. The Lynn Sage Cancer Center has been designated as a Center of Excellence by the Avon Foundation (the largest corporate philanthropy organization for breast cancer in the United States). The breast center program, designated as a *Specialized Program of Research Excellence* (SPORE) in breast cancer, also is very active in research on digital mammography and ultrasound. A special program for women at high risk also is available.

To make an appointment, call or visit `www.nmh.org/`.

John Wayne Cancer Institute: Santa Monica, CA

Internet: `www.jwci.org/`

Phone: 800-262-6259

John Wayne Cancer Center is home to the Joyce Eisenberg Keefer Breast Center. This center pioneered the *sentinel node biopsy procedure* (see Chapter 5), which is now being adopted by cancer centers nationwide as a method of diagnosing the degree of spread of breast cancer. This center is also the leader in ongoing studies exploring the need for further surgery after a positive sentinel node biopsy, and in research to find ways to predict when breast cancer will recur.

To make an appointment, call or visit the Web site.

Dana-Farber/Harvard Cancer Center: Boston, MA

Internet: `www.dfci.harvard.edu`

Phone: 866-408-3324

The Dana-Farber Cancer Institute joined with Harvard Medical School and four of its affiliated hospitals, Brigham, Women's, Massachusetts General Hospital, and Harvard School of Public Health, to create the Dana-Farber/Harvard Cancer Center, the largest and most comprehensive cancer center in the world. More than 780 senior scientists have access to all the academic and research facilities and resources to promote collaborative learning, teaching, treatment, and research. The center also has several SPOREs, including one on breast cancer. The goal of the Breast Cancer SPORE is promoting interdisciplinary research that results in better prevention, diagnosis, and treatment of breast cancer. Research in the breast cancer program focuses on understanding the causes of breast cancer, improving diagnosis and screening, and finding and evaluating many novel therapies to treat breast cancer with minimal side effects.

To make an appointment online, go to www.dana-farber.org/pat/becoming/. A new-patient coordinator will contact you within 24 hours.

Sidney Kimmel Comprehensive Cancer Center at Johns Hopkins: Baltimore, MD

Internet: www.hopkinsmedicine.org/breastcenter

Phone: 410-995-8964

The Johns Hopkins Kimmel Cancer Center is the only NCI Comprehensive Cancer Center in the state of Maryland, and is home to the Johns Hopkins Breast Center. The Johns Hopkins Breast Center has a breast cancer SPORE and is a leader in breast cancer research and treatment. The research focus is on antihormonal therapy, and the center is a leader in investigating the role of ovarian hormones in breast cancer in young women.

Patients at this center are able to access the most advanced tests and treatments, and the survival rates among women with early stage breast cancer are often higher than the national rates. Premenopausal women with breast cancer who are treated here have a 10 percent higher survival rate at ten years when compared to the national average.

To make an appointment, call or visit the Web site.

University of Michigan: Ann Arbor, MI

Internet: www.cancer.med.umich.edu/

Phone: 800-865-1125

The University of Michigan Cancer Center sees more cancer patients than any other hospital in Michigan. Its 200 cancer clinicians and researchers work in multidisciplinary teams, bringing the latest research into their treatment. This program is well known for its important work in discovering newer methods of breast imaging, postmastectomy radiation, and other aspects of breast radiation.

Most of this center's appointments are made by a referral from a physician, so if you want to receive treatment here, ask your doctor to assist you with that.

The Mayo Clinic: Rochester, MN

Internet: www.mayoclinic.org/about/

Phone: 507-284-2111

Mayo Clinic is a not-for-profit organization based in Rochester, Minnesota, with its own breast cancer program. Its collaboration with the other Mayo Clinics in Scottsdale, Arizona, and in Jacksonville, Florida, results in shared knowledge and resources. Mayo Clinic, Saint Mary's Hospital, and Rochester Methodist Hospital together form an integrated medical center that provides comprehensive care and access to the latest clinical trials. Researchers from the Mayo Clinic have contributed greatly by their research into prophylactic (preventive) mastectomy, clinical trials of adjuvant therapy (chemotherapy in early stage breast cancer discussed in Chapter 12), and finding ways to alleviate symptoms.

To make an appointment, ask your doctor for a referral or call between 8 a.m. and 5 p.m. central time, Monday through Friday.

UCLA's Jonsson Comprehensive Cancer Center: Los Angeles, CA

Internet: www.cancer.mednet.ucla.edu/

Phone: 310-206-6909

For the third consecutive year, UCLA's Jonsson Comprehensive Cancer Center ranks as the best cancer center in the western United States. It received its National Cancer Institute designation more than 25 years ago, and as such has a long established tradition of excellence. More than 230 doctors and scientists conduct research and provide treatment, including hundreds of clinical trials looking at the latest in experimental cancer treatments. The center is famous for its development of Herceptin, the first therapy that interrupts the HER-2 oncogene (gene that causes cancer.) This center has also greatly contributed to our understanding of quality of life among survivors, during treatment and beyond.

Chapter 23

Ten-Plus Helpful Resources

In This Chapter

▶ Finding out you're not alone

▶ Getting information, receiving referral, survivor's support

*O*ne thing you can be sure of is that you're not alone. Many sources of support, information, referrals, programs, and much more are available. In fact, finding out just to whom you need to turn and where you need to start can seem overwhelming. We've selected resources that we know you and your family will need.

This list is by no means a complete one, but it provides you with a great start. Choose the resources that fit your needs, and they'll lead you to others that you may want or need. You'll find a home among at least a few of these wonderful resources.

CANCERLIT

www.cancer.gov/cancerinfo/literature

The "LIT" portion of CANCERLIT refers to literature, and this site is *the one* to go to whenever you want to find any cancer articles published in scientific journals, books, meetings, or reports.

Families USA

www.familiesusa.org

Families USA is a national nonprofit organization whose mission is to achieve high-quality, affordable health and long-term care for all Americans and to serve as the consumer watchdog on behalf of health-care consumers. This organization is on your side, so it's worth a visit.

Health Insurance Association of America

www.hiaa.org

The Health Insurance Association of America represents almost all health insurance companies within the United States. The association's Web site includes insurance guides, a survey of hospitals, and other educational and insurance industry information.

Hospice Net

www.hospicenet.org

Geared toward the patient and her family, you can find answers to all your questions about hospice care. The site also shows you where to find a hospice and features a professional staff that provides answers to your questions via e-mail. You'll seldom meet a more dedicated group of people.

National Alliance of Breast Cancer Organizations

www.nabco.org

800-806-2226

"The More You Know, the less you fear" is the driving motto of the National Alliance of Breast Cancer Organizations (NABCO). This coalition of more than 370 breast cancer organizations is the leading nonprofit information and educational resource on breast cancer in the United States, featuring links to virtually everything that you ever wanted to know about breast cancer.

National Cancer Institute

cancer.gov

The National Cancer Institute (NCI) is an institute of the National Institutes of Health, the federal government organization that is responsible for funding cancer research. It's huge and has many divisions; the following are probably the ones that will be of most help to you.

Cancer Information Service

```
cancer.gov/cis
```
800-426-6237

The NCI's Cancer Information Service (CIS) is the place to call when you want someone to explain the latest research in simple to understand, nontechnical language. Yes, that can be done! Call or visit the Web site.

Clinical Trials

```
cancertrials.nci.nih.gov
```

Find out everything you need to know about clinical trials through a link to the NCI's database of all its current clinical trials. By clicking on this link (CancerNet/NCI database), you can search for clinical trials by state, city, and type of cancer. The NCI Web site also provides insurance information — the cost of the trials and how to find out whether your insurance will cover it. Simply type the word `Insurance` into the site's search feature and follow the prompts.

National Center for Complementary and Alternative Medicine

```
nccam.nih.gov
```

The National Center for Complementary and Alternative Medicine is one of the 27 Institutes that make up the National Institutes of Health. The center's mission is to conduct research on complementary and alternative medicine (CAM), train practitioners in CAM, and educate the public on which CAM methods work, which don't, and why. Discussion about the latest research on CAM can be found at the center's Web site.

The Susan G. Komen Foundation

```
www.komen.org
```
800-462-9273

The Susan G. Komen Foundation is a private fundraising foundation that raises awareness and awards grants for research and programs to fulfill its mission of preventing breast cancer through research, education, and screening. Call the toll-free helpline for information.

Visiting Nurse Associations of America

www.vnaa.org

A well-established nonprofit organization, the Visiting Nurse Associations of America (VNA) provides information, education, and other resources for accessing nurses and other health-care professionals who can provide care in your home. Information about insurance coverage is provided.

Y-ME National Breast Cancer Organization

www.y-me.org

800-221-2141

Y-ME National Breast Cancer Organization wants to ensure that no one faces breast cancer alone. It provides information, support, and a 24-hour-a-day hotline for whenever you need to talk — any time of day or night.

Young Survival Coalition

www.youngsurvival.org

212-577-6259

If you're younger than 40 and have been diagnosed with breast cancer, the Young Survival Coalition (YSC) is the place for you. It's an international network of breast cancer survivors who are dedicated to the concerns and issues unique to young women (younger than 40) and breast cancer. In addition to its focus on advocacy and awareness, this group serves as a point of contact for young women living with breast cancer.

Chapter 24

Ten-Plus American Cancer Society Resources

● ●

In This Chapter

▶ Networking with ACS and cancer survivors

▶ Coping with your diagnosis

▶ Hooking up with many and varied ACS programs

● ●

*T*he American Cancer Society (ACS) offers almost everything you'll ever need that's cancer-related. You can get answers to all your questions and receive support, information, training, and other benefits from ACS programs. Local offices are situated throughout the United States and its territories.

I (Ronit Elk, a coauthor of this book) can honestly say, that in all my years (and there have been many of them!), I have never had the opportunity to work in such a caring and compassionate organization. The ACS is the place I would turn to for information, advice, and support, and this is the organization I would recommend for anyone going through the cancer experience.

American Cancer Society

www.cancer.org

800-227-2345

The ACS programs, some of which are described in the sections that follow, are free and are designed to meet your needs. Programs are culturally appropriate, and information is available in many languages. The ACS also has a well-respected program that funds cancer research nationwide (you'll find me there!) If the ACS can't meet your needs, its staffers will find the right place to refer you.

Cancer Survivors Network

www.acscsn.org

877-333-4673

The Cancer Survivors Network is a virtual community created by and for cancer survivors and their families. It's the place to go to when you want to reach out, talk with other survivors, get information, listen to Web-based interviews (I've done a few of those), and give and get support.

Hope Lodge

www.cancer.org

800-227-2345

Hope Lodge is a home away from home for cancer patients and their caregivers. You can stay free at one of the 20 such lodges around the country. Call the toll-free number or go to the ACS Web site, type Hope Lodge into Search function, and click on "Go" to find out more about the various Hope Lodges around the country.

1 Can Cope

www.cancer.org

"I Can Cope" is an ACS course that helps people diagnosed with cancer and their families discover how to deal with and cope with cancer, gaining knowledge and a sense of control over their lives. Go to the ACS Web site, type I Can Cope into the Search function, and click on "Go."

Look Good . . . Feel Better

www.lookgoodfeelbetter.org

800-395-5665

In partnership with the National Cosmetic Association and the Cosmetic, Toiletry and Fragrance Association Foundation, the American Cancer Society provides a service known as "Look Good . . . Feel Better" for women with cancer. This free service shows you ways to restore your appearance, apply makeup so that your lack of eyebrows and lashes isn't obvious, and don a scarf or hat with aplomb. Call the toll-free number to find a program nearest you. Try it; it'll make you feel worlds better.

National Cancer Information Center

800-227-2345

The National Cancer Information Center is an ACS call center that's open 24/7 and is staffed with professionals who can answer all your questions about cancer — symptoms, diagnosis, treatment options, treatment centers, where to find clinical trials, support groups, or breast prostheses. The center will guide you to the appropriate locations to receive any help that you may need. Call anytime, day or night.

Reach to Recovery

800-227-2345

No one can understand you, the person stricken with cancer, as well as someone who's walked in your shoes before and is now on the other side — a survivor! Reach to Recovery is an ACS program that matches survivors with women just diagnosed with breast cancer. These volunteers are trained to share their knowledge and experience in a supportive and nonintrusive way. Contact the toll-free Reach to Recovery phone number for information about the program nearest you.

tlc (Tender Loving Care) magazine/catalog

www.tlccatalog.org

800-850-9445

tlc is an ACS-sponsored magazine/catalog that combines information with products for women who are coping with cancer. Wigs, hairpieces, breast forms, hats, accessories, and more are available. You can order on-line or call for a free catalog. This program is self-supporting and profits are reinvested in the program to make it more accessible to people in need.

Relay for Life

800-227-2345

Relays for Life are ACS events designed to celebrate survivorship and raise money for ACS research and programs in literally thousands of communities. The event honors cancer survivors, who always take the first lap, graced with a purple sash, with literally thousands of people cheering them on. Relay for Life is the place to be to feel connected with other survivors and to celebrate your journey. To find out about the Relay for Life in the area where you live, call the toll-free number.

ACS CAN

800-227-2345

ACS CAN is a sister organization to the American Cancer Society. The ACS Cancer Action Network is a national advocacy organization (nonpartisan and not-for-profit). This program shows you how to approach your local legislators, applying positive pressure aimed at providing more funding for cancer research, ensuring that everyone has access to treatment, and enhancing the many other ways that government can support the fight against cancer. To join, go to the American Cancer Society Web site (www.cancer.org) and type ACS CAN in the search engine.

Finding a Clinical Trial through ACS

www.cancer.org

In Chapter 23, we suggest several ways of finding clinical trials. One of the easiest ways is through the American Cancer Society. At the home page on the ACS Web site, under "Patients, Family and Friends" click on "clinical trials" which takes you to a page that explains *everything* you ever wanted to know about clinical trials. Finding a clinical trial is easy. Simply click on "Find a Clinical Trial" and a free, confidential service (supported by the ACS and EmergingMed, a company that keeps track of the trials and does the matching) finds a clinical trial that's right for you. Click on "Use Our Matching Service," which takes you to a small questionnaire where you answer a few questions about your cancer. Once that information is entered, you can find clinical trials matching your specific profile. You can get to this page directly at: clinicaltrials.cancer.org/.

Index

• *D* •

• T •

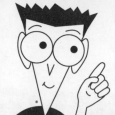
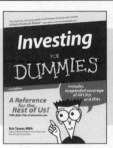
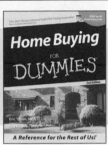
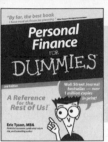
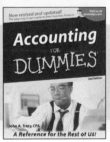
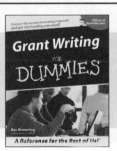
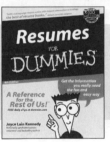
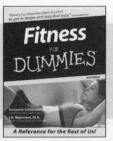
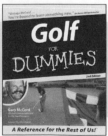
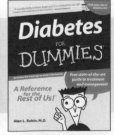
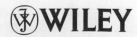

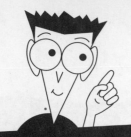
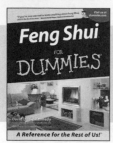
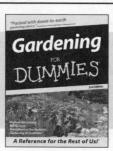
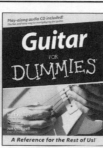
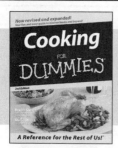
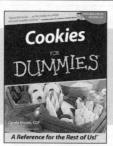
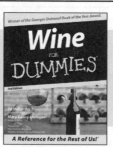
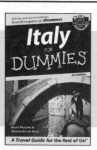
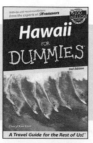
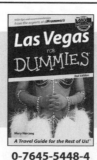

FOR DUMMIES®

Plain-English solutions for everyday challenges

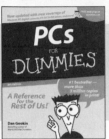
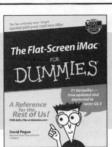
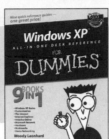
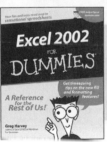
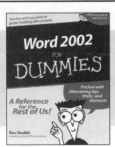
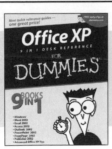
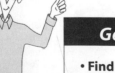

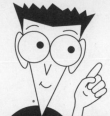

FOR DUMMIES®

Helping you expand your horizons and realize your potential

INTERNET

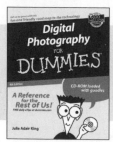

The Internet FOR DUMMIES
A Reference for the Rest of Us!

0-7645-0894-6

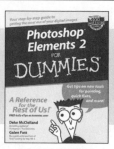

The Internet ALL-IN-ONE DESK REFERENCE FOR DUMMIES
9 BOOKS IN 1

0-7645-1659-0

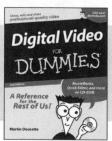

eBay FOR DUMMIES
A Reference for the Rest of Us!

0-7645-1642-6

Also available:

America Online 7.0 For Dummies
(0-7645-1624-8)

Genealogy Online For Dummies
(0-7645-0807-5)

The Internet All-in-One Desk Reference For Dummies
(0-7645-1659-0)

Internet Explorer 6 For Dummies
(0-7645-1344-3)

The Internet For Dummies Quick Reference
(0-7645-1645-0)

Internet Privacy For Dummies
(0-7645-0846-6)

Researching Online For Dummies
(0-7645-0546-7)

Starting an Online Business For Dummies
(0-7645-1655-8)

DIGITAL MEDIA

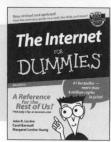

Digital Photography FOR DUMMIES
A Reference for the Rest of Us!

0-7645-1664-7

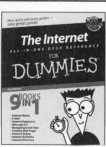

Photoshop Elements 2 FOR DUMMIES
A Reference for the Rest of Us!

0-7645-1675-2

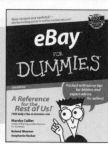

Digital Video FOR DUMMIES
A Reference for the Rest of Us!

0-7645-0806-7

Also available:

CD and DVD Recording For Dummies
(0-7645-1627-2)

Digital Photography All-in-One Desk Reference For Dummies
(0-7645-1800-3)

Digital Photography For Dummies Quick Reference
(0-7645-0750-8)

Home Recording for Musicians For Dummies
(0-7645-1634-5)

MP3 For Dummies
(0-7645-0858-X)

Paint Shop Pro "X" For Dummies
(0-7645-2440-2)

Photo Retouching & Restoration For Dummies
(0-7645-1662-0)

Scanners For Dummies
(0-7645-0783-4)

GRAPHICS

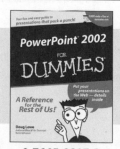

PowerPoint 2002 FOR DUMMIES
A Reference for the Rest of Us!

0-7645-0817-2

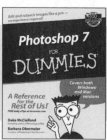

Photoshop 7 FOR DUMMIES
A Reference for the Rest of Us!

0-7645-1651-5

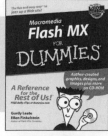

Macromedia Flash MX FOR DUMMIES
A Reference for the Rest of Us!

0-7645-0895-4

Also available:

Adobe Acrobat 5 PDF For Dummies
(0-7645-1652-3)

Fireworks 4 For Dummies
(0-7645-0804-0)

Illustrator 10 For Dummies
(0-7645-3636-2)

QuarkXPress 5 For Dummies
(0-7645-0643-9)

Visio 2000 For Dummies
(0-7645-0635-8)

FOR DUMMIES®

The advice and explanations you need to succeed

SELF-HELP, SPIRITUALITY & RELIGION

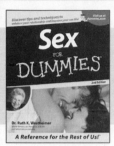
0-7645-5302-X

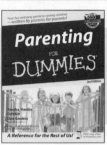
0-7645-5418-2

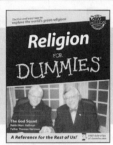
0-7645-5264-3

Also available:

The Bible For Dummies
(0-7645-5296-1)

Buddhism For Dummies
(0-7645-5359-3)

Christian Prayer For Dummies
(0-7645-5500-6)

Dating For Dummies
(0-7645-5072-1)

Judaism For Dummies
(0-7645-5299-6)

Potty Training For Dummies
(0-7645-5417-4)

Pregnancy For Dummies
(0-7645-5074-8)

Rekindling Romance For Dummies
(0-7645-5303-8)

Spirituality For Dummies
(0-7645-5298-8)

Weddings For Dummies
(0-7645-5055-1)

PETS

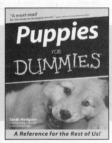
0-7645-5255-4

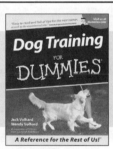
0-7645-5286-4

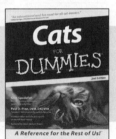
0-7645-5275-9

Also available:

Labrador Retrievers For Dummies
(0-7645-5281-3)

Aquariums For Dummies
(0-7645-5156-6)

Birds For Dummies
(0-7645-5139-6)

Dogs For Dummies
(0-7645-5274-0)

Ferrets For Dummies
(0-7645-5259-7)

German Shepherds For Dummies
(0-7645-5280-5)

Golden Retrievers For Dummies
(0-7645-5267-8)

Horses For Dummies
(0-7645-5138-8)

Jack Russell Terriers For Dummies
(0-7645-5268-6)

Puppies Raising & Training Diary For Dummies
(0-7645-0876-8)

EDUCATION & TEST PREPARATION

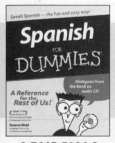
0-7645-5194-9

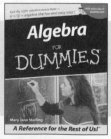
0-7645-5325-9

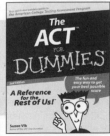
0-7645-5210-4

Also available:

Chemistry For Dummies
(0-7645-5430-1)

English Grammar For Dummies
(0-7645-5322-4)

French For Dummies
(0-7645-5193-0)

The GMAT For Dummies
(0-7645-5251-1)

Inglés Para Dummies
(0-7645-5427-1)

Italian For Dummies
(0-7645-5196-5)

Research Papers For Dummies
(0-7645-5426-3)

The SAT I For Dummies
(0-7645-5472-7)

U.S. History For Dummies
(0-7645-5249-X)

World History For Dummies
(0-7645-5242-2)

Available wherever books are sold. Go to www.dummies.com or call 1-877-762-2974 to order direct.

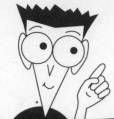
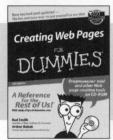
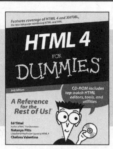
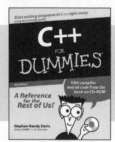
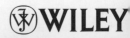